Lecture Notes in Biomathematics 95

Managing Editor:
S. A. Levin

Editorial Board:
Ch. DeLisi, M. Feldman, J. B. Keller, M. Kimura
R. May, J. D. Murray, G. F. Oster, A. S. Perelson
L. A. Segel

W0042522

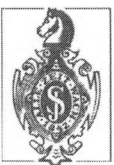

Herbert W. Hethcote   James W. Van Ark

Modeling HIV Transmission and AIDS in the United States

Springer-Verlag Berlin Heidelberg GmbH

Authors

Herbert W. Hethcote
Department of Mathematics
University of Iowa
Iowa City, IA 52242
USA

James W. Van Ark
Department of Mathematics
University of Detroit Mercy
Detroit, MI 48221
USA

Mathematics Subject Classification (1980): 92A15, 92C60, 92D30

ISBN 978-3-540-55904-7   ISBN 978-3-642-51477-7 (eBook)
DOI 10.1007/978-3-642-51477-7

© Springer-Verlag Berlin Heidelberg 1992
Originally published by Springer-Verlag Berlin Heidelberg in 1992.
Typesetting: Camera-ready by authors
46/3140-543210 - Printed on acid-free paper

FOREWORD

The disease that came to be called acquired immunodeficiency syndrome (AIDS) was first identified in the summer of 1981. By that time, nearly 100,000 persons in the United States may have been infected with human immunodeficiency virus (HIV). By the time the routes of transmission were clearly identified and HIV was established as the cause of AIDS in 1983, over 300,000 people may have been infected. That number has continued to increase, with approximately 1,000,000 Americans believed to be infected in 1991. The epidemic is of great public health concern because HIV is infectious, causes severe morbidity and death in most if not all of those infected, and often occurs in relatively young persons. In addition, the cost of medical care for a person with HIV disease is high, and the medical care needs of HIV–infected persons place a severe burden on the medical care systems in many areas.

Understanding and controlling the HIV epidemic is a particularly difficult challenge. The long and variable period between HIV infection and clinical disease makes it difficult both to forecast the future magnitude of the epidemic, which is important for health care planning, and to estimate the number infected in the last several years, which is important for monitoring the current status of the epidemic. Furthermore, because the common routes of HIV transmission (nonmonogamous sexual contact (both homosexual and heterosexual), and needle–sharing by injecting drug users) evoke controversy, it has been difficult to gather information about the prevalence of behaviors that result in high risk for HIV transmission. In such a situation, mathematical and statistical modeling are especially important.

The work in this monograph represents a major contribution to the mathematical modeling of the HIV epidemic. The authors have carefully organized and used the known relevant information. They draw important qualitative conclusions, including identifying factors that affect the spread of HIV in a population and emphasizing the importance of social structure in that spread. These conclusions provide guidance on what data are most important for understanding the spread of HIV. The authors also demonstrate that, if enough reliable data are available (such as in San Francisco), mathematical models can help us understand the historical dynamics of the HIV epidemic and the factors affecting it. Appropriate modifications of this model could help public health officials decide which behavior modifications are most promising in controlling the epidemic.

Our discussions with the authors during their work on this project emphasized to us how hard it is to formulate, implement and evaluate a good mathematical model for HIV transmission and disease. A great deal of information must be incorporated, and reliable estimates are still needed for some important parameters. Model predictions need to be validated with external information, such as the results of seroprevalence surveys, before quantitative results can be regarded as reliable. We thank the authors for their contribution to our understanding of the HIV epidemic and for the many discussions that helped clarify our understanding of this epidemic.

John M. Karon, Ph.D.
Senior Statistician
National Center for Infectious Diseases
Centers for Disease Control

James W. Curran, M.D., M.P.H.
Associate Director
Centers for Disease Control
Director of HIV/AIDS Programs

PREFACE

Acquired immunodeficiency syndrome (AIDS) was first identified as a distinct new disease syndrome in 1981 in the United States. In 1983 the human immunodeficiency virus (HIV) was identified as the causative agent for AIDS. There are several rather unusual aspects of HIV and AIDS which make this new disease different from previous diseases. For example, the mean time from HIV infection to AIDS is approximately 10 years, which is much longer than the infectious periods of less than 10 days for measles, mumps and chicken pox. Moreover, because HIV infected individuals do not recover, they continue to be infectious throughout their lives. Modeling approaches have been useful in analyzing previous infectious diseases, so it is natural to use models to study the epidemiology of HIV/AIDS.

This monograph describes the results of a project to use mathematical modeling and computer simulations to analyze HIV transmission dynamics and AIDS in various risk groups in the United States (U.S.). This research project started in 1987 and has been supported by contract 200–87–0515 from the Division of HIV/AIDS, Center for Infectious Diseases, Centers for Disease Control (CDC), Atlanta, Georgia. Although some results have been described in journal articles (Hethcote, 1987; Hethcote, 1989; Hethcote, Van Ark and Longini, 1991; Hethcote, Van Ark and Karon, 1991; Hethcote and Van Ark, 1992), many results in this monograph have not appeared before or have only appeared in reports to CDC. Our modeling approach to HIV/AIDS has been similar to the approach to gonorrhea (Hethcote and Yorke, 1984); namely, to use simple models to answer specific questions and to emphasize conceptual understanding through reconstruction of the HIV epidemics. A detailed discussion of the purposes and limitations of epidemiological modeling is given in Section 1.6.

The epidemiology of HIV/AIDS and general aspects of modeling HIV/AIDS are described in Chapter 1. The model formulated in Chapters 2 and 3 is analyzed mathematically in Chapter 4 and applied to the population of homosexual/bisexual men in San Francisco in Chapters 5 and 6. This group has been chosen as the first population to be analyzed because there is more information available on HIV/AIDS in these homosexual men than for any other group in the world. This model is expanded in Chapter 7 to encompass the five major risk groups in the U.S. It is shown in Chapter 8 that the HIV epidemics in homosexual men and intravenous drug users (IVDUs) are not crucially linked by homosexual IVDUs so that they can be modeled as separate epidemics. Chapter 9 considers relationships between AIDS incidence data in related risk groups and racial/ethnic groups in the Northeast region of the U.S. and its subregions. In Chapter 10 the modeling approach is used to compare HIV and AIDS in the five major risk groups in 15 subregions of the U.S. and then the similarities and differences revealed by these comparisons are discussed.

Because some injections (e.g., steroids) are not intravenous, the term *intravenous drug user* or IVDU has been changed in some recent publications to *injecting drug user* or IDU. Moreover, the term *homosexual/bisexual men* has recently often been replaced by *men who have sex with men*. Since much of the work presented here was done before the terminology changed, we have not converted to the new terms. If the reader prefers the new terminology, then the reader can mentally convert the old terms to the new terms throughout this manuscript.

As described in Section 1.4, AIDS is a worldwide problem, so it would be desirable to extend the modeling approach used here to other continents and countries. Some aspects of the model developed here would be useful for other countries, but other aspects would not. In the U.S. the dominant modes of transmission are through homosexual contact and needle–sharing between IVDUs. In many other parts of the world the dominant mode of transmission is through heterosexual contact. Here we have focused on HIV/AIDS in the U.S. since better AIDS incidence data is available in the U.S. than in most other countries.

We hope that the mathematical modeling and computer simulations of HIV/AIDS in this monograph will be useful to epidemiologists, scientists, mathematicians and students who are interested in the epidemiology of HIV/AIDS or in how modeling can contribute to the understanding of disease transmission in populations. Modeling has become a widely used tool in epidemiology. One indication of the increased importance of epidemiological modeling is the workshop, "A National Effort to Model AIDS Epidemiology", held at Leesburg, Virginia on July 25–28, 1988, which was sponsored by the Office of Science and Technology Policy, Executive Office of the President of the U.S. (OSTP, 1988).

We wish to express our gratitude to the many people in San Francisco, New York City and other areas who have participated in studies, collected data and reported the results. Without their efforts, the parameter estimation for the simulation modeling would not have been possible. We are grateful for valuable data, suggestions and comments from Nancy Hessol, Robert Kohn and George Lemp (San Francisco Department of Public Health), Peter Bacchetti and Andrew Moss (San Francisco General Hospital), William Lang and Michael Samuel (San Francisco Men's Health Study), James Wiley (University of California at Berkeley), Larry Bye (Communication Technologies), Michael Aldrich (California AIDS Intervention Training Center), James Fordyce and Rand Stoneburner (New York City Department of Health), Don Des Jarlais (New York State Division of Substance Abuse Services) and Ira Longini (Emory School of Public Health).

We thank the personnel of the Division of HIV/AIDS, National Center for Infectious Diseases, Centers for Disease Control, Atlanta, Georgia. This AIDS modeling project would not have been possible without their willingness to supply data, discuss concepts, and consider new ideas. During our visits there, we have consulted with Ruth Berkelman, Robert Byers, James Curran, William Darrow, Owen Devine, Lynda Doll, Timothy Dondero, Timothy Green, Marta Gwinn, Debra Hanson, Harold Jaffe, John Karon, W. Meade Morgan, Tom O'Brien, Marguerite Pappaioanou, Glen Satton, Richard Selik and John Ward. We especially appreciate the cooperation of James Curran, Director of the Division of HIV/AIDS and John Karon, Statistics and Data Management Branch.

We thank Director Jay Semel and Administrator Lorna Olson at the University of Iowa Center for Advanced Studies for cheerfully providing support services while we were working on this project.

TABLE OF CONTENTS

CHAPTER 1

BACKGROUND ON THE EPIDEMIOLOGY AND MODELING OF HIV/AIDS

Before modeling any disease it is crucial to understand the epidemiological features of the disease. The first four sections of this chapter present epidemiological information on the human immunodeficiency virus (HIV) and the acquired immune deficiency syndrome (AIDS) including transmission mechanisms, data, and historical, biological and clinical aspects. The last three sections discuss not only advantages and disadvantages of various approaches to modeling HIV/AIDS, but also the purposes and limitations of epidemiological modeling.

1.1 HIV Transmission Mechanisms

The three known modes of transmission of HIV are sexual contact, direct contact with HIV–infected blood or fluids and perinatal transmission from an infected mother to her child. There is no evidence of spread from toilet seats, by insects or by casual contact. There are indications that the transmissibility of HIV infection varies greatly during the multi–year course of infection in an individual (Goedert, Eyster et al., 1987; Longini et al., 1990). Transmission may be more likely during the early flu–like illness, which occurs just after HIV infection and before the body develops an antibody response. Since the HIV virus level in the blood decreases during the asymptomatic period, the transmissibility appears to be lower in this period. Then the transmissibility seems to increase again as the CD4⁺ cell count gets low, the HIV virus level in the blood increases, and symptoms appear.

In homosexual partners the most important route of transmission seems to be receptive anal intercourse. The likelihood of transmission seems to be less for insertive anal intercourse and for insertive or receptive orogenital contact (Kaslow and Francis, 1989, p. 98). In heterosexual partners engaging in penile–vaginal intercourse, both male–to–female and female–to–male transmissions do occur. However, a recent study in the U.S. suggests that male–to–female HIV transmission is much more likely than female–to–male transmission (Padian et al., 1991). Although HIV has been isolated in saliva, there is strong evidence against HIV transmission by kissing (Kaslow and Francis, 1989, p. 99).

The transfer of blood from an HIV–infected person to another person has been clearly established as a mode of transmission. In the U.S. this has been an important transmission mechanism for the needle–sharing IVDUs. In Africa nonsterile needles used for injection of medications have resulted in numerous HIV infections. Before blood screening began in the U.S. in 1985, some HIV infections resulted from blood transfusions with HIV–infected blood and from HIV–infected blood factor concentrate for hemophiliacs. Other sources of HIV infection in this category are transplanted organs such as kidneys and semen for artificial insemination. Transmission of HIV by arthropod vectors such as mosquitoes has not been observed and seems very unlikely.

Perinatal transmission from an HIV–infected mother to her child at a time before, during, or after birth is the third transmission mode. The exact times of transmission and the role of breast feeding have not been established, but approximately 30% of the children of HIV–infected mothers are infected.

1.2 Biological and Clinical Aspects of HIV Infection

The retrovirus called *human immunodeficiency virus* (HIV) was established in 1983 as the causative agent of AIDS. Isolates of HIV are molecularly and biologically heterogeneous, with some isolates being more virulent. Moreover, the HIV virus can change rapidly, even within an individual. The HIV infects a subpopulation of thymus–derived T lymphocytes called CD4⁺ lymphocytes or T4 cells, which are helper/inducer cells. These T cells perform recognition and induction functions as part of the immune response to foreign stimuli. The HIV integrates into the CD4⁺ host cell DNA, where it can remain dormant for a long time. The CD4⁺ T lymphocytes are eventually killed by the HIV while the HIV reproduces itself, so that the number of CD4⁺ cells gradually decreases from the normal number of about 900/ml (Kaslow and Francis, 1989). This leads to severe immunodeficiency in persons infected with HIV. Thus the natural history of HIV infection is a gradual depletion of CD4⁺ cells, progressive unresponsiveness of the immune system and increased susceptibility to opportunistic infections such as Pneumocystis Carinii pneumonia and malignancies such as Kaposi's sarcoma.

Transmission of HIV infection can be through the transfer of either cell–free HIV virus or HIV–infected lymphocytes. The probability of transmission appears to depend on the stage of HIV infection. In the first few weeks following infection, more HIV has been isolated from blood plasma than in the asymptomatic stage, so that people in the pre–antibody stage may be more infectious than people in the asymptomatic stage. In the late stages of HIV infection and AIDS, the cell–free HIV virus is found more frequently in blood plasma, so that these people may also be more infectious.

The enzyme–linked immunoassay (ELISA) test for HIV antibodies is inexpensive and useful for screening large numbers of samples; this test has almost no false negatives, but it is very sensitive (i.e., it has false positives at the rate of about 2 per 1000). Samples which are positive by the ELISA test are then tested by the Western blot assay. This immunoblot method is very specific (i.e., false positives occur in no more than 0.001% of the samples). Another test used is an indirect immunoflorescent antibody test involving microscopic examination of infected cell spots on glass slides. The combination of these and other tests such as PCR (polymerase chain reaction) are quite accurate in identifying HIV–positive individuals (Kaslow and Francis, 1989).

There are many different clinical manifestations of HIV infection and AIDS. Acute HIV infection occurs just after infection in some patients and is characterized as an acute febrile illness with fever, sweats, lethargy, muscle ache, headache and sore throat. These symptoms may last 2 to 3 weeks. About 2 months after infection, the immune system has generated antibodies which are recognized by the ELISA test. After an asymptomatic period of about 5 years, an HIV–infected person may develop some symptoms such as oral candidiosis (thrush), hairy leukoplakia, herpes zoster, weight loss, diarrhea, persistent generalized lymphadenopathy, neurologic diseases (dementia, myelopathy, polyneuropathy) and tuberculosis. The HIV–infected person may die of these diseases, but most get one or more of the opportunistic infections or neoplasms which characterize AIDS. These include cytomegalovirus infection, *Pneumocystis Carinii* pneumonia, toxoplasmosis of the brain and Kaposi's sarcoma. The original definition of AIDS was revised in 1985 (CDC, 1985c) and again in 1987 (CDC, 1987j). Now there are plans to change the AIDS definition again to include all HIV–positive people with CD4+ cell count below 200; this would approximately double the number of people satisfying the AIDS definition.

1.3 HIV and AIDS in the United States

The history of AIDS in the United States (U.S.) is interesting. In June 1981 the Centers for Disease Control (CDC) reported on five homosexual men in Los Angeles with an uncommon *Pneumocystis carinii* pneumonia (PCP) who had a cellular immune disfunction (CDC, 1981a). The next month CDC reported that 26 homosexual men in New York and California had Kaposi's sarcoma (KS), a rare skin cancer (CDC, 1981b). In August 1981 CDC reported more PCP and KS among homosexual men with immunosuppression (CDC, 1981c). Further study of some men with KS revealed that they had greatly reduced CD4+ T lymphocytes and that KS cases in these homosexual men were associated with a large number of sexual partners and a history of sexually transmitted diseases (Friedman–Klein et al., 1982). In 1982, the name *acquired immunodifficiency syndrome* (AIDS) was used to describe the people with this new condition. The clinical syndrome of AIDS was also recognized in heterosexual intravenous drug users (IVDUs) in the early 1980s (CDC, 1982). The retrovirus which causes AIDS was identified in 1983 and was called the *human T–lymphotropic virus* (HTLV–III) or *lymphadenopathy– associated virus* (LAV); it is now called the *human immunodeficiency virus* (HIV) or HIV–1 since an HIV–2 has been identified (CDC, 1986h). Thus important aspects of HIV transmission and AIDS in the U.S. were identified within a few years after the first cases were reported. Namely, that HIV was a virus which could be transmitted sexually and by needle–sharing IVDUs, that the immune system deteriorated due to the decline of CD4+ cells and that opportunistic infections and cancers occurred in the late stage of the disease.

Note that the *incidence* of a disease or condition is the number of new cases occurring per month (or year or other time interval), and that the *prevalence* is the total number of cases which exist at a given time. In an equilibrium situation for a disease such as measles, the prevalence is equal to the incidence times the average duration of the disease, but that this formula does not work for HIV or AIDS, since an equilibrium has not been reached and the duration of HIV infection is long and variable.

The yearly AIDS incidence in the U.S. has increased every year since 1980 and was about 44,000 in 1991 so that 22% of the 200,000 AIDS cases through 1991 occurred in 1991. The AIDS incidence is not uniform throughout the U.S. Figure 1.1 shows the 1991 annual case rates for the states. The incidence of AIDS is also not uniformly spread among people in the U.S., but is focused in certain risk groups and occurs more commonly in certain racial/ethnic groups.

So far, most of the AIDS cases in the U.S. have occurred in homosexual men with homosexual intercourse as the transmission mechanism. There have also been many AIDS cases in intravenous drug users (IVDUs) and some AIDS cases in homosexual men who are also IVDUs.

4

AIDS annual rates per 100,000 population, for cases reported in 1991, United States

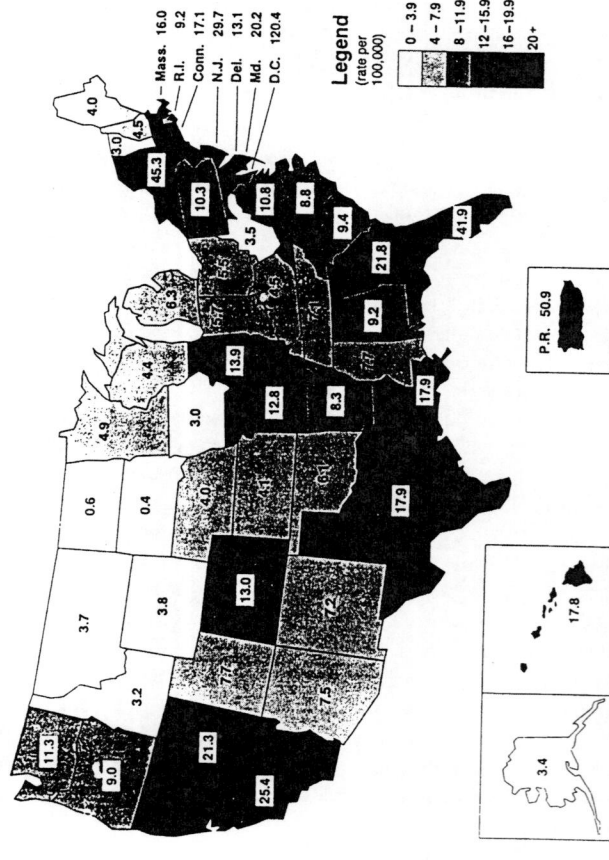

Mass. 16.0
R.I. 9.2
Conn. 17.1
N.J. 29.7
Del. 13.1
Md. 20.2
D.C. 120.4

Legend
(rate per 100,000)

0 – 3.9
4 – 7.9
8 – 11.9
12 – 15.9
16 – 19.9
20 +

P.R. 50.9

17.8

3.4

Figure 1.1. The geographical distribution of AIDS case rates in the United States. Source: CDC (1992, p. 3).

Most of the heterosexual AIDS cases in the U.S. are in the risk group of heterosexual partners of IVDUs. These four risk groups account for 94% of the AIDS cases in the U.S. in adults with a known risk of HIV infection. In children (<13 years old) 78% of AIDS cases with known risk of infection have occurred in children whose mother is an IVDU or a heterosexual partner of an IVDU (CDC, 1992). Since these are the major risk groups in the U.S., they are the groups analyzed by modeling in this monograph. Figure 1.2a shows the AIDS case rates by age group and sex in the U.S. The case rate in men is higher than in women because of homosexual and needle–sharing transmission (approximately three fourths of IVDUs with AIDS are men). Figure 1.2b shows the reported adult/adolescent AIDS cases by exposure category.

Blood–transfusion–acquired HIV infections are now very rare. Since 1985 all blood in the U.S. has been screened for HIV antibodies, with positive units being discarded. The risk group of being a recipient of a blood transfusion, blood component or tissue accounts for about 2% of all AIDS cases in the U.S., but this is primarily the result of those infected before screening started.

Many hemophiliacs in the U.S. were infected in the early 1980s by blood factor concentrate which was produced by pooling 5 to 10 thousand units of blood. Approximately three fourths of the 14,000 hemophiliacs in the U.S. have been infected with HIV. After HIV was identified, the blood factor concentrate was heat–treated to kill the HIV starting in late 1984. Hemophiliacs account for about 1% of AIDS cases in adults.

Other categories with small percentages of AIDS cases are heterosexual partners of people born in pattern II countries and children of women born in pattern II countries. Pattern II countries as described in the next section are those such as Haiti and many African countries, where heterosexual transmission predominates.

The primary source of data on AIDS in the U.S. is the Centers for Disease Control (CDC). All 50 states, the District of Columbia, U.S. dependencies and possessions and other related nations report AIDS cases to CDC using a uniform case definition and case report form. CDC compiles the data and reports it monthly in the publication, HIV/AIDS Surveillance Report. These reports include Tables of AIDS incidence in the states, large cities, adults, men, women, children, racial/ethnic groups and age groups. Tables 1.1, 1.2, and 1.3 are from the January 1992 HIV/AIDS Surveillance Report (CDC, 1992) which gives data through December 1991. These Tables give the numbers and percentages of AIDS cases in the various risk groups.

Note that 90% of AIDS cases in adults occur in men. Among white men, most AIDS cases occur in homosexual men, but among black and Hispanic men, the number of AIDS cases in homosexual men and in IVDUs are about equal. Among women, most cases occur in IVDUs, but many cases also occur in heterosexual partners of IVDUs. Observe that 29% of all AIDS cases occur in blacks, who constitute about 12% of the U.S. population, and 16% of all AIDS cases occur in Hispanics, who are about 8% of the U.S. population.

Reporting delays of AIDS cases are significant; about half of all AIDS cases are reported within 3 months of diagnosis, but about 15% are reported more than 1 year after diagnosis. Various methods are used for adjusting for reporting delays, but CDC uses a procedure developed by Karon, Devine and Morgan (1989). AIDS incidence data must be adjusted for reporting delays in order to see trends over time. Figure 1.3 shows AIDS incidences adjusted for reporting delays

ACQUIRED IMMUNODEFICIENCY SYNDROME (AIDS) — Annual rates per 100,000 adult population, by selected age group and sex for reported cases, United States, 1990

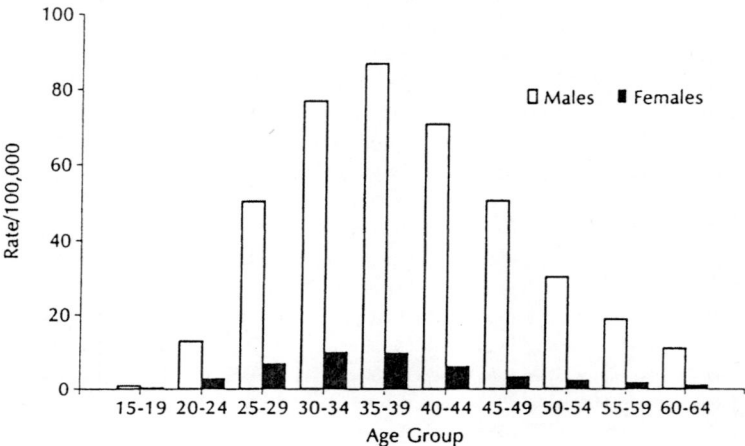

ACQUIRED IMMUNODEFICIENCY SYNDROME (AIDS) — Reported adult/adolescent cases, by exposure category, United States, 1990

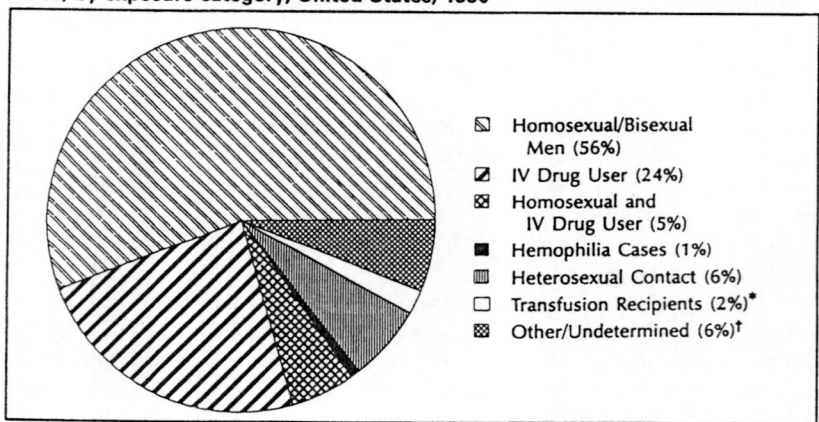

Figure 1.2 a) AIDS case rates by age and sex, b) AIDS case rates by exposure category.
Source: CDC (1990, p. 16).

Table 1.1 Male adult/adolescent AIDS cases by exposure category and race/ethnicity, reported through December 1991.
Source: CDC (1992, p. 11).

Male exposure category	White, not Hispanic		Black, not Hispanic		Hispanic		Asian/Pacific Islander		American Indian/Alaska Native		Total[4]	
	No.	(%)	No.	(%)	No.	(%)	No.	(%)	No.	(%)	No.	(%)
Men who have sex with men	83,205	(80)	20,540	(44)	13,240	(46)	936	(81)	172	(64)	118,362	(65)
Injecting drug use	7,017	(7)	16,798	(36)	11,083	(39)	40	(3)	33	(12)	35,048	(19)
Men who have sex with men and inject drugs	7,547	(7)	3,578	(8)	1,925	(7)	28	(2)	41	(15)	13,135	(7)
Hemophilia/coagulation disorder	1,373	(1)	127	(0)	137	(0)	18	(2)	8	(3)	1,671	(1)
Heterosexual contact:	813	(1)	3,307	(7)	548	(2)	9	(1)	3	(1)	4,687	(3)
Sex with injecting drug user	483		1,077		313		5		3		1,882	
Sex with person with hemophilia	7		1		2		–		–		10	
Born in Pattern-II[1] country	8		1,779		11		2		–		1,805	
Sex with person born in Pattern-II country	40		48		9		1		–		98	
Sex with transfusion recipient with HIV infection	43		19		16		–		–		79	
Sex with HIV-infected person, risk not specified	232		383		197		1		–		813	
Receipt of blood transfusion, blood components, or tissue[2]	1,938	(2)	418	(1)	259	(1)	55	(5)	1	(0)	2,679	(1)
Other/undetermined[3]	2,287	(2)	2,269	(5)	1,432	(5)	67	(6)	11	(4)	6,114	(3)
Male subtotal	104,180	(100)	47,037	(100)	28,624	(100)	1,153	(100)	269	(100)	181,696	(100)

8

Table 1.2 Female adult/adolescent AIDS cases by exposure category and race/ethnicity, reported through December 1991.
Source: CDC (1992, p. 11).

Female
exposure category

Injecting drug use	2,268 (41)	6,185 (55)	2,191 (50)	16 (15)	25 (56)	10,705 (50)
Hemophilia/coagulation disorder	29 (1)	10 (0)	3 (0)	–	–	42 (0)
Heterosexual contact:	1,700 (31)	3,784 (34)	1,694 (39)	37 (35)	10 (22)	7,249 (34)
Sex with injecting drug user	*859*	*2,244*	*1,343*	*14*	*7*	*4,484*
Sex with bisexual male	*343*	*216*	*78*	*11*	*1*	*651*
Sex with person with hemophilia	*78*	*10*	*4*	*2*	*–*	*94*
Born in Pattern-II country	*5*	*709*	*3*	*–*	*–*	*718*
Sex with person born in Pattern-II country	*10*	*63*	*2*	*–*	*–*	*76*
Sex with transfusion recipient with HIV infection	*102*	*28*	*28*	*2*	*–*	*161*
Sex with HIV-infected person, risk not specified	*303*	*514*	*236*	*8*	*2*	*1,065*
Receipt of blood transfusion, blood components, or tissue	1,055 (19)	349 (3)	220 (5)	35 (33)	5 (11)	1,668 (8)
Other/undetermined	414 (8)	828 (7)	292 (7)	17 (16)	5 (11)	1,561 (7)
Female subtotal	5,466 (100)	11,156 (100)	4,400 (100)	105 (100)	45 (100)	21,225 (100)

Table 1.3 Pediatric (< 13 years old) AIDS cases by exposure category and race/ethnicity, reported through December 1991.
Source: CDC (1992, p. 10).

Pediatric (<13years old) exposure category

Hemophilia/coagulation disorder	112 (15)	22 (1)	26 (3)	3 (18)	—	163 (5)
Mother with/at risk for HIV infection:	465 (63)	1,704 (92)	742 (87)	8 (47)	8(100)	2,936 (85)
Injecting drug use	*224*	*833*	*365*	*2*	*2*	*1,430*
Sex with injecting drug user	*91*	*269*	*238*	*2*	*1*	*603*
Sex with bisexual male	*22*	*24*	*14*	*1*	—	*61*
Sex with person with hemophilia	*9*	*3*	*1*	—	—	*13*
Born in Pattern-II country	*1*	*241*	*2*	—	—	*244*
Sex with person born in Pattern-II country	—	*13*	—	—	—	*14*
Sex with transfusion recipient with HIV infection	*4*	*4*	*4*	—	—	*13*
Sex with HIV-infected person, risk not specified	*30*	*70*	*40*	*1*	*2*	*144*
Receipt of blood transfusion, blood components, or tissue	*22*	*25*	*13*	—	—	*60*
Has HIV infection, risk not specified	*62*	*222*	*65*	*2*	*3*	*354*
Receipt of blood transfusion, blood components, or tissue	152 (21)	65 (4)	66 (8)	6 (35)	—	289 (8)
Undetermined	10 (1)	53 (3)	20 (2)	—	—	83 (2)
Pediatric subtotal	739(100)	1,844 (100)	854(100)	17 (100)	8(100)	3,471(100)
Total	**110,385**	**60,037**	**33,878**	**1,275**	**322**	**206,392**

a. Total cases, cases among homosexual/bisexual men[†], and cases among women and heterosexual men reporting intravenous (IV)-drug use

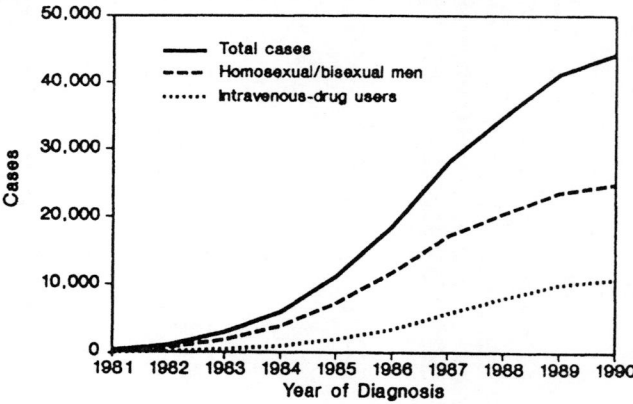

b. Cases among persons reporting heterosexual contact with persons with, or at high risk for, HIV infection

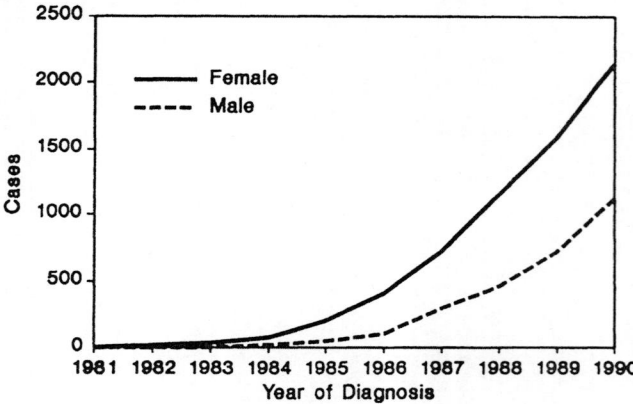

Figure 1.3. AIDS cases adjusted for reporting delays by year of diagnosis. a) total cases, homosexual/bisexual men, and IVDUs, b) heterosexual cases. Source: CDC (1991, p. 360).

c. Perinatally acquired pediatric AIDS cases

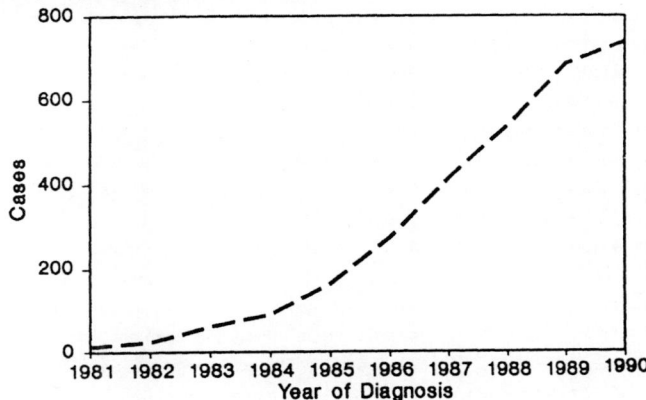

d. Cases among recipients of transfusions of blood or blood products

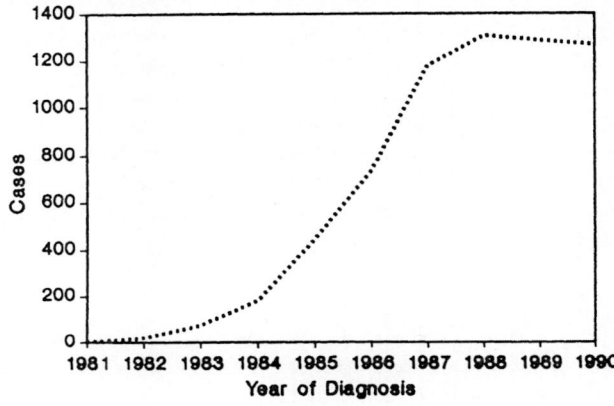

Figure 1.3. AIDS cases adjusted for reporting delays by year of diagnosis. c) perinatal cases, d) transfusion cases. Source: CDC (1991, p. 361).

for various risk groups (CDC, 1991b). From Figure 1.3a it appears that AIDS cases in homosexual men may be slowing down or leveling off. Also, AIDS incidence in IVDUs started later and continues to increase. In Figure 1.3b AIDS incidence in people reporting heterosexual contact started even later, but is now rising very rapidly. Pediatric AIDS cases in Figure 1.3c also continue to go up; the change in the last year may not be significant and due to reporting changes. The trend in recipients of transfusions of blood or blood products in Figure 1.3d is clear; AIDS cases in this group are now declining. This trend is not surprising since almost no new HIV infections occurred as a result of transfusions after blood screening started in early 1985.

Although national time trends in AIDS cases give some information, they often do not tell the whole story. Figure 1.4 shows that AIDS cases in homosexual men in New York City (NYC), San Francisco (SF), and Los Angeles (LA) appear to be leveling off after 1987, but AIDS cases in homosexual men in all other regions continue to increase at least through 1989 (Karon and Berkelman, 1991). Even this graph does not reveal the complete picture. Figure 1.5 shows AIDS incidence trends in NYC, LA, and SF; AIDS incidence appears to have started to decrease in NYC and has slowed down in LA and SF, but may not have leveled off yet in LA and SF. Karon and Berkelman (1991) also show that the trends in NYC, LA and SF are primarily due to changes in AIDS incidence in white homosexual men with smaller changes in blacks and Hispanics. In many other regions the AIDS incidence is increasing for both whites and non–whites. The take–home lesson from this analysis of AIDS in homosexual men is that it is often necessary to look beyond national data into regions, cities, and racial/ethnic groups to discover trends.

Data on HIV incidence and prevalence is relatively sparse and definitely less reliable than the AIDS incidence data. Some data on HIV incidence and prevalence is available from blood samples saved for other purposes; see Section 5.4.1 on San Francisco. But generally, there is no information on HIV incidence or prevalence in previous years. Even now it is very difficult to get information on HIV incidences or prevalences. Due to nonresponse bias and other factors, data from national surveys are often considered to be inaccurate. The widely–used value of 1 million HIV–infected people in the U.S. is based on a variety of estimates such as the back calculation method described in Section 1.5 (CDC, 1991b).

1.4 HIV and AIDS in the World

The AIDS pandemic is now entering its second decade. Although projections of its future are uncertain, it is clear that the world–wide epidemic is still in its early stages. In the 1990s millions of people who are already infected with HIV will develop AIDS and die. The World Health Organization (WHO) estimates that about 5 to 6 million men and 3 to 4 million women in the world have been infected with HIV. So far over 1 million have progressed to AIDS and an equal number have HIV–related illness. Worldwide, WHO forecasts that the cumulative number of HIV–infections will be 30 to 40 million by the year 2000. WHO projects that there will be 1 million adult AIDS cases and deaths per year, with about 1/2 million in Africa and 1/4 million in Asia (WHO, 1991).

13

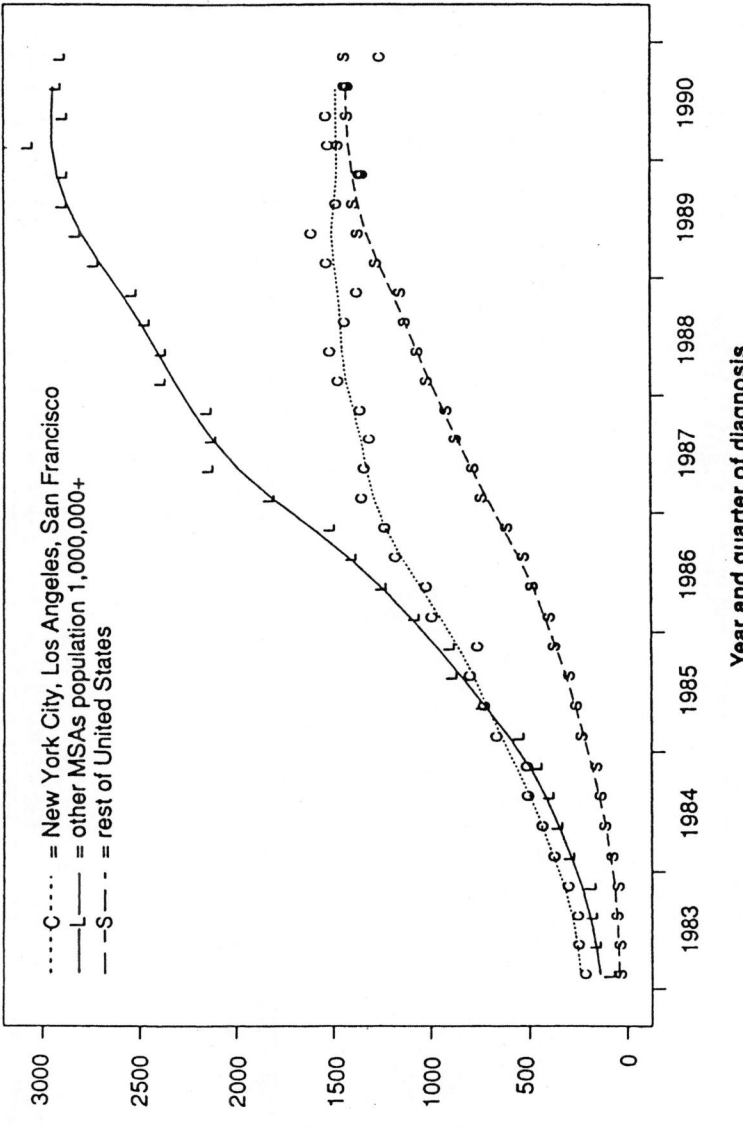

Figure 1.4. AIDS incidence adjusted for reporting delays in homosexual/bisexual men in the U.S. Source: Karon and Berkelman (1991).

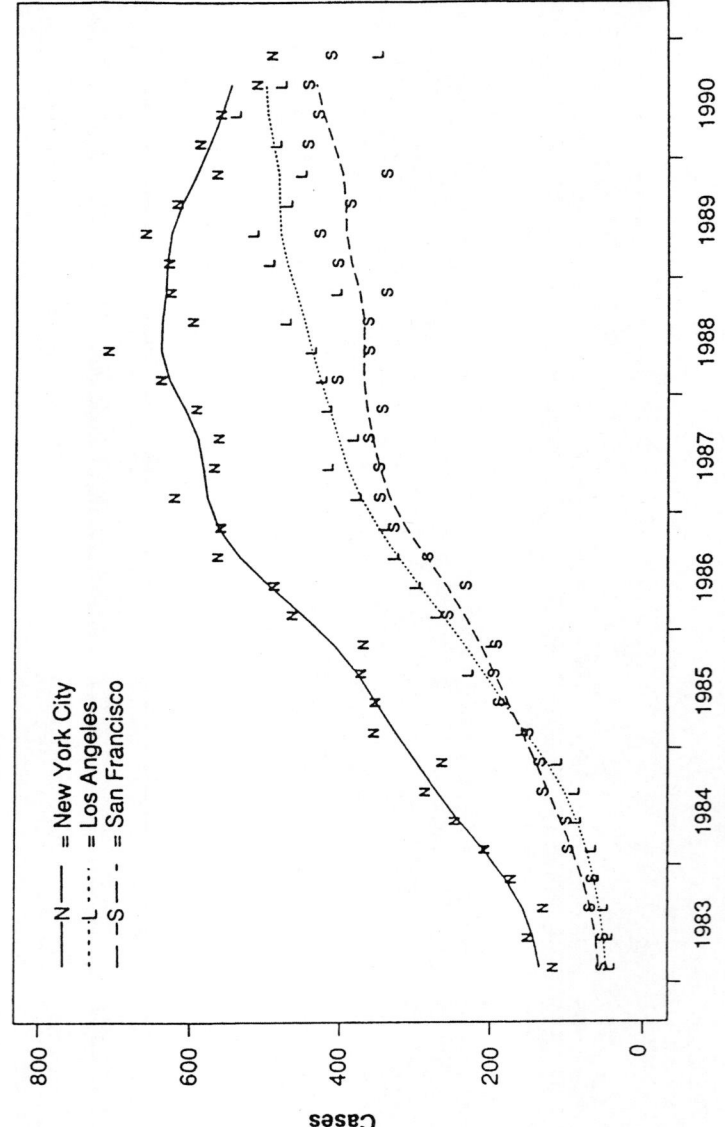

Figure 1.5. AIDS incidence adjusted for reporting delays in homosexual/bisexual men in three major cities (NYC, LA, SF) in the U.S. Source: Karon and Berkelman (1991).

The WHO has identified three basic patterns of HIV infection and AIDs in the world. Pattern I for AIDS occurs in North America, Western Europe, Australia and New Zealand. In these areas, the predominant modes of transmission are homosexual contact and needle–sharing by IVDUs, but there is some heterosexual and perinatal transmission. The male–to–female ratio is 10:1 to 15:1. There is no transmission by blood transfusion since blood is now screened. WHO suggests that the annual incidence of HIV infections in these areas may have peaked in the first half of the 1980s when there was rapid spread among homosexual men and IVDUs. The annual HIV incidences seem to have now decreased, presumably due to the reduction of risky behavior in these high risk groups. Heterosexual transmissions may increase, but WHO predicts that AIDS incidence will remain stable in the 1990s (WHO, 1991).

Pattern II for AIDS occurs in much of Africa and in parts of the Caribbean. In these areas the spread is primarily by heterosexual contact, and the male–to–female ratio is about 1:1. Some HIV transmission occurs during homosexual contact and by blood transfusion or medical uses of needles and syringes. Perinatal transmission is significant since there are many infected women. In sub–Sahara Africa the HIV epidemic grew in the 1970s and 1980s. The optimistic prediction of WHO is that the annual HIV incidence in this region will peak in the mid–1990s (WHO, 1991). Their prediction for Latin America, where the HIV incidence has been less, is similar, although there is the potential for high infection rates in Brazil.

Pattern III for AIDS occurs in the remainder of the world, including Asia, the Middle East and North Africa, where the HIV virus has arrived more recently. There is some HIV and AIDS in these areas; some HIV infections were acquired in other areas and some occurred within these areas. The AIDS incidence in these regions has been low so far, but there is the potential for increased incidence. In Asia, HIV transmission began in the late 1980s in a few countries, but HIV infection has spread rapidly since then. WHO predicts that annual HIV incidence in Asia will continue to rise until the early part of the next century, and by the end of the 1990s the annual incidence in Asia will exceed that in Africa (WHO,1991).

Worldwide, heterosexual transmission is responsible for two–thirds of all HIV infections so far, and this fraction is expected to increase. About one out of three children born to an HIV–infected mother is HIV–infected and dies of AIDS, usually by age five. The other two children become orphans when their mother dies of AIDS. So far, there have been about 1 million HIV–infected infants born, over half of whom died of AIDS. There are now approximately 2 million uninfected children who are or will become orphans. WHO predicts that there will be 10 to 15 million AIDS orphans by the year 2000, most of them in sub–Sahara Africa (WHO, 1991).

The social and economic consequences of AIDS in developing countries will be stunning. Elderly people will not only be left without support as their grown children die, but also will become responsible for their surviving grandchildren. The costs of caring for people with HIV–related diseases will overwhelm the health care resources of many developing countries. There will be a decrease in the productivity of the workforce as young and middle–aged adults die from AIDS.

Meeting the challenge of AIDS requires extraordinary efforts throughout the world. Governments need to make AIDS prevention and control a top priority. They need to get all agencies and organizations involved in preventing HIV infections. They need to counter discrimination against HIV-infected persons and to fight complacency and denial about AIDS. The social conditions which put people at risk of HIV infection, such as multiple sexual partners, occur throughout the world. No racial and ethnic groups seem to have greater susceptibility or resistance to HIV infection. The prospects during the 1990s for developing a vaccine to prevent HIV infection or prevent AIDS are uncertain. Thus the primary means of prevention is through education of the people about the risks and possible preventative measures.

1.5 Three Approaches to Modeling HIV/AIDS

The objective of this section is to present descriptions and cite the literature on the main approaches to HIV/AIDS modeling. Surveys of mathematical models for HIV transmission and AIDS have been given by Isham (1988) and Anderson (1988b). An annotated bibliography of statistical methodology for study of HIV/AIDS has been published by Fusaro et al. (1989). Schwager, Castillo–Chavez and Hethcote (1989) have reviewed both statistical and mathematical approaches in HIV/AIDS modeling.

The first and most direct approach to predicting AIDS cases in the future is extrapolation (Morgan and Curran, 1986; Karon et al., 1988, 1989). This method is to fit an assumed form of the AIDS incidence curve to the AIDS incidence data in recent years and then to extend this curve for several years as a prediction of AIDS cases in the future. This method assumes that the current trends will continue for at least a few years into the future. Often separate curves and extrapolations are done for various risk groups. Advantages of extrapolation are its simplicity and ease of use. The extrapolation method has been a good predictor of AIDS incidence for a few years into the future, but it is not good for longer forecasts since it does not consider changes in the HIV epidemic due to factors such as behavioral changes or saturation in the high risk groups . Another disadvantage is that it does not give any information on HIV incidence or any understanding of the HIV transmission mechanisms. Extrapolation has been used on United Kingdom data by Healy and Tillett (1988) and on European data by Downs et al. (1987). Extrapolation has not worked as well in recent years because there have been clear changes in trends with a decreasing rate of growth and the incidence has reached a plateau in some risk groups.

The second approach to modeling AIDS incidence is usually called back calculation (Brookmeyer and Gail, 1986, 1988; Gail and Brookmeyer, 1988; Brookmeyer and Damiano, 1989). The total number of cases of AIDS at time t is the summation up to time t of the product of the HIV incidence at time τ and the probability of developing AIDS within $t - \tau$ years after infection. Thus if the HIV incidence and the distribution of the AIDS incubation period were known up to time t, then the cumulative AIDS cases would be calculated in a straight-forward way using the convolution summation above. Back calculation is a deconvolution process; it uses a given AIDS incidence up to time t and an estimated distribution for the AIDS incubation period to estimate the HIV incidence up to time t. This HIV incidence up to time t and its extrapolation for a few years are then used to forecast the AIDS incidence for a few years. The distribution of the incubation period for AIDS can be estimated parametrically or nonparametrically. The back calculation procedure is often applied to separate risk groups.

Back calculation has been used for forecasting AIDS incidence for a few years and does have the advantage that it also yields estimates of HIV incidence; however, there are several disadvantages. It does not yield any information on the HIV transmission dynamics or estimates of parameter values. Estimated distributions for the AIDS incubation period are uncertain and the back calculation procedure is very sensitive to the distribution used (Brookmeyer and Damiano, 1988; Hyman and Stanley, 1988). The instability of the back calculation process implies that the confidence intervals of the estimates of HIV incidence and future AIDS incidence are very wide.

The third approach to modeling AIDS is to use HIV transmission dynamics models which include the progression to AIDS. These models often have the population divided into compartments consisting of those who are susceptible, in each of the infectious stages, or in the AIDS phase. In deterministic transmission models, the movements between these compartments by becoming infected, progressing to the next stage or AIDS, migrating or dying are specified by systems of difference or differential equations. The models of this type used in this monograph are formulated in Chapters 3 and 7. Dynamic models and computer simulations are experimental tools for comparing regions or risk groups, testing theories, assessing quantitative conjectures and answering questions. For example, in Chapter 6 we determine the relative importance of saturation in the high risk group and behavior changes in changing the AIDS incidence in homosexual men in San Francisco. Modeling can also be used to theoretically evaluate, compare or optimize various detection, prevention, intervention or control programs. A detailed discussion of the purposes and limitations of dynamic epidemiological modeling is given in the next section.

Some HIV transmission dynamics models are stochastic with probabilities of moving to the next stage at each time step. Mode et al. (1989) investigated the relationship between Monte Carlo simulations of a stochastic HIV/AIDS model and solutions of a deterministic model using the expected values. Tan (1991) looks at general stochastic models for the simulation of HIV transmission and AIDS. In the book (Tan, 1992) the stochastic analog of the deterministic model used in Chapters 5 and 6 is analyzed and the results are compared with those for the deterministic model. A special issue (vol 107, No 2, December 1991) of the journal *Mathematical Biosciences* contains six papers on stochastic models for HIV/AIDS.

Both deterministic and stochastic dynamic epidemiological models have been used to analyze many diseases including measles, rubella, mumps, chicken pox, poliomyelitis, smallpox, gonorrhea, schistosomiasis, malaria, cholera and rabies. For examples, see the books by Bailey (1975), Anderson (1982), Anderson and May (1982, 1991) and Hethcote and Yorke (1984). Many dynamic models have been analyzed mathematically; see Hethcote (1989a) for an introduction to mathematical epidemiology or Hethcote et al. (1981) and Hethcote and Levin (1989) for surveys of mathematical results.

In recent years there has been a tremendous number of modeling papers which use dynamic models of HIV transmission and progression to AIDS. Surveys of these modeling papers are cited at the beginning of this section. Two authors who have contributed to HIV/AIDS modeling are Anderson and May (e.g., Anderson, 1988; Anderson and May, 1988; May, 1988); some of their modeling results are incorporated into their encyclopedic book (Anderson and May, 1991), which is built from their numerous epidemiological papers during the past ten years. Their models have covered not only homosexual and heterosexual populations in the United States and United Kingdom, but also heterosexual populations in Africa. They have estimated reproduction numbers (contact numbers), doubling times and demographic consequences.

Some of the multigroup models for HIV/AIDS are similar in formulation to the multigroup models developed for gonorrhea, which is another sexually transmitted disease (STD) (Lajmanovich and Yorke, 1976; Hethcote and Yorke, 1984). Multigroup models are appropriate for STDs because people are heterogeneous in their behaviors and contact rates with others. The contacts can be homosexual, heterosexual or needle–sharing contacts. The models in this monograph in Chapters 3 and 7 are multigroup models.

Proportionate mixing in multigroup models was used in gonorrhea modeling by Nold (1980) and Hethcote and Yorke (1984). They also used a convex combination of internal contacts and proportionate mixing, which has been named *preferred mixing* by Jacquez et al. (1988) and *biased mixing* by Hyman and Stanley (1988, 1989). Jacquez et al. (1988) used multigroup compartmental models for HIV with constant recruitment into susceptible classes and variable infectivity in the infectious stages to analyze the effects of different mixing patterns. This analysis has been extended to more complicated mixing structures by Jacquez et al. (1989) and Koopman et al. (1989). Castillo–Chavez and coauthors (Blythe and Castillo–Chavez, 1989; Busenberg and Castillo–Chavez, 1989; Castillo–Chavez et al., 1989) have focused on the theoretical analysis of diverse mixing structures in HIV/AIDS models.

Hyman and Stanley (1988, 1989) have considered both continuous and discrete HIV/AIDS models with heterogeneity and different mixing structures. They have analyzed the spread from high to low risk groups, the effects of variable infectivity and the instability of the back calculation procedure. An innovative approach to dynamic modeling of HIV/AIDS has been developed by Dietz and Hadeler (Dietz, 1988; Dietz and Hadeler, 1988; Hadeler et al., 1988). Their models explicitly consider the dynamics of pairs of individuals and the duration of their partnerships. These pair formation and dissolution models are distinctly different from the *contact rate mixing matrix* models used by many other modelers.

We have not attempted to give a complete survey of HIV/AIDS modeling; other papers are cited in later chapters. For more information the reader is referred to the survey articles cited earlier or the collection of papers edited by Castillo–Chavez (1989). The primary features which distinguish the approach in this monograph are the use of the deterministic dynamic simulation models as a framework for the interpretation of data, the efforts to estimate parameter values from data, the fitting of the model to HIV and AIDS incidence data and comparisons obtained by fitting the same model in fifteen different subregions of the U.S.

1.6 Purposes and Limitations of Epidemiological Modeling

Epidemiology is the study of the distribution and determinants of disease prevalence in humans. Epidemiologists study both infectious diseases and chronic diseases such as cancer and cardiovascular disease. One function of epidemiology is to describe the distribution of the disease, *i.e.*, find out who has how much of what, where and when. Another function is to identify the causes or risk factors for diseases in order to find out why everyone doesn't have the same thing uniformly. A third function of epidemiology is to build and test theories. A fourth function is to plan, implement and evaluate detection, control and prevention programs.

Epidemiological modeling can play an important role in the last two functions above. Here we focus on modeling infectious diseases in human populations and do not consider models for chronic diseases such as cancer. In most of this section "epidemiological modeling" refers to dynamic modeling where the population is divided into compartments based on their health status (e.g. susceptible, infectious, recovered) and the movements between compartments by becoming infected, progressing, recovering or migrating are specified by differential or difference equations. First, fifteen purposes of epidemiological modeling are described and then three limitations are considered; they are all summarized in Table 1.4. One cannot infer from the numbers of purposes and limitations that the advantages overwhelm the limitations since the first limitation is very broad.

A primary reason for infectious disease modeling is that it leads to clear statements of the assumptions about the biological and social mechanisms which influence disease spread. The model formulation process is valuable to epidemiologists and modelers because it forces them to be precise about the relevant aspects of transmission, infectivity, recovery and renewal of susceptibles. Epidemiological modelers need to formulate models clearly and precisely using parameters which have well–understood epidemiological interpretations such as a contact rate or an average duration of infection (Hethcote, 1976, 1989a). Complete statements of assumptions are crucial so that the reasonableness of the model can be evaluated in the process of assessing the conclusions.

An advantage of mathematical modeling of infectious diseases is the economy, clarity and precision of a mathematical formulation. A model using difference, differential, integral or functional differential equations is not ambiguous or vague. Of course, the parameters must be defined precisely and each term in the equations must be explained in terms of mechanisms, but the resulting model is a definitive statement of the basic principles involved. Once the mathematical formulation is complete, there are many mathematical techniques available for determining the threshold, equilibrium, periodic solutions, and their local and global stability. Thus the full power of mathematics is available for analysis of the equations. Moreover, information about the model can also be obtained by numerical simulation on digital computers of the equations in the model. The mathematical analyses and computer simulations can identify important combinations of parameters and essential aspects or variables in the model. In order to choose and use epidemiological modeling effectively on specific diseases, one must understand the behavior of the available formulations and the implications of choosing a particular formulation.

Table 1.4. Purposes and Limitations of Epidemiological Modeling

---

Fifteen Purposes of Epidemiological Modeling

1. The model formulation process clarifies assumptions, variables and parameters.

2. The behavior of precise mathematical models can be analyzed using mathematical methods and computer simulations.

3. Modeling allows explorations of the effect of different assumptions and formulations.

4. Modeling provides concepts such as a threshold, reproduction number, etc.

5. Modeling is an experimental tool for testing theories and assessing quantitative conjectures.

6. Models with appropriate complexity can be constructed to answer specific questions.

7. Modeling can be used to estimate key parameters by fitting data.

8. Models provide structures for organizing, coalescing and cross–checking diverse pieces of information.

9. Models can be used in comparing diseases of different types or at different times or in different populations.

10. Models can be used to theoretically evaluate, compare or optimize various detection, prevention, therapy and control programs.

11. Models can be used to assess the sensitivity of results to changes in parameter values.

12. Modeling can suggest crucial data which needs to be collected.

13. Modeling can contribute to the design and analysis of epidemiological surveys.

14. Models can be used to identify trends, make general forecasts, or estimate the uncertainty in forecasts.

15. The validity and robustness of modeling results can be assessed by using ranges of parameter values in many different models.

Three Limitations of Epidemiological Modeling

1. An epidemiological model is not reality; it is an extreme simplification of reality.

2. Deterministic models do not reflect the role of chance in disease spread and do not provide confidence intervals on results.

3. Stochastic models incorporate chance, but are usually harder to analyze than the corresponding deterministic model.

Thus mathematical epidemiology provides a foundation for the applications (Hethcote et al., 1981; Hethcote and Levin, 1989).

Modelers are able to explore and examine the effects of different assumptions and formulations. For example, they can compare an ordinary differential equations model, which corresponds to a negative exponential distribution for the infectious period, with a delay–differential equations model, which assumes that everyone has the same fixed, constant–length infectious period. They can examine the impact of assuming homogeneous mixing instead of heterogeneous mixing. They can study the influence of different mixing patterns between groups on the spread of a disease in a heterogeneous population (see Jacquez et al., 1988; Castillo–Chavez et al., 1989). They can decide if models with and without an exposed class for people in the latent period behave differently. The results of exploring different formulations may provide insights for epidemiologists and are certainly useful to modelers who are choosing models for specific diseases. For example, if the essential behaviors (thresholds and asymptotic behaviors) are the same for a formulation using ordinary differential equations and a formulation using delay differential equations, then the modeler would probably choose to use the ordinary differential equations model since it is simpler (Hethcote and Tudor, 1980).

Epidemiologists need to understand the concept of a threshold which determines whether the disease persists or dies out. They need to know that the reproduction number is a combination of parameters which gives the number of secondary cases "reproduced" by a typical infective during the infectious period in a population where everyone is susceptible. They need to be aware that this reproductive number is the same as the contact number, which is the average number of adequate contacts of an infective person during the infectious period (Hethcote and Van Ark, 1987). They need to realize that the average replacement number is one at an endemic equilibrium because, in an average sense, each infective replaces itself by one new infective in an equilibrium situation. Probably the most valuable contributions of mathematical modeling to epidemiologists are concepts like those above. Mathematical models serve as a framework to explain causes, relationships and ideas. Mathematical models are very useful in obtaining conclusions that have an easily understood interpretation. Helping epidemiologists internalize conceptual and intuitive understandings of disease processes, mechanisms and modeling results is an essential aspect of the work of mathematical modelers.

Epidemiological modeling is an important part of the epidemiologist's function to build and test theories. Mathematical and computer simulation models are the fundamental *experimental tools* in epidemiology. Experiments with infectious diseases in actual populations are often unethical or very expensive or impractical. Thus modeling is essential for exploratory work. The only data usually available are from naturally occurring epidemics or from the natural incidence of endemic diseases; unfortunately, even these data are not complete since many cases are not reported. Since repeatable experiments and accurate data are usually not available in epidemiology, mathematical and computer simulation models must be used to perform needed theoretical experiments with different parameter values and different data sets. It is easy in a computer simulation to find out what happens if one or several parameters are changed.

Another advantage of epidemiological modeling is the availability of models to assess quantitative conjectures. For example, models can be used to check the claim that a two–dose vaccination program for measles would lead to herd immunity whereas a one–dose program would not (Hethcote, 1983). With a model one could see if the AIDS virus would eventually disappear in a population of homosexual men if half of them became celibate or practiced safer sex. Although it is understood how an infective can transmit the infection by contacts with others and how a disease spreads through a chain of infections, it is not easy to comprehend the large scale dynamics of disease spread in a community or to evaluate quantitative theories without the formal structure of a mathematical model. An epidemiological model connects the microscopic description or role of an infectious individual to the macroscopic spread of the infection in a community. Mathematical models are a formal, quantitative way of building and testing theories.

When formulating a model for a particular disease, it is necessary to decide which factors to include and which to omit. This choice will often depend on the particular question that is to be answered. Simple models have the advantage that there are only a few parameters, but have the disadvantage of possibly being naive and unrealistic. Complex models may be more realistic, but they may contain many parameter values for which estimates cannot be obtained. The art of epidemiological modeling is to make suitable choices in the model formulation so that it is as simple as possible and yet is adequate for the question being considered. It is important to recognize both the capabilities and limitations of epidemiological modeling. Many important questions cannot be answered using a given class of models. The most difficult problem for a modeler is to find the right combination of available data, an interesting question and a mathematical model which can lead to the answer.

For AIDS one can ask whether needle–sharing is more important for transmission than sexual activity. How important are homosexual intravenous drug users in linking the epidemics in the homosexual/bisexual men and intravenous drug users? Is there a "core" group for AIDS as there was for gonorrhea and is it the same core group? How important are bisexuals and prostitutes in the transmission process? How rapidly does HIV infection spread from high risk groups to low risk groups? Why do AIDS cases in many populations increase initially as a cubic function of time? Hyman and Stanley (1988) suggest that this cubic growth could be explained by the spread of infection from high contact–rate groups down through lower contact–rate groups. Is sustained transmission likely in the heterosexual population with frequent partner changes? What effect will therapy with zidovudine (AZT) have on the average survival time with AIDS and on the transmission? There are many relevant questions to ask about AIDS.

By fitting the incidence predicted by a model to actual incidence data (number of new cases per month), it is possible to estimate key parameters such as contact numbers or average durations. Contact numbers (reproduction numbers) are estimated for various directly–transmitted diseases in Anderson and May (1982, 1991). Hethcote and Van Ark (1987) present methods for estimating contact numbers for the groups in a multigroup model for disease transmission.

In AIDS modeling, fitting the predicted HIV prevalence and AIDS incidence to data on both can lead to estimates of the average number of new partners per month and the probability of HIV transmission per new partner (see Chapter 6). Since these parameters have already been estimated from the literature, the modeling provides a check on these *a priori* estimates. Thus the model is a way of coalescing parameter estimates and other pieces of data to see if they fit into a consistent framework. The model can serve as the conceptual and quantitative unifier of all the available information.

Comparisons can lead to a better understanding of the process of disease spread. It may be enlightening to compare the same disease at different times, the same disease in different populations or different diseases in the same population. One method for comparing diseases is to estimate parameter values for the diseases and then compare the parameter values. For example, in Anderson and May (1982, 1991) and Hethcote (1989a) estimates of contact numbers (also called reproduction numbers) are given for various diseases such as measles, whooping cough, chicken pox, diphtheria, mumps, rubella, poliomyelitis and smallpox. These numbers lead to fractions of the population which must be immune in order to achieve herd immunity for these diseases. Childhood diseases are compared in rural and urban areas in Anderson (1982). The level of HIV infection in homosexual men in San Francisco is compared at various times and the changes in behavior in this population are given in Chapter 6.

A very important reason for epidemiological modeling is the value of models for theoretical evaluations and comparisons of detection, prevention, therapy and control programs. Epidemiologists and politicians need to understand the effects of different policy decisions. Qualitative predictions of infectious disease models are always subject to some uncertainty since the models are idealized and the parameter values can only be estimated. However, quantifications of the relative merits of several control methods or of control versus no control are often robust in the sense that the same conclusions hold for a broad range of parameter values and a variety of models. Control strategies for gonorrhea such as screening, rescreening, infectee tracing, infector tracing and potential vaccines for both women and men were compared in Hethcote and Yorke (1984). Various vaccination strategies for rubella and measles have been compared using modeling (Hethcote, 1983, 1989b; Anderson and May, 1982).

Sometimes an optimization method can be used on some aspect of an epidemiological model. Hethcote and Waltman (1973) used dynamic programming to find an optimal vaccination strategy to control an epidemic at least cost. Longini et al.(1978) determined the best age or social groups to vaccinate for Hong Kong and Asian influenza when there was a limited amount of vaccine available. Hethcote (1988) found theoretical optimal ages of vaccinations for measles in three geographic locations. See Wickwire (1977) for a survey of modeling papers on the control of infectious diseases.

Predictions or quantitative conclusions of a model are said to be sensitive to a parameter if a small change in the parameter causes a large change in the outcome. A model is insensitive to a parameter if the outcomes are the same for a wide range of values of that parameter. An important reason for epidemiological modeling is the determination of the sensitive and insensitive parameters since this information provides insight into the epidemiological processes. Once the sensitive parameters are identified, it may be possible to make special efforts to gather data to obtain better estimates of these parameters. Thus the modeling process can help identify crucial data that should be collected. If the data and information are insufficient to estimate parameters in a model or to piece everything together, then the model formulation process can identify the missing information which must be gathered.

Modeling can enhance an epidemiological survey by providing a framework for the analysis of the survey results. In the design phase modeling can help identify important questions that need to be asked in order to have adequate data to obtain results. The statistical aspects of a survey design are now analyzed before the survey is conducted. Similarly, those design aspects relevant to parameter estimation in models should be analyzed before the survey is conducted to see if all significant data are being collected.

Another purpose of epidemiological modeling is to make forecasts about the future incidence of a disease. Although people often think of prediction as the first or only purpose of epidemiological modeling, the purposes given above are more important. Accurate forecasts are usually not possible because of the idealization in the models and the uncertainty in the parameter values. However, possible forecasts under various scenarios can sometimes be given or trends can be identified. One purpose of epidemiological modeling is to reduce the uncertainty in future incidence projections. For example, improved estimates of the number of HIV infections and AIDS cases in future years are needed in order to provide appropriate public health programs and adequate medical care for patients with HIV-related medical conditions and AIDS. Although simple extrapolations for 2 or 3 years of the time trends for numbers with AIDS or in a final stage of HIV infection are often adequate, better estimates are obtained with models which consider population changes due to the disease transmission process.

The validation of models and modeling results is difficult since there are rarely enough good data to adequately test or compare different models with data (Anderson and May, 1991). However, when the same concept or result is obtained for a variety of models and by several modelers, then the confidence in the validity of the result is increased. For example, three different papers using different approaches to comparing two rubella vaccination strategies agree on the criteria determining situations when each strategy is best (Hethcote, 1989b). Similarly, when a quantitative result holds for a wide range of parameter values, then this result has some robustness. For example, if the same relative values of a variety of control procedures are obtained for wide ranges of parameter values, then the relative values may be robust even though the absolute values may vary (see Hethcote and Yorke, 1984).

After discussing the purposes and advantages of epidemiological modeling, it is imperative to also discuss the limitations. Epidemiologists and policy makers need to be aware of both the strengths and weaknesses of the epidemiological modeling approach.

The first and most obvious limitation is that all epidemiological models are simplifications of reality. For example, it is often assumed that the population is uniform and homogeneously mixing; this is always a simplification, but the deviation of reality from this simplification varies with the disease and the circumstances. This deviation from reality is rarely testable or measurable; however, it can sometimes be estimated intuitively from an understanding of the disease epidemiology. As described in the introduction, part of the reason for the differences between the model's behavior and the actual spread of the disease is that transmission is based on the interactions of human beings, and homo sapiens have highly variable behavior and interactions. People do not behave in reasonably predictable ways like molecules or cells or particles.

Because transmission models are simplifications with usually unknown relationships to actual disease spread, one can never be completely certain about the validity of findings obtained from modeling such as conceptual results, experimental results, answers to questions, comparisons, sensitivity results and forecasts. Even when models are made more complicated in order to better approximate actual disease transmission, they are still abstractions. For example, multigroup models based on risk groups or sexual activity levels or age structure still assume that the distinctions between groups are clear and sharp and that the mixing between groups follows some assumed pattern. The modeler must always exercise judgment in deciding which factors are relevant and which are not when analyzing a specific disease or question.

The modeler needs to know that an SIR model is usually adequate since the behavior is essentially the same for the SEIR model where E is the latent period class. The notation SEIR for a model means that susceptibles (S) move to an exposed class (E) (when they are in a latent period; i.e., they are infected, but not yet infectious), then move to an infectious class (I), and finally to a removed class (R) when they recover and have permanent immunity. The modeler must realize that assuming that the infectivity is constant during the infectious period is reasonable for diseases like measles with a short infectious period (about 8 days), but is not reasonable for a disease like the human immunodeficiency virus (HIV) where the average time from HIV infection to AIDS is about 10 years. To incorporate age structure, the modeler must decide whether to use a model with time and age as continuous variables or to use discrete compartments corresponding to age brackets; the former requires the estimation of birth, death and aging rate coefficients as functions of time while the latter requires the estimation of birth, death and transfer rate constants. The modeler needs to decide whether the disease is epidemic in a short time period so that vital dynamics (births and deaths) can be excluded or the disease is endemic over a long time period (many years) so that vital dynamics must be included. The modeler must be aware that as the complexity of a model is increased so that it better approximates reality, the number of parameters increases so that it becomes increasingly difficult to estimate values of all of these parameters. Thus the modeler must (consciously or unconsciously) make many decisions regarding the relevant aspects in choosing a model for a specific disease or question.

When describing the purposes for epidemiological modeling, we have been thinking primarily of deterministic models, but the purposes also apply to stochastic epidemiological models. Deterministic models are those which use difference, differential, integral or functional differential equations to describe the changes in time of the sizes of the epidemiological classes. Given the starting conditions for a well—posed deterministic model, the solutions as a function of time are unique. In stochastic models, there are probabilities at each time step of moving from one epidemiological class to another. When these models are simulated with the probabilities calculated using random number generators, the outcomes of different runs are different so that this approach is often called Monte Carlo simulation; conclusions are obtained by averaging the results of many computer simulations. Simple deterministic models for epidemics have a precise threshold which determines whether an epidemic will or will not occur. In contrast, stochastic models for epidemics yield quantities such as the probability that an epidemic will occur and the mean time to extinction of the disease. Thus the approach, concepts and appropriate questions are quite different for stochastic models (Bartlett, 1960; Ludwig, 1974; Bailey, 1975; Nasell, 1985; Becker, 1989).

Both deterministic and stochastic epidemiological models have other limitations besides being only approximations of reality. Deterministic models do not reflect the role of chance in disease spread. Sometimes parameter values in deterministic models are set equal to the mean of observed values and the information on the variance is ignored. A set of initial conditions leads to exactly one solution in a deterministic model; thus no information is available on the reliability of or the confidence in the results. When quantities such as the contact number, replacement number, average infectious period, etc. are estimated by fitting output to data, confidence intervals on these estimates are not obtained. Confidence intervals also can not be found for comparisons and forecasts. Some understanding of the dependence on parameter values is obtained through a sensitivity analysis where the effects of changes in parameter values on results are found. If the variance of the observed value of a parameter is high and the results are sensitive to that parameter, then the confidence in the results would be low. However, the lack of precise confidence intervals implies that the reliability of the results is uncertain.

Stochastic epidemiological models incorporate chance, but it is usually harder to get analytic results for these models. Moreover, computational results are also harder since Monte Carlo simulations require many computer runs (25 to 100 or more) in order to detect patterns and get quantitative results. Even for stochastic epidemiological models where parameters are estimated by fitting the mean of the simulations to data, it may not be possible to find confidence intervals on these parameter estimates.

1.7 Expectations of Modeling HIV Transmission Dynamics and AIDS

In June 1988 the Presidential Commission on the HIV Epidemic recommended that "the research community should be actively engaged in developing innovative models that better describe and explain the transmission of HIV within the population." On July 25–29, 1988 the AIDS Modeling and Epidemiology Workshop was held in Leesburg, Virginia. Ninety scientists in the fields of mathematics, statistics, epidemiology, data management, biology, behavioral sciences and social sciences participated. "The purpose of the Workshop was to examine the current status of AIDS and HIV modeling, to assess the potential benefits from mathematical and statistical analysis, and to make recommendations for a program of research." The conclusions from this meeting given below are from the report of the Office of Science and Technology Policy, Executive Office of the President (OSTP, 1988).

> "The major findings of the workshop are
>
> 1.   "Mathematical modeling and statistical analysis must be brought to bear fully on the AIDS epidemic. The success of

mathematical techniques in other fields of application and the presence of modern computational capability argue strongly for this added approach to AIDS and HIV analysis and projection. The modeling of the gonorrhea epidemic earlier this decade, cost—benefit analysis of rubella in England, and predictions of the spread of Hong Kong flu have exhibited that modeling and statistical projections of epidemics can make key contributions."

2.   "Mathematical and statistical methods that have been used for sexually transmitted diseases and other epidemics are only partially applicable to AIDS and HIV. The basic structure will be similar but empirical parameters and functions that characterize the new disease are required: intra— and inter—risk group mixing, partner relationships and duration, and biological transmissibility and infectivity during the period between HIV and AIDS. Progress has been made in formulating these parameters, but more data are required and a diverse set of modeling techniques and models are appropriate."

3.   "Given a supply of biological and behavioral data of good quality, modeling and advanced statistical analysis can provide better estimates of AIDS and HIV prevalence than are now available and eventually of HIV incidence. Cost—benefit assessments of prevention and intervention strategies and estimates of health care costs can be made. All of these depend on the accuracy and the coverage of the data. The mathematical studies can, in turn, point toward data needs and to insufficiencies in data quality."

4.   "AIDS incidence data allow short—term projections (3 to 5 years). HIV prevalence is difficult to estimate. Statistical extrapolations have shown that AIDS appears to be increasing as the third power of the time. Dynamic model analysis has been used to exhibit the subgroup behavior accounting for this dependence. HIV prevalence has been obtained by back—calculation for special risk groups and the general population. However, error ranges are large for this kind of calculation. HIV incidence can only be measured in special groups."

5.   "The quality of AIDS case data is good. Some selected risk group data are of special value. Improvements in the quality of HIV prevalence data require that the currently planned seroprevalence surveys, including those of the general population and the special family of surveys, proceed if they are found to be feasible."

6.   "Progress toward long—range predictions for AIDS and HIV prevalence requires new biological and behavioral data and collaborative efforts between modelers, statisticians, epidemiologists, and behavioral, social and data management scientists."

7.   "Collaboration has increased in the past year, and this has begun to increase the number of scientific results. In the past year there have been a number of meetings in which mathematical scientists, modelers, and statisticians have worked together with epidemiologists. Collaborative work has been funded by the National Institute for Drug Abuse (NIDA) on the advanced statistical analysis of AIDS among IV drug users at several universities."

8.   "There is a good supply of high—quality, motivated mathematical researchers, applied mathematicians, and statisticians to conduct the modeling effort. There are currently about 20 people involved in all of the mathematics work, several of whom work in PHS. The work to be done will require a total of 60 people in the next several years."

9.   "However, funding for the modeling effort is not adequate.
Few of those now doing modeling are supported. Funding required to
support those now working on modeling and the additional scientists
required to carry out the needed research would amount to $6 million
by 1991."

10.   "Access to AIDS and HIV data must be improved. As data
are collected, they must be made available to researchers.   A
comprehensive directory of data sources is required to bring modelers,
epidemiologists, and behavioral and social scientists to the data.
Large—population, public—use databases must continue to be made
more available in terms of the kinds of data released.   Small—
population datasets need to be made easier to access. A research
environment that facilitates sharing of data needs to be promoted.
However, all of these measures must be taken in a way that preserves
confidentiality and maintains individual anonymity."

The ten conclusions of this 1988 Workshop are quite interesting. Despite the fact that the
past contributions of epidemiological modeling cited in conclusion 1 are primarily conceptual,
conclusion 3 emphasizes the use of mathematical modeling for forecasting. Although we are
enthusiastic about the value of dynamic transmission modeling for conceptual understanding, we
are more cautious about its value for forecasting future AIDS incidence and HIV prevalence and
incidence. It may be difficult to do better forecasting than done by the extrapolation and back
calculation techniques mentioned in conclusion 4 and described in more detail in the previous
section. Dynamic transmission modeling can explore possible future incidences under different
scenarios, but the predictions are likely to be similar to those obtained by short—term forecasting
using simple direct methods such as extrapolation. We are disappointed that the Workshop
findings put so much emphasis on the use of mathematical modeling to give forecasts. Most of the
other findings seem valid since they address such issues as data and personnel availability,
collaboration and funding.

Two more recent publications have concluded that mathematical models for HIV
transmission and AIDS have great potential for forecasting, but that the data are not currently
available for parameter estimation in these models.

In *AIDS: Sexual Behavior and Intravenous Drug Use* (Turner et al., 1989) published by the
National Academy Press, it is stated on p. 74 that

"...promising mathematical models of the dynamics of the spread of
HIV infections require data on a wide range of sexual behaviors; these
data currently are not available. ... There are currently no reliable
data on sexual contacts for the national population; there are also no
such data for groups with elevated risks of transmitting or contracting
HIV infections (e.g., men who have sex with men, IV drug users,
heterosexuals with many sexual partners). Indeed, there is no reliable
information on the size of the nonmonagamous heterosexual population.
The lack of such data makes predictions about the future spread of
AIDS extremely uncertain."

In *AIDS Forecasting*, published by the General Accounting Office (1989), four types of
forecasting models are presented and analyzed. In their conclusions, they state on pp. 84—85 that

"...micro–simulation models were judged most comprehensive in the sense that they measured six components of the epidemic. These models explicitly consider HIV transmission and the development of AIDS and show how these contribute to past, current, and forecasted levels of the epidemic. In addition, projected future occurrences for individual components can be adjusted by the forecaster, allowing assessments of the effect of potential changes. But, unfortunately, the empirical basis of these models was extremely weak, due to lack of available information on specific components of the AIDS epidemic.

If knowledge about AIDS transmission were improved, the most comprehensive (micro–simulation) models would be deemed superior to the others in the sense that micro–simulation models make explicit the forces that contribute to the forecast."

We agree with the two quotations above; currently there are inadequate data to estimate the parameters in dynamic transmission simulation models well enough so that they will provide accurate forecasting. As better data become available, the forecasts of future HIV and AIDS incidences will improve, but it will be very difficult to estimate the accuracy of these forecasts. The social mixing, sexual interactions and needle–sharing behavior in our society are very complicated so that some simplifications are necessary in a model. The forecasts depend on the model used and it is difficult to decide how to choose a model with the appropriate amount of complexity. One guiding philosophy is to include the minimum structure to give reasonable fits to the data. Once the model is specified, it is then necessary to estimate the values of the parameters in the model. Even if the complete current and past sexual and needle–sharing behavior were known for each person in the United States, the problem would still remain of deciding on a reasonable model and then deciding how to summarize, group, categorize and condense the data in order to estimate parameter values in the model. Transmission dynamics models can be used to help identify trends, make general forecasts or estimate the uncertainty in the forecasts, but they are not more likely than other approaches to give accurate AIDS forecasts in the U.S. or elsewhere in the world. Both of the quotations above have focused on forecasting as the reason for AIDS modeling. We believe that the other benefits of epidemiological modeling described in the previous section are very important and are the aspects where mathematical modeling and computer simulations of HIV/AIDS can make the biggest contributions. In this monograph we emphasize conceptual understanding by the reconstruction of HIV/AIDS epidemics instead of forecasting future AIDS cases.

CHAPTER 2

MODELING THE PROGRESSION OF HIV–INFECTED PERSONS TO AIDS

Since people who are infected with HIV seem to progress through various stages or phases towards AIDS and death due to AIDS (Redfield et al., 1986; Seligman et al., 1987), a natural model for this progression is through a sequence of five phases (Hethcote, 1987, 1989; Longini et al., 1989, 1990). The first phase is the pre–antibody period, in which a person is infected, but not antibody seropositive. Some people in this first phase have acute illness. The second phase includes persons who are infected and antibody seropositive, but are asymptomatic. The third phase (symptomatic) occurs when the person develops an abnormal hematologic indicator and/or prodromal illnesses such as persistent generalized lymphadenopathy or oral candidiasis. The fourth phase is clinical AIDS, and the fifth phase is death due to AIDS. In Section 2.1 the asymptomatic and symptomatic phases are subdivided into stages in order to provide enough flexibility to match the HIV prevalence and AIDS incidence data in SF. If the number m of infectious stages is even, then the numbers of asymptomatic and symptomatic stages are equal to $(m-2)/2$; otherwise, they are $(m-3)/2$ and $(m-1)/2$, respectively.

As information about the effects of HIV on the immune system has accumulated, it has become clear that the progress towards AIDS coincides with a decline in the number of $CD4^+$ T–lymphocytes (T4 cells). Thus T4 cell count intervals can be used as stages and the progression through these stages can be measured. Longini et al. (1991) have used a continuous–time Markov process to model the decline of T4 cells in HIV–infected persons. The stages and mean waiting times are given in Section 2.2. This second staged progression model is probably more precise since it is based on quantitative laboratory measurements instead of the clinical symptoms involved in the first progression model.

The progression of HIV–infected children to AIDS is significantly different from that of adults (Auger et al., 1988). Some children progress rapidly, while others progress more slowly. In Section 2.3 a staged progression model for children with fast and slow tracks is formulated and parameter values are estimated. This model for the progression of children is used in later chapters for the children of female intravenous drug users (IVDUs) and female heterosexual partners of male IVDUs.

2.1 Staged Progression Based on Clinical Phases

The AIDS incubation period is the time from HIV infection until the development of AIDS. A variety of distributions such as the Weibull, gamma and normal have been used to fit AIDS incubation period data (Lui et al.,1988; Medley et al., 1987; Rees, 1987); however, a staged progression model is more useful for simulations. The model here results in a generalized gamma distribution for the AIDS incubation period (Longini et al., 1989,1990).

This staged progression model has five phases: pre–antibody, asymptomatic, symptomatic, AIDS and death. Longini et al. (1989) estimated the transition rate constants between these phases from censored data on 603 individuals who have HIV infections by using a

Table 2.1. Transition rate constants and mean waiting times in clinical phases.

Clinical phase	estimates ± std. error in months^{-1}	mean waiting time in months(years)	median waiting time in months (years)
pre–antibody	0.4571±0.1381	2.2 (0.2)	1.5 (0.1)
asymptomatic	0.0190±0.0022	52.6 (4.4)	36.5 (3.0)
symptomatic	0.0159±0.0018	62.9 (5.2)	43.6 (3.6)
AIDS	0.0424±0.0044	23.6 (2.0)	16.3 (1.4)

five–phase, time–homogeneous, Markov model with a negative exponential waiting time in each phase. Their estimates (Table 2.1) yield a mean incubation period from HIV infection to AIDS of 9.8 years (117.7 months), with a 95% confidence interval of [8.4; 11.2] years.

Payne et al. (1989) reported a median survival time of 12.5 months for 4524 AIDS patients in SF between July 1981 and December 1987. Survival time is the time from diagnosis of AIDS to death. Lemp et al. (1990) reported a median survival time of 12.1 months for patients in the SF Vaccine Trial Cohort; but this was 14.4 months for patients diagnosed in 1986 and 1987 (presumably due to therapy or better care). Thus the median survival time of AIDS patients (without therapy) seems to be approximately one year. The median survival time of 16.3 months in Table 2.1 may be longer because some of the AIDS patients were lost to follow–up, and their deaths were not recorded. Consequently, a 12.5 month median survival time is used; this corresponds to a mean survival time of 18.0 months, and a transition rate constant equal to 0.0555. This transition rate constant has no effect on AIDS incidence, but it does affect the AIDS prevalence and the AIDS death rate. The incidence of a condition such as HIV infection or developing AIDS is the number of persons contracting the condition per unit time, which is not the same as the prevalence, which is the number of people with the condition at the given time.

The asymptomatic and symptomatic phases are subdivided into stages so that the cumulative distribution function for the AIDS incubation period matches the data. For example, if m = 7, the transition rate constants are γ_1 = 0.4571 for the pre–antibody stage, $\gamma_2 = \gamma_3$ = 2 x 0.0190 for the two asymptomatic stages, $\gamma_4 = \gamma_5 = \gamma_6$ = 3 x 0.0159 for the three symptomatic stages and γ_7 = 0.0555 for the AIDS stage. The staged progression model for m = 7 is shown in Figure 2.1.

Figure 2.2 shows the graphs for 5, 6, and 7 stages of the fraction who have developed AIDS as a function of time since HIV infection, i.e., the cumulative distribution functions. Figure 2.2 also shows data on fractions progressing to AIDS from three additional sources with smaller data sets than used in Longini et al. (1989). Lifson et al. (1990) used data on 268 men in the San Francisco City Clinic Cohort (SFCCC) to estimate the fraction who developed AIDS each year after infection; their median AIDS incubation period is between 9 and 10 years. From an analysis of the hepatitis B vaccine trial cohort in the SFCCC, Bacchetti and Moss (1989) found that 20.8% developed AIDS within the first 6 years and 51.2% within 10 years; their median

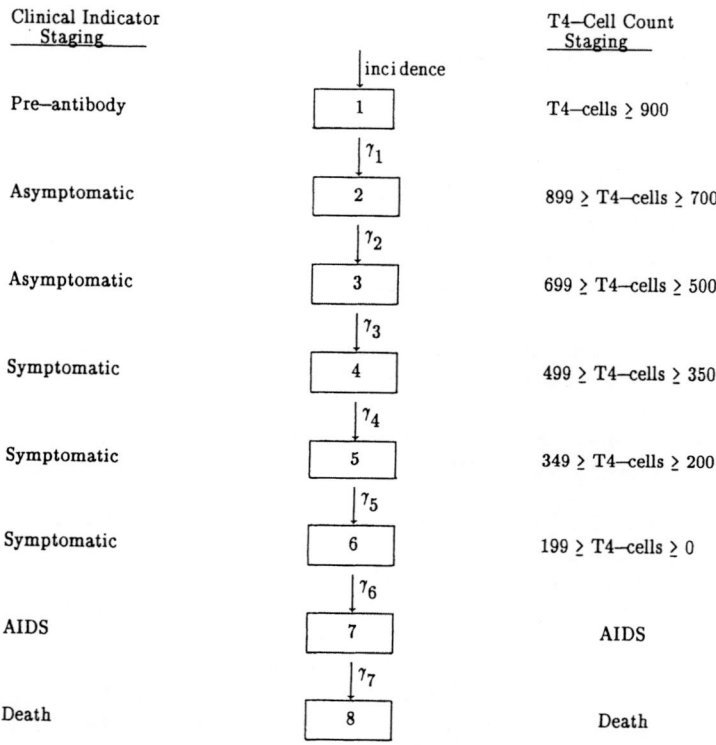

Clinical Indicator Staging		T4–Cell Count Staging
	incidence	
Pre–antibody	1	T4–cells $\geq$ 900
	γ_1	
Asymptomatic	2	$899 \geq$ T4–cells ≥ 700
	γ_2	
Asymptomatic	3	$699 \geq$ T4–cells ≥ 500
	γ_3	
Symptomatic	4	$499 \geq$ T4–cells ≥ 350
	γ_4	
Symptomatic	5	$349 \geq$ T4–cells ≥ 200
	γ_5	
Symptomatic	6	$199 \geq$ T4–cells ≥ 0
	γ_6	
AIDS	7	AIDS
	γ_7	
Death	8	Death

Figure 2.1. The staged model based on clinical indicators or T4–cell counts for progression to AIDS and death when there are 7 infectious stages (6 stages before AIDS).

AIDS incubation period is 9.8 years. Hessol et al. (1989) used data on 135 hepatitis B vaccine trial participants to get a Kaplan–Meier survival curve of the cumulative proportions of men with AIDS by duration of HIV infection.

The cumulative distributions of Lifson et al. (1990) and Bacchetti and Moss (1989) agree with each other in Figure 2.2, but the Hessol et al. (1989) distribution does not. Their cumulative distribution curves are roughly consistent with the $m = 5, 6, 7$ curves based on the data in Longini et al. (1989), except that their curves are lower at 10 and 11 years. Their estimates are probably low at longer times because therapy with zidovudine and pentamidine has delayed the onset of AIDS for many treated patients in their cohorts.

33

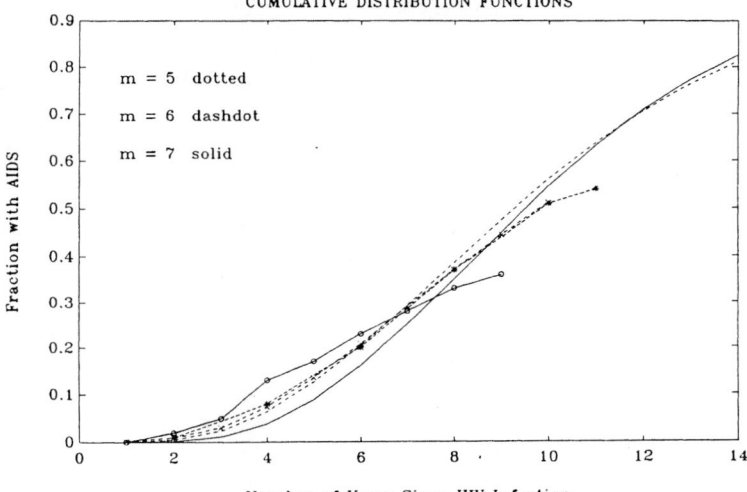

Figure 2.2. Cumulative distribution functions for developing AIDS based on data of Longini et al. (1989), where the number of infectious stages is $m = 5$, 6, or 7. The symbol o is used for the data of Hessol et al. (1990), $*$ for that of Lifson et al. (1990), and x for that of Bacchetti and Moss (1989).

2.2 Staged Progression Based on T4 Cell Counts

The CD4$^+$ T–lymphocytes (T4 cells) are a primary target of HIV in the host, and the decline in T4 cells is an important indicator of progression towards AIDS. Thus it is logical to use T4 cell decline in a staged progression model. Longini et al. (1991) defined six stages of HIV infection for individuals who have not yet been diagnosed with AIDS (technically, who have developed an opportunistic infection corresponding to the Walter Reed stage six (Redfield et al., 1986). These six stages correspond to T4 cell count intervals given in Table 2.2. The transition rates between these stages were estimated from data on 1796 HIV–positive individuals in the United States Army using a continuous–time Markov process model. The transition rate constants and mean waiting times are given in Table 2.2.

Since T4–cell levels in individuals can vary due to measurement error and changing physiological conditions, Longini et al. (1991) use a persistance criteria that two consecutive measurements are needed to confirm a true reduction in T4–cell count. The estimated mean waiting time from seroconversion to when the T4 cell count is persistently below 500 is 4.1 years, the mean waiting time until it is below 200 is 8.0 years, and the mean waiting time from seroconversion to AIDS diagnosis (technically, diagnosis with Walter Reed stage 6 opportunistic infection) is 9.6 years. The data were also analyzed for three age groups ($\leq$ 25, 26–30, and

Table 2.2   Estimated parameters, γ, and mean waiting times, μ, in each stage of infection with no cofactors. Standard errors are in parentheses.

Stage i	T4–cell count interval	Transition rate $\hat{\gamma}_i$ in months^{-1}	Mean waiting time $\hat{\mu}_i$ in years	Cum. waiting time in years
1	> 899	0.0764 (0.0051)	1.1 (0.1)	1.1 (0.1)
2	700 – 899	0.0665 (0.0033)	1.3 (0.1)	2.4 (0.1)
3	500 – 699	0.0499 (0.0021)	1.7 (0.1)	4.1 (0.1)
4	350 – 499	0.0429 (0.0019)	1.9 (0.1)	6.0 (0.1)
5	200 – 349	0.0408 (0.0022)	2.0 (0.1)	8.0 (0.2)
6	1 – 199	0.0529 (0.0035)	1.6 (0.1)	9.6 (0.2)

> 30), and although the progression rates were the same for T4 cell counts $\geq$ 500, the two older groups progressed faster when T4 cell counts were < 500. Although age is a cofactor, it is not considered in our model.

It seems likely that T4 cell counts will become the most widely used marker for HIV progression. They are currently used as indicators for starting zidovudine, other antiviral treatments and PCP prophylaxis with aerosol pentamidine. The T4 cell counts will probably also be used as surrogate endpoints in clinical trials of therapies and vaccines. Under certain conditions, the use of surrogate endpoints can significantly shorten the clinical trials needed for testing and approval of drugs and vaccines (Machado et al., 1990).

2.3 Staged Progression for Children

Auger et al. (1988) give the AIDS incubation cumulative distribution function for 215 pediatric AIDS patients. The mean incubation period is shorter for these children and there is an initial steep rise followed by a slower increase. They found that approximately 20% develop AIDS in the first year of life and the remainder develop AIDS at a nearly constant rate of 8% per year. Thus a reasonable model might have a subgroup of fast progressers and a second subgroup of slower progressers.

The progression model for adults is modified as shown in Figure 2.3 so that a fraction p of pediatric HIV infecteds progress rapidly through one stage with a negative exponential waiting time and a removal (to AIDS) rate constant b. The fraction $1-p$ move through six stages with rate constants in each stage given by $a\gamma_i$ where γ_i is the rate constant for the corresponding adult stage given in Table 2.2. Thus the mean incubation period for those who progress rapidly is $1/b$ and the mean incubation period for those who progress more slowly is $(9.8/a)$ years.

The best fit to the data of Auger et al. (1988) has parameter values of $p = 0.34$, $b = 0.08$, $m = 7$, and $a = 1.55$ so the mean incubation periods are 12.5 months and 6.3 years for those who progress rapidly and slowly, respectively. Note that about one–third of the children progress

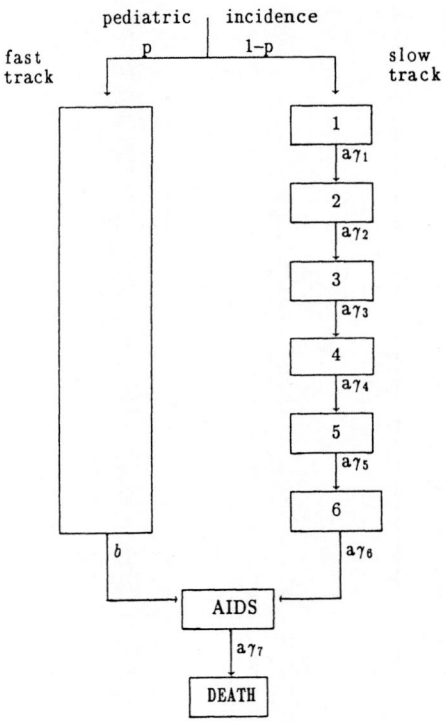

Figure 2.3. Progression of children to AIDS and death showing slow and fast tracks.

rapidly and two–thirds progress slowly. The data points and cumulative distribution function for the parameters above are shown in Figure 2.4.

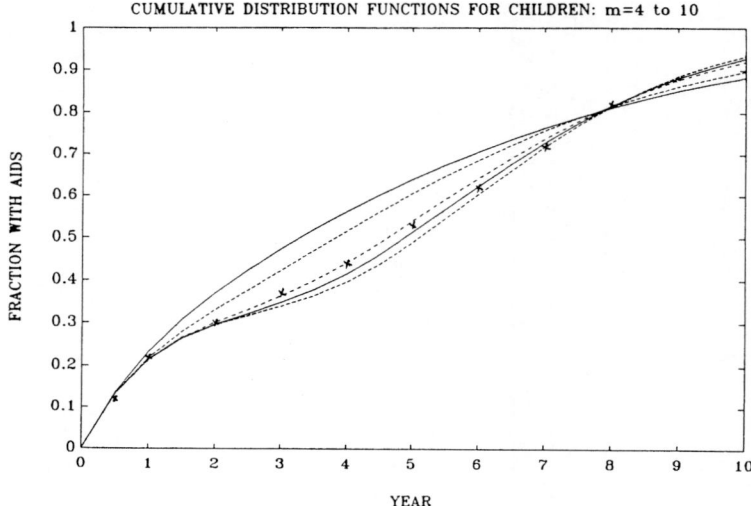

CUMULATIVE DISTRIBUTION FUNCTIONS FOR CHILDREN: m=4 to 10

YEAR

Figure 2.4. Cumulative distribution functions for developing AIDS in pediatric HIV–infected patients with parameters $a = 1.55$, $p = 0.34$, $b = 0.08$, and $m = 4$ (top) to 10 (bottom). The $m = 7$ curve matches the data points * of Auger et al. (1988).

CHAPTER 3

FORMULATION OF THE SIMULATION MODEL FOR HOMOSEXUAL MEN

Transmissions of HIV have occurred after exposure to people in the pre–antibody period (Peterman et al., 1985). The latent period (i.e., from infection to infectiousness) for HIV infection is short enough to be ignored in a model. The infectious period is unknown, but the virus seems to persist in the host indefinitely since it can be isolated from the blood for many years after the infection (Curran et al., 1988). No evidence to the contrary exists; therefore HIV infectivity is assumed to continue for life. Since individuals are either susceptible to HIV infection or infectious, HIV is an SI (susceptible-infected) disease (Hethcote, 1978, 1989c). In contrast, gonorrhea is an SIS disease since people can recover and return to the susceptible class.

3.1 The Compartmental Model with Two Sexual Activity Levels

In modeling gonorrhea, the population was divided by level of sexual activity (Hethcote et al., 1982; Hethcote and Yorke, 1984). The population considered here consists of homosexual men who change male sex partners frequently, i.e., at least once every few years. This group is subdivided into men who have many different male sex partners (very active) and those who have only a few different partners (active). Although some modelers have used more sexual activity levels or risk groups in theoretical studies (Jacquez et al., 1988; Blythe and Anderson, 1988; Castillo–Chavez et al., 1989; Kaplan and Lee, 1990), the two activity levels used here do not introduce lots of parameters which cannot be estimated and are consistent with the existence of a small fraction of homosexual men who are very active sexually. The mixing structure, sexual activity level and progression to AIDS in a population may depend on the age of the individuals, but there is currently not enough data available to justify the incorporation of age structure into the model; see Busenberg and Castillo–Chavez (1991) for an age–structured HIV/AIDS model.

Consider the flow diagram for homosexual men shown in Figure 3.1. Table 3.1 contains a list of the parameters and variables used in the model. The number m of infectious stages shown in Figure 3.1 is four for simplicity, but in Section 2.1, we found that $m = 6$ or 7 gives best fits to the AIDS incubation data. The population size is Q, the number of very active men is $QV = F \times Q$, and the number of active men is $QA = (1-F) \times Q$. The numbers of susceptible persons are SV and SA for the very active and active groups, respectively. The five compartments X(I) in Figure 3.1 correspond to four stages in the progression to AIDS and death among very active people while the compartments Y(I) are analogous for active people. The sum of the left column of compartments in Figure 3.1 is always QV and the sum of the middle column is QA so that the very active and active population sizes are conserved.

Men in the first three Z(I) compartments are those who have moved from the region after they were infected with HIV. When men in these three Z(I) compartments eventually develop AIDS, they are placed in the ZAIDS compartment. The compartment Z(4) consists of those who emigrated from the region after they had AIDS but who would still be counted as local AIDS cases. The compartments X(5), Y(5) and Z(5) contain men who have died of AIDS, and the

38

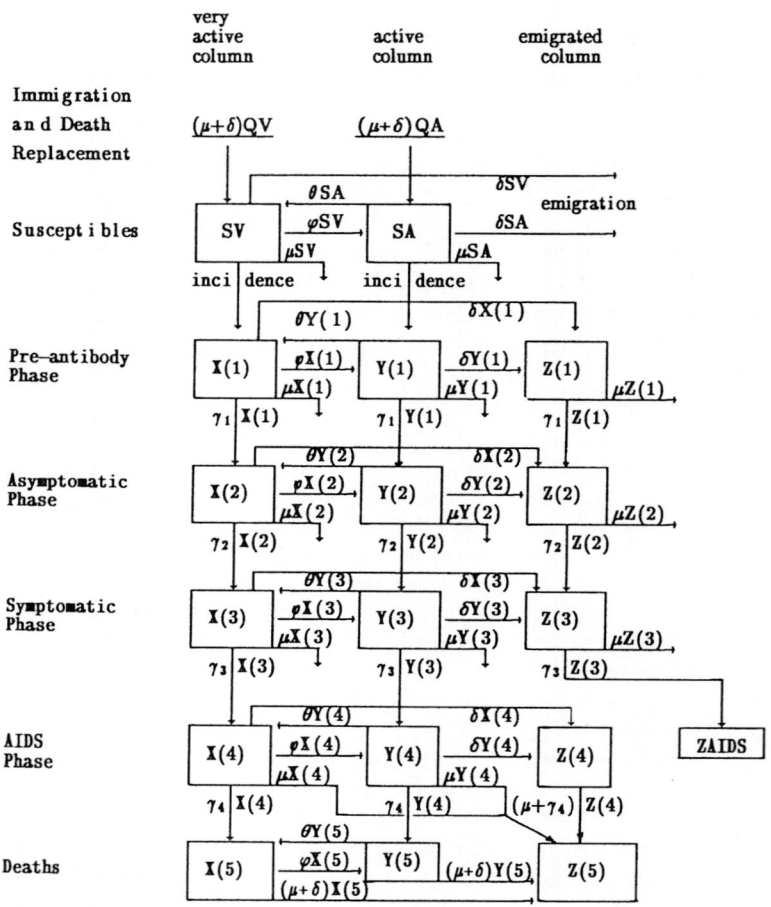

Figure 3.1. Diagram with compartments and transfers in the simulation model.

transfers between these compartments are merely to balance the flows so that the total very active and active populations remain constant. Since men who have died of AIDS are included in the total very active and active population sizes, the fraction of these populations which are still alive and sexually active will decrease as more men in those populations die.

Natural deaths (not related to HIV infection) occur in each compartment with rate constant μ with balancing inflows μQV and μQA into the susceptible compartments. Let δ be the turnover rate constant corresponding to the normal migration of sexually active

Table 3.1. List of parameters and variables.

Population Size and Turnover Rate Constants.

Q = total population size
F = fraction of population who are sexually very active
R = ratio of partnership rates for very active and active men
μ = natural mortality rate constant
δ = migration rate constant
ϕ = transfer rate constant from very active to active states

Stages of the Infection

m = number of infectious stages
γ_k = rate constant for progression from stage k to stage $k+1$
ω_k = relative infectivity of stage k men compared with asymptomatic men
ρ_k = relative sexual activity of stage k men compared with asymptomatic men

Sexual Activity

STD = starting date of the epidemic
QH = probability of transmission to partners by infected asymptomatic men
PAS = average number of partners per month at start
STR = starting date for reduction in average number of partners per month
STP = stopping date for reductions
RDN = yearly reduction factor
η = fraction of new partnerships distributed by proportionate mixing

Variables (functions of time)

SV = number of susceptible very active men
SA = number of susceptible active men
$X(k)$ = number of very active men in stage k
$Y(k)$ = number of active men in stage k
$Z(k)$ = number of emigrated men in stage k

---

homosexual men. The emigrations from the very active and active groups are balanced by immigration δQV and δQA into the very active and active susceptibles. In addition to geographic migration, the turnover could also be due to initiation or cessation of homosexual activity. The transfer rate constant φ corresponds to the natural movement of homosexual men from sexually very active status to active status. There are balancing transfers from the active to the very active compartments with a transfer rate constant of $\theta = \phi \cdot QV/QA$.

As in Chapter 2, the parameters γ_1, γ_2, γ_3 and γ_4 in Figure 3.1 govern the movement through the stages of HIV infection to AIDS and death due to AIDS. These transfer rate constants correspond to negative exponential waiting times in the compartments with mean waiting times equal to $1/\gamma_1, 1/\gamma_2, 1/\gamma_3$ and $1/\gamma_4$, respectively.

The monthly change in the number of people in a compartment in Figure 3.1 is equal to the monthly inflows minus the monthly outflows. Thus the model consists of simultaneous nonlinear difference equations given in Figure 3.2, which correspond to the compartments in

$$\frac{\Delta S V}{\Delta t} = (\delta+\mu)(QV-SV) - V_{\text{incidence}} - \varphi SV + \theta SA$$

$$\frac{\Delta S A}{\Delta t} = (\delta+\mu)(QA-SA) - A_{\text{incidence}} + \varphi SV - \theta SA$$

$$\frac{\Delta X(1)}{\Delta t} = V_{\text{incidence}} - (\gamma_1+\mu+\delta+\varphi)X(1) + \theta Y(1)$$

$$\frac{\Delta Y(1)}{\Delta t} = A_{\text{incidence}} - (\gamma_1+\mu+\delta+\theta)Y(1) + \varphi X(1)$$

$$\frac{\Delta Z(1)}{\Delta t} = \delta(X(1)+Y(1)) - (\gamma_1+\mu)Z(1)$$

$$\frac{\Delta X(2)}{\Delta t} = \gamma_1 X(1) + \theta Y(2) - (\gamma_2+\mu+\delta+\varphi)X(2)$$

$$\frac{\Delta Y(2)}{\Delta t} = \gamma_1 Y(1) + \varphi X(2) - (\gamma_2+\mu+\delta+\theta)Y(2)$$

$$\frac{\Delta Z(2)}{\Delta t} = \delta(X(2)+Y(2)) + \gamma_1 Z(1) - (\gamma_2+\mu)Z(2)$$

$$\frac{\Delta X(3)}{\Delta t} = \gamma_2 X(2) + \theta Y(3) - (\gamma_3+\mu+\delta+\varphi)X(3)$$

$$\frac{\Delta Y(3)}{\Delta t} = \gamma_2 Y(2) + \varphi X(3) - (\gamma_3+\mu+\delta+\theta)Y(3)$$

$$\frac{\Delta Z(3)}{\Delta t} = \delta(X(3)+Y(3)) + \gamma_2 Z(2) - (\gamma_3+\mu)Z(3)$$

$$\frac{\Delta Z\text{AIDS}}{\Delta t} = \gamma_3 Z(3)$$

$$\frac{\Delta X(4)}{\Delta t} = \gamma_3 X(3) + \theta Y(4) - (\gamma_4+\mu+\delta+\varphi)X(4)$$

$$\frac{\Delta Y(4)}{\Delta t} = \gamma_3 Y(3) + \varphi X(4) - (\gamma_4+\mu+\delta+\theta)Y(4)$$

$$\frac{\Delta Z(4)}{\Delta t} = \delta(X(4)+Y(4)) - (\gamma_4+\mu)Z(4)$$

$$\frac{\Delta X(5)}{\Delta t} = \gamma_4 X(4) + \theta Y(5) - (\mu+\delta+\varphi)X(5)$$

$$\frac{\Delta Y(5)}{\Delta t} = \gamma_4 Y(4) + \varphi X(5) - (\mu+\delta+\theta)Y(5)$$

$$\frac{\Delta Z(5)}{\Delta t} = \delta(X(5)+Y(5)) + (\gamma_4+\mu)Z(4) + \mu(X(4)+Y(4)+X(5)-Y(5))$$

Figure 3.2 The difference equations for the model in Figure 3.1.

Figure 3.1. The HIV epidemic starts with one infected person entering the very active pre–antibody compartment on the starting date STD and then progresses in one–month time steps.

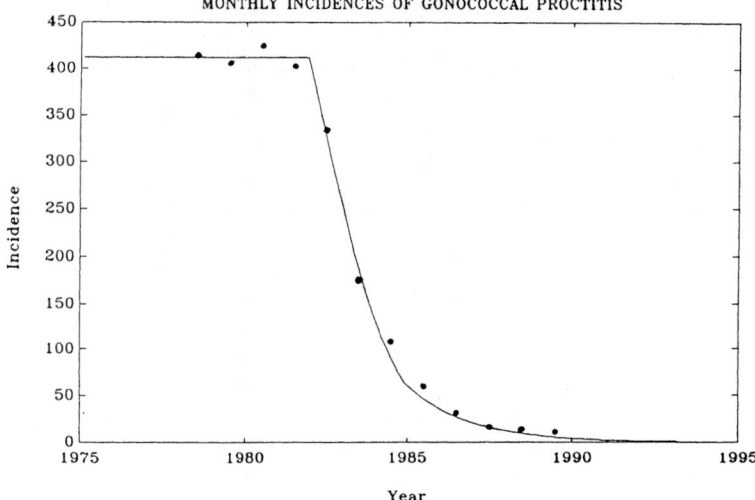

Figure 3.3. The curve with • symbols indicates the incidence of gonococcal proctitis in San Francisco, and the solid curve is the incidence in the gonorrhea simulation.

3.2 Modeling the Incidence of HIV Infection

Individuals in some phases cease sexual activity or adopt protective measures when they learn of their HIV status because of a desire to avoid infecting others; others cease sexual activity because they are ill due to HIV–related symptoms. Let PA be the average number of partners per month for asymptomatic infected men. Let ρ_k be the relative sexual activity of those in stage k compared to asymptomatic infected men, so $\rho_k PA$ is the average number of homosexual partners per month for stage k infected men.

The infectiousness of individuals in the phases leading to AIDS seems to vary. People in the pre–antibody, symptomatic and AIDS phases seem to be more infectious than people in the asymptomatic phase (Longini et al., 1989). If QH is the probability of transmission of HIV infection to a partner by an infected asymptomatic man and ω_k is the relative infectivity of those in stage k, normalized so $\omega_k = 1$ for asymptomatics, then the probability of transmission for infected persons in stage k is $\omega_k QH$. All of the ω_k are equal for men in the symptomatic stages. Since there are many types of sexual interactions in a homosexual partnership, QH is a simplified composite or average of many factors such as the numbers and types (anal, oral, receptive, insertive, unprotected, safer) of contacts per partner. Although very active people may tend to have shorter length partnerships with fewer contacts than active people, the contacts of very active people may have higher risk of transmission. The quantity QH is really the proportion of partners of infected asymptomatic men who are infected, but it is usually called the probability of transmission.

Data on sexual behavior and gonococcal proctitis for homosexual men in large cities suggest that partnership formation rates for homosexual men have changed (CDC, 1990a, 1990c). A simple way to model this phenomenon is to assume that the average number PA of different partners per month is first constant, then decreases as a geometric sequence, and then is constant again. A geometric sequence is the discrete approximation to a negative exponential decrease in partnership rates suggested by the gonococcal proctitis data in Figure 3.3. In the model, the number of partners per month before reduction starts is PAS, the date at which reduction starts is STR, the date at which reduction stops is STP, and the yearly reduction factor is RDN.

The number of different partners per month is $PH = PA/(1+F(R-1))$ for the fraction $1-F$ of the population which is active and $R \times PH$ for the fraction F which is very active. The monthly effective contact rate is the product of the contact rate (the number of different partners per month) and the proportion of partnerships resulting in transmission.

One method of specifying the contact rates between subpopulations in an epidemiologic model is with proportionate mixing (Hethcote and Yorke, 1984; Nold, 1980; Dietz and Schenzle, 1985b; Hethcote and Van Ark, 1987). In this method each group has a sexual activity level, and the new partners of a person are distributed among the groups in proportion to the activity levels of the groups. Alternatively, a person may be more likely to choose a sexual partner with the same level of sexual activity. This situation occurred in the gonorrhea modeling of Hethcote and Yorke (1984, p.83) in which 20% of the contacts were internal to the activity level groups and 80% were external contacts governed by proportionate mixing. This is now called preferred mixing (Jacquez et al.,1988; Blythe and Castillo–Chavez, 1989).

Since data have not been found on mixing patterns in SF, the more general form of mixing is used here. Let η be the fraction of the new partnerships distributed by proportionate mixing among all groups so that the fraction $1-\eta$ of new partnerships occur internally to each group. Since some of the contacts of a group governed by proportionate mixing are contacts with others in the same group, these proportionate–mixing contacts are really internal to the group, so that not all of the proportionate–mixing contacts are external to the group. Nevertheless, it is convenient to use the term *internal* for the fraction $1-\eta$ of the partnerships which must be within the group and to use the term *external* for the fraction η governed by proportionate mixing. The incidences of HIV infection in the active and very active groups due to the internal mixing in each group are, respectively,

$$\left[\sum_{i=1}^{m} (1-\eta) \times \rho_i \times PH \times \omega_i \times QH \times Y(i) \right] \times \frac{SA}{QA-Y(m+1)} ,$$

$$\left[\sum_{i=1}^{m} (1-\eta) \times \rho_i \times R \times PH \times \omega_i \times QH \times X(i) \right] \times \frac{SV}{QV-X(m+1)} .$$

Now consider the fraction η of new partnerships distributed by proportionate mixing among all groups (Hethcote and Van Ark, 1987, eq. 6.6). The activity levels for the active and very active subpopulations are the numbers of partners per month, PH and R ꞏ PH, respectively. The average number of partnership formations in the population per month is

$$C = PH \text{ ꞏ } (QA - Y(m+1)) + R \text{ ꞏ } PH \text{ ꞏ } (QV-X(m+1))$$

so that the incidences in the active and very active subpopulations due to proportionate mixing are, respectively,

$$\sum_{i=1}^{m} \eta \text{ ꞏ } \rho_i \text{ ꞏ } PH \text{ ꞏ } \omega_i \text{ ꞏ } QH \text{ ꞏ } [R \text{ ꞏ } X(i)+Y(i)] \text{ ꞏ } \frac{PH \text{ ꞏ } SA}{C} ,$$

$$\sum_{i=1}^{m} \eta \text{ ꞏ } \rho_i \text{ ꞏ } PH \text{ ꞏ } \omega_i \text{ ꞏ } QH \text{ ꞏ } [R \text{ ꞏ } X(i)+Y(i)] \text{ ꞏ } \frac{R \text{ ꞏ } PH \text{ ꞏ } SV}{C} .$$

The total incidences in the active and very active subpopulations are the sums of the internal incidences and the external proportionate mixing incidences.

CHAPTER 4

MATHEMATICAL ANALYSIS OF THE MODEL FOR HOMOSEXUAL MEN

For systems of linear differential and difference equations, it is possible to find explicit solutions (see introductory differential and difference equations textbooks). The difference equations in Figure 3.2 are nonlinear because the incidences involve products of susceptible fractions and the numbers of infectives . For systems of nonlinear differential and difference equations, it is not generally possible to find explicit solutions, but it is possible to find numerical solutions as a function of time. The numerical solutions of the system of nonlinear difference equations in Figure 3.2 are called the simulations of the HIV transmission dynamics model in Figure 3.1.

The value of the threshold quantity in an epidemiological model determines whether the disease persists or dies out. For single population models the threshold quantity is usually the *contact number*, which is the average number of adequate contacts of an infective during the infectious period (Hethcote, 1976; 1989a). This contact number is also called a *reproduction number* since it gives the number of secondary cases "reproduced" by a typical infective during the infectious period in a population in which everyone is susceptible (Anderson and May, 1991). For models in which the population is subdivided into groups with contacts between the groups given by a matrix, the threshold quantity is the *stability modulus* (i.e., the largest real part of an eigenvalue) of the contact matrix (Lajmanovich and Yorke, 1976; Hethcote, 1978; Hethcote and Yorke, 1984). The disease dies out if the stability modulus is below zero and the disease persists if the stability modulus is above zero. This threshold condition is equivalent to the *spectral radius* (i.e., the maximum absolute value of an eigenvalue) of a transmission matrix being less than one or greater than one (Hethcote and Van Ark, 1987). A general formulation of the reproduction number as a spectral radius has been applied to many models by Diekmann et al. (1990).

Even though explicit solutions of the nonlinear differential or difference equations corresponding to the model in Figure 3.1 cannot be found, it is possible to determine the threshold quantity as the *spectral radius* of a certain matrix. For the differential or difference equations for a simplification of the model in Figure 3.1 in which there is only one sexual activity level, the threshold can be found explicitly. The explicit expression for the *contact number* σ (the threshold quantity) given in equation (4.7) is useful because one can see how each parameter affects the threshold and hence affects whether the disease persists or dies out. In the mathematical analysis of an epidemiological model, often the goals are to determine the threshold quantity, to prove rigorously that *below the threshold* the disease prevalence goes to zero, and that *above the threshold* there is a unique, positive *equilibrium state* and the disease prevalence approaches this positive (endemic) equilibrium state (see Hethcote, 1976, 1989a). In this chapter we obtain some of these results for HIV dynamics models related to Figure 3.1. Those interested primarily in the application of the model to HIV/AIDS and not interested in the mathematical analysis may go directly to Chapter 5.

The *equilibria* of the model are the points with the property that solutions starting at these points stay there. First a differential equations analog of the difference equations model formulated in Chapter 3 for homosexual men is analyzed mathematically by finding the equilibria and their stability. This model can have both a *disease–free* equilibrium (DFE) and a unique *endemic* equilibrium (EE). Threshold results are obtained for this model which determine whether the disease dies out (approaches the DFE) or remains endemic (approaches the EE). This differential equations model analyzed in Sections 4.1 to 4.3 has one sexual activity level. In Section 4.4 it is shown that the threshold results obtained for the differential equations model also hold for the difference equations model with one sexual activity level. Although the thresholds and stability for the models with two sexual activity levels cannot be determined explicitly, the Jacobian is found in Section 4.5 for the difference equations model with two sexual activity levels corresponding to Figure 3.1. For the parameter sets occurring in Section 6.2, the eigenvalues of this Jacobian are found numerically in order to determine the stability of the DFE by finding the value of the *spectral radius* relative to the threshold one.

Another HIV/AIDS model with multiple groups has been studied by Jacquez et al. (1988; 1989), Sattenspiel and Simon (1988), Koopman et al. (1989), Lin (1991), and Simon and Jacquez (1992). Their differential equations model is similar to the model considered in Section 4.1, but their model has constant recruitment into each group and the group population sizes can vary. In contrast to our model, their model does not have transfers between the groups, their waiting times are the same in all stages, and people with AIDS are assumed to be sexually inactive. The model in Section 3.1 has constant recruitment into the two activity groups at a rate proportional to the group sizes and the sizes of the active and very active groups are constant; this also leaves a variable number of people still active in the population. Other multiple–group models for HIV/AIDS have been considered by Hyman and Stanley (1989), May and Anderson (1989), Blythe and Castillo–Chavez (1989), Castillo–Chavez et al. (1989) and Kaplan et al. (1989). See the survey papers of Isham (1987) and Schwager et al. (1989) for more details and references.

4.1 Equilibria for the Differential–Equations Model with One Sexual Activity Level.

The first model considered is a differential equations analog of the difference–equations models in Chapter 3. This model is for a homogeneous population with only one activity level. Let Y_k represent the number of people in stage k where stage 0 people are susceptible (not HIV–infected), stage 1 people are in the first infectious stage (see Chapter 2), $\cdots$, stage m people have AIDS, and stage $m+1$ people have died after having AIDS. Therefore, with N being the (constant) number of people in the population, the variables satisfy $Y_0+\cdots+Y_{m+1} = N$. Define λ_j, $j = 1,2, \cdots, m$ to be the average number of sexual contacts that a person in infectious stage j has with all people that are sufficient to cause HIV infection in susceptible persons. This value is a composite of several parameters defined for the model in Chapter 3.

The system of differential equations for this model corresponding to Figure 3.1 is

$$Y'_0 = (\delta + \mu)(N - Y_0) - (\sum_{j=1}^{m} \lambda_j Y_j)(Y_0 / \sum_{k=0}^{m} Y_k) \, ,$$

$$Y'_1 = (\sum_{j=1}^{m} \lambda_j Y_j)(Y_0 / \sum_{k=0}^{m} Y_k) - (\delta + \mu + \gamma_1)Y_1 \, , \tag{4.1}$$

$$Y'_k = \gamma_{k-1} Y_{k-1} - (\delta + \mu + \gamma_k)Y_k \, , \, 2 \leq k \leq m+1$$

where primes denote derivatives with respect to time and $\gamma_{m+1} = 0$. In (4.1) the $-(\delta + \mu)Y_k$ terms represent emigration and natural deaths, while $(\delta + \mu)N$ represents the immigration and other inflow to replace the losses. The *incidence term* is the sum of the contact rates and the numbers infected in the stages times the susceptible fraction. The model (4.1) can be simplified by converting from numbers in the stages to the fractions in the stages. Let $I_j = Y_j/N$ be the *fraction of the population in infectious stage* j, $0 \leq j \leq m+1$. The model can then be written

$$I'_1 = g(I) I_0 - \xi_1 I_1 \, , \tag{4.2}$$

$$I'_k = \gamma_{k-1} I_{k-1} - \xi_k I_k \, , \, 2 \leq k \leq m+1$$

where $g(I) = (\sum_{j=1}^{m} \lambda_j I_j)/(1 - I_{m+1})$, $\xi_k = (\delta + \mu + \gamma_k)$, $\gamma_{m+1} = 0$, and $I_0 = 1 - \sum_{j=1}^{m+1} I_j$. By examining (4.2) on each face, it can be shown that the region

$$D = \{(I_1, \cdots, I_{m+1}) | \ 0 \leq I_k \leq 1; I_1 + \cdots + I_{m+1} \leq 1\} \tag{4.3}$$

is positively invariant. The right side is Lipschitz continuous for $I_{m+1} < 1$ so that unique solutions of initial value problems exist on a maximal interval which must be $[0, \infty)$ since solutions remain in D (Miller and Michel, 1982). Thus the initial value problem is mathematically well—posed. The system (4.2) is epidemiologically reasonable since solutions remain in $[0, 1]^{m+1}$.

At equilibrium points, the right sides of the system (4.2) are zero. There are two possible equilibrium points for this model: the trivial or disease—free equilibrium (DFE), and an endemic equilibrium (EE) which is explicitly derived below. The DFE, with $I_0 = 1$ and $I_k = 0$ for $1 \leq k \leq m+1$, is always in the region D. The EE below is in D when the parameter values satisfy the condition of being *above the threshold*. To obtain the EE, work backwards from the $(m+1)^{st}$ equilibrium equation, solving for I_{k-1} in terms of I_k to get:

$$I_k = \left[\prod_{j=k}^{m} \xi_{j+1}/\gamma_j \right] \times I_{m+1} \, , \, 1 \leq k \leq m \, . \tag{4.4}$$

The $I'_1 = 0$ equation gives I_0 in terms of the other I_k values; using (4.4), simplification gives

$$I_0 = \frac{\xi_1 I_1}{g(I)} = \frac{\left[1 - I_{m+1} \right]}{\sum_{j=1}^{m} \lambda_j I_j} \xi_1 I_1 = \frac{\left[1 - I_{m+1} \right] \times I_{m+1} \left[\prod_{j=1}^{m+1} \xi_j \right]}{\sum_{j=1}^{m} \lambda_j \prod_{k=j}^{m} (\xi_{k+1}/\gamma_k) I_{m+1} \left[\prod_{j=1}^{m} \gamma_j \right]} \, ,$$

$$I_0 = \left[1 - I_{m+1} \right] \div \left[\sum_{j=1}^{m} \left[\prod_{k=1}^{j-1} (\gamma_k/\xi_k) \right] (\lambda_j/\xi_j) \right] \tag{4.5}$$

Using $I_0 + \cdots + I_{m+1} = 1$, the I_{m+1} term at endemic equilibrium satisfies

$$I_{m+1}^e = \frac{\left[\sum_{j=1}^{m}\left[\prod_{k=1}^{j-1}\frac{\gamma_k}{\xi_k}\right]\frac{\lambda_j}{\xi_j}\right] - 1}{\left\{\left[\sum_{j=1}^{m}\left[\prod_{k=1}^{j-1}\frac{\gamma_k}{\xi_k}\right]\frac{\lambda_j}{\xi_j}\right]\left[\sum_{j=1}^{m}\left[\prod_{k=j}^{m}\frac{\xi_{k+1}}{\gamma_k}\right] + 1\right] - 1\right\}}. \tag{4.6}$$

Using I_{m+1}^e given in (4.6), the equilibrium values I_k^e and I_0^e are given by (4.4) and (4.5).

Define the *contact number* σ as

$$\sigma = \left[\sum_{j=1}^{m}\left[\prod_{k=1}^{j-1}\frac{\gamma_k}{\xi_k}\right]\frac{\lambda_j}{\xi_j}\right] \tag{4.7}$$

In many epidemiological models a contact number serves as the threshold quantity with 1 as the threshold value (Hethcote, 1976; Hethcote and Van Ark, 1987). In the following sections we show that the contact number σ given by (4.7) is the *threshold quantity* which determines whether the disease dies out ($\sigma \leq 1$) or remains endemic ($\sigma > 1$). However, we first give a heuristic interpretation of the contact number σ which explains why it is a reasonable threshold quantity. The quotient $\gamma_k/\xi_k = \gamma_k/(\delta + \mu + \gamma_k)$ is the probability that an infective leaving stage k goes into the next infectious stage $(k+1)$ instead of migrating out of the community or dying. Thus the product of the γ_k/ξ_k up through $(j-1)$ in the expression (4.7) for σ is the probability that an infective reaches stage. j. The contact rate of infectives in stage j is λ_j and the mean waiting time in stage j is $1/\xi_j$ so that λ_j/ξ_j is the mean number of adequate contacts (sufficient for transmission of HIV infection) of an infective while in stage j. Thus the summation in the expression (4.7) for σ is the sum over all infectious stages j of the probability of reaching stage j times the mean number of adequate contacts while in stage j. Hence the contact number σ is the average number of adequate contacts of an infective during all of the infectious stages. Since the contact number σ is the average number of new infectives produced by an infective during its infectious stages in a totally susceptible population, it is sometimes called the basic reproductive number (Anderson and May, 1991). It is intuitively reasonable that if $\sigma < 1$, then each infective is replaced with less than one new infective so that the disease dies out (the DFE is asymptotically stable). However, if $\sigma > 1$ so that the average infective in a totally susceptible population is replaced with more than one new infective, then the disease should persist (the DFE is unstable). Below and in the following sections we show that when $\sigma > 1$ the disease persists, there is a unique endemic equilibrium and all solutions approach the endemic equilibrium.

Lemma 4.1 *If $\sigma > 1$, then the endemic equilibrium given by (4.6) and (4.4) is a distinct equilibrium in D and is the only equilibrium in D other than the DFE.*

proof If $\sigma > 1$, then I_{m+1}^e given by (4.6) is positive and $1/I_{m+1}^e$ is 1 plus a positive quantity so $I_{m+1}^e < 1$. Thus all of the I_k^e for $0 \leq k \leq m$ are positive by (4.4) and (4.5). Since the sum of these positive I_k^e values adds to 1, each of them must be less than one, and this equilibrium is an

EE in D. If $\sigma = 1$, then the EE given by (4.6) and (4.4) is the DFE. If $\sigma < 1$, then I_{m+1}^e is negative, and this equilibrium is not in D.∎

4.2 Stability of the Disease–Free Equilibrium.

The local and global stability of the DFE are now analyzed. Recall that the incidence $\mathcal{I}$ (rate of new infections) is

$$\mathcal{I} = g(I)I_0 = \left[\sum_{j=1}^{m} \lambda_j I_j\right]\left[1 - \sum_{k=1}^{m+1} I_k\right](1 - I_{m+1})^{-1}.$$

The second and third factors of $\mathcal{I}$ are

$$\left[1 - \sum_{k=1}^{m+1} I_k\right]\left[1 + I_{m+1} + I_{m+1}^2 + I_{m+1}^3 + \cdots \right] = \left[1 - \sum_{k=1}^{m} I_k - I_{m+1}\sum_{k=1}^{m} I_k - I_{m+1}^2\sum_{k=1}^{m} I_k - \cdots \right]$$

so that

$$\mathcal{I} = \sum_{j=1}^{m} \lambda_j I_j - G(I) , \tag{4.8}$$

where $G(I) = (\sum_{j=1}^{m} \lambda_j I_j)(\sum_{i=1}^{m} I_i)(\sum_{k=1}^{\infty} I_{m+1}^k)$. $G(I)$ is $o(I)$, i.e., $\lim_{I \to 0} G(I)/|I| = 0$, so to linearize the model, we replace the incidence term $\mathcal{I}$ by $\mathcal{I}_L = \sum_{j=1}^{m} \lambda_j I_j$. To check for stability by linearization, define $I = [I_1, I_2, \cdots , I_{m+1}]^T$, $G(I)$ as above, and the $m+1 \times m+1$ matrix A as

$$A = \begin{bmatrix} \lambda_1 - \zeta_1 & \lambda_2 & \lambda_3 & \cdots & \lambda_m & 0 \\ \gamma_1 & -\zeta_2 & 0 & \cdots & 0 & 0 \\ 0 & \gamma_3 & -\zeta_3 & \cdots & 0 & 0 \\ \vdots & & & \ddots & & \vdots \\ 0 & 0 & \cdots & & \gamma_m & -\zeta_{m+1} \end{bmatrix}$$

The model (4.2) becomes

$$I' = AI + [G(I), 0, \cdots , 0]^T . \tag{4.9}$$

The linearization of this is

$$I' = AI . \tag{4.10}$$

The local stability of the DFE is determined by examining the eigenvalues of A at the DFE.

Lemma 4.2. For the above matrix A, the eigenvalue with largest real part is an algebraically simple real eigenvalue.

proof Let E_k be the $k \times k$ identity matrix. Then the characteristic equation of A is $|\alpha E_{m+1} - A| = (\alpha - \zeta_{m+1})|\alpha E_m - A_m|$, where A_m is the $m \times m$ matrix obtained by crossing off the last row and column of A, i.e., expanding around the last column of A. The eigenvalue already obtained is $\alpha = -\zeta_{m+1} = -(\delta + \mu) < 0$, and the remaining m eigenvalues of A are the eigenvalues of A_m. Define the *stability modulus* $s(A)$ to be the maximum of the real parts of the eigenvalues of A and the *spectral radius* $\rho(A)$ to be the maximum of the absolute values of the eigenvalues of A. Let $\tau = \max\{\xi_1{-}\lambda_1,\ \xi_2,\ \xi_3,\ \cdots,\ \xi_m\} + 1 > 0$, and $B = A_m + \tau E_m$. Therefore, B is a non–negative matrix with eigenvalues $\beta_k = (a_k + \tau)$, $k = 1,\ \cdots,\ m$, where $\{a_1,\ a_2,\ \cdots,\ a_m\}$ are the eigenvalues of A_m. Since infection in any stage I_k can spread the infection throughout the population, the matrix A_m (hence the matrix B also) is *irreducible* [Hethcote, 1978]. Since B is irreducible and nonnegative, $\rho(B) = s(B)$ is an eigenvalue of B which is real and geometrically and algebraically simple, and there exists a positive eigenvector ω for $s(B)$ [Horn and Johnson, 1985, p 508]. Therefore, $s(A_m) = (s(B) - \tau)$ is a real, simple eigenvalue of A.■

By a similar approach [Horn and Johnson, 1985, p 492] we find bounds on $s(A_m)$ given by

$$\min_{1 \leq k \leq m} \{\lambda_k{-}\delta{-}\mu\} \leq s(A_m) \leq \max_{1 \leq k \leq m} \{\lambda_k{-}\delta{-}\mu\}.$$

Lemma 4.3. *The eigenvalues of the matrix* A_m *above are the roots of the characteristic equation* $p_m(a) = \det[aE_m - A_m]$, *where*

$$p_m(a) = \prod_{j=1}^{m}(\xi_j + a) - \sum_{k=1}^{m}\left[\prod_{j=1}^{k-1}\gamma_j\right](\lambda_k)\left[\prod_{i=k+1}^{m}(\xi_i + a)\right]$$

$$= \left[\prod_{j=1}^{m}(\xi_j + a)\right]\left[1 - \sum_{k=1}^{m}\left[\prod_{i=1}^{k-1}\frac{\gamma_i}{\xi_i + a}\right]\frac{\lambda_k}{\xi_k + a}\right], \qquad (4.11)$$

$\left(with\ \prod_{j=1}^{0}(\cdot) = 1\right).$

proof The proof is by induction on m. Observe that

$$|aE_2 - A_2| = \begin{vmatrix} a + \xi_1 {-} \lambda_1 & -\lambda_2 \\ \gamma_1 & a + \xi_2 \end{vmatrix} = (a + \xi_1)(a + \xi_2) - \lambda_1(a + \xi_2) - \lambda_2\gamma_2,$$

so (4.11) is true for $m = 2$.

Assume that the induction hypothesis is true for m. Note that

$$|aE_{m+1} - A_{m+1}| = \begin{vmatrix} a + \xi_1 {-} \lambda_1 & -\lambda_2 & -\lambda_3 & \cdots & & -\lambda_{m+1} \\ -\gamma_1 & a + \xi_2 & 0 & 0 & \cdots & 0 \\ 0 & -\gamma_2 & a + \xi_3 & 0 & \cdots & 0 \\ & & & & & \\ 0 & \cdots & & -\gamma_{m-1} & a + \xi_m & 0 \\ 0 & \cdots & & & 0 & -\gamma_m & a + \xi_{m+1} \end{vmatrix}$$

Expanding around the last column gives

$$|aE_{m+1} - A_{m+1}| = (-1)^{m+1}\lambda_{m+1}\prod_{j=1}^{m}(-\gamma_j) + (a + \xi_{m+1})p_m(a)$$

$$= -\left[\prod_{j=1}^{m}\gamma_j\right]\lambda_{m+1} + \prod_{j=1}^{m+1}(\xi_j + a) - \sum_{k=1}^{m}\left[\prod_{j=1}^{k-1}\gamma_j\right](\lambda_k)\left[\prod_{i=k+1}^{m+1}(\xi_i + a)\right]$$

$$= \prod_{j=1}^{m+1}(\xi_j + a) - \sum_{k=1}^{m+1}\left[\prod_{j=1}^{k-1}\gamma_j\right](\lambda_k)\left[\prod_{i=k+1}^{m+1}(\xi_i + a)\right] = p_{m+1}(a).■$$

Notice that $p_m(0) = \prod\limits_{j=1}^{m}(\xi_j) - \sum\limits_{k=1}^{m}\left[\prod\limits_{j=1}^{k-1}\gamma_j\right](\lambda_k)\left[\prod\limits_{i=k+1}^{m}(\xi_i)\right]$, and $|A_m| = (-1)^m p_m(0)$.

By Lemma 4.1, $s(A)$ is the real simple eigenvalue with largest positive (or least negative) real root for $p(a) = 0$, so if $s(A) < 0$, then all eigenvalues of A have negative real parts, and if $s(A) > 0$, at least one eigenvalue of A has positive real part. In the former case, the DFE is locally asymptotically stable, and in the latter case, it is unstable. The Theorem below gives a threshold condition on this property. The following Lemma will be used in the proof of the Theorem.

Lemma 4.4. Let $p_m(a)$ be given by (4.11) and σ be as in (4.7). Then $\sigma < 1$ implies that $p_m(a)$ has no nonnegative real roots.

proof Notice that

$$p_n(a) = (\xi_n + a)p_{n-1}(a) - \lambda_n \prod\limits_{j=1}^{n-1}\gamma_j , \qquad (4.12)$$

so that $p_n' = p_{n-1} + (\xi_n + a)p_{n-1}'$. The proof is by induction on $p_n(0) > 0$ and $p_n'(a) > 0$ for $a > 0$ with $1 \leq n \leq m$. For $n = 1$, $\sigma < 1$ implies that $\lambda_1 - \xi_1 < 0$. Then $p_1(0) = -\lambda_1 + \xi_1 > 0$, and p_1' is $1 > 0$, so the induction hypothesis is true for $n = 1$.

Now assume that the induction hypothesis is true for $n \leq m - 1$. Now $\sigma < 1$ for $n + 1$ implies

$$p_{n+1}(0) = \left[\prod\limits_{j=1}^{n+1}(\xi_j)\right]\left[1 - \sum\limits_{k=1}^{n+1}\left[\prod\limits_{j=1}^{k-1}\frac{\gamma_j}{\xi_j}\right]\frac{\lambda_k}{\xi_k}\right] > 0.$$

Also $p_{n+1}'(a) = p_n(a) + (\xi_{n+1} + a)p_n'(a) > 0$ for $a > 0$, since $p_n(a) > 0$ and $p_n'(a) > 0$ for $a > 0$. Thus the induction hypothesis is true for m so that $p_m(a)$ has no nonnegative real roots. ∎

Theorem 4.5. Let σ be given by (4.7). Then the DFE for the model (4.2) is locally asymptotically stable if $\sigma < 1$, and the DFE is unstable if $\sigma > 1$.

proof The characteristic polynomial is $|aE - A| = (\xi_{m+1} + a)p_m(a) = 0$. Notice that $|aE - A|$ is a polynomial in a with leading coefficient $+1$, so that as $a \to \infty$, $|aE - A| \to +\infty$.

Evaluating $|aE - A|$ at $a = 0$ yields $\prod\limits_{j=1}^{m+1}(\xi_j)(1-\sigma)$, which has the same sign as $1 - \sigma$.

Therefore, if $1 - \sigma < 0$ there exists $\hat{a} > 0$ such that $|\hat{a}E - A| = 0$, so that $\hat{a}$ is a real eigenvalue of A, and the DFE is unstable. On the other hand, if $\sigma < 1$, Lemma 4.4 implies that $p_m(a)$ has no roots for $a \geq 0$, and the remaining root is $-\xi_{m+1} = -(\delta + \mu) < 0$. Since Lemma 4.1 proves that $s(A)$, the eigenvalue of A with largest real part, is real, the argument above proves that $s(A) < 0$, so that the DFE is locally asymptotically stable [Miller and Michel, 1982, p 261]. ∎

Theorem 4.6. *For $\sigma \leq 1$, the DFE for the model (4.2) is globally asymptotically stable.*

proof The transpose A^T of the matrix A in (4.9) is irreducible with nonnegative off–diagonal elements, so it has a positive eigenvector w corresponding to the eigenvalue $s(A) = s(A^T)$ (Hethcote, 1978). Note from the proof of Theorem 4.5 that $\sigma \leq 1$ is equivalent to $s(A) \leq 0$. As in Lajmanovich and Yorke [1976] or Hethcote [1978], consider the Liapunov function $V = w \cdot I$ with derivative given by

$$V' = w \cdot I' = w(AI - [G(I),0, \cdots ,0]^T) = A^T w \cdot I - w_1 G(I) = s(A)w \cdot I - w_1 G(I) \leq 0.$$

By Liapunov theory [Miller and Michel, 1982, p 227], all solutions approach the largest invariant subset of the set M in which $V' = 0$. For the Liapunov function V above, this subset M is the origin, so all solutions approach the DFE where the I_k are zero for $1 \leq k \leq m + 1$. ∎

4.3 Stability of the Endemic Equilibrium.

The local stability of the endemic equilibrium (EE) given by (4.4) and (4.6) is proved by methods similar to those in the previous Section.

Theorem 4.7. *If $\sigma > 1$, then the endemic equilibrium of (4.2) is locally asymptotically stable.*

proof The Jacobian of (4.2) evaluated at the EE given by (4.4) and (4.6) is

$$B = \begin{bmatrix} \tau_1-\xi_1 & \tau_2 & \tau_3 & \cdots & \tau_m & \tau_{m+1} \\ \gamma_1 & -\xi_2 & 0 & \cdots & 0 & 0 \\ 0 & \gamma_2 & -\xi_3 & \cdots & 0 & 0 \\ \vdots & & & & -\xi_m & 0 \\ 0 & 0 & \cdots & & \gamma_m & -\xi_{m+1} \end{bmatrix} \tag{4.13}$$

where $\tau_i = \lambda_i/\sigma - g(I)$ for $1 \leq i \leq m$ and $\tau_{m+1} = -(1 - 1/\sigma)g(I)$. From the proof of Lemma 4.3, we find that the characteristic equation corresponding to the matrix B is

$$|\alpha E - B| = q_{m+1}(\alpha) = 0$$

where $q_{m+1}(\alpha)$ is the same as $p_{m+1}(\alpha)$ defined by (4.10) with λ_k replaced by τ_k. The proof is by induction on $q_n(0) > 0$ and $q'_n(\alpha) > 0$ for $\alpha > 0$, with $1 \leq n \leq m + 1$. For $n = 1$, $q_1(\alpha) = \alpha - \tau_1 + \xi_1$, so $q'_1 = 1 > 0$ and $q_1(0) = \xi_1[1 - (\lambda_1/\xi_1)/\sigma + g(I)] > 0$ since $\sigma > \lambda_1/\xi_1$ by (4.7).

Assume that the induction hypothesis is true for $q_n(\alpha)$. If $n < m$, then

$$q_{n+1}(0) = \left[\prod_{j=1}^{n+1}(\xi_j) \right] \left[1 - \sum_{k=1}^{n+1} \left[\prod_{j=1}^{k-1} \frac{\gamma_j}{\xi_j} \right] \frac{\tau_k}{\xi_k} \right]$$

$$= \left[\prod_{j=1}^{n+1}(\xi_j) \right] \left[1 - \left[\sum_{k=1}^{n+1} \left[\prod_{j=1}^{k-1} \frac{\gamma_j}{\xi_j} \right] \frac{\lambda_k}{\xi_k} \right] / \sigma + \sum_{k=1}^{n+1} \left[\prod_{j=1}^{k-1} \frac{\gamma_j}{\xi_j} \right] \frac{g(I)}{\xi_k} \right] > 0.$$

The positivity follows because the denominator σ in the second term is greater than or equal to the numerator. If $n = m$, then

$$q_{m+1}(0) = \left[\prod_{j=1}^{m+1}(\zeta_j)\right]\left[\sum_{k=1}^{m}\left[\prod_{j=1}^{k-1}\frac{\gamma_j}{\zeta_j}\right]\frac{g(I)}{\zeta_k} + \prod_{j=1}^{m}\frac{\gamma_j}{\zeta_j}\frac{(1 - 1/\sigma)g(I)}{\zeta_{m+1}}\right] > 0.$$

As in the proof of Lemma 4.4,

$$q_{n+1}'(\alpha) = q_n(\alpha) + (\zeta_n + \alpha)q_n'(\alpha) > 0$$

by the induction hypothesis for q_n. Thus $q_{m+1}(0) > 0$ and $q_{m+1}'(\alpha) > 0$ so $q_{m+1}(\alpha) > 0$ for $\alpha \geq 0$, and $q_{m+1}(\alpha)$ has no nonnegative real roots. If $q_{m+1}(\alpha)$ had a complex conjugate pair of roots with nonnegative real parts, then the graph of q_{m+1} would have a local minimum for some nonnegative α. This is impossible since $q_{m+1}'(\alpha) > 0$, so $q_{m+1}(\alpha)$ has no complex roots with nonnegative real part. Thus the endemic equilibrium is locally asymptotically stable. ∎

4.4 Stability of the Difference Equations Model with One Sexual Activity Level.

In Sections $4.1 - 4.3$ thresholds and stability of equilibria are analyzed for the differential–equations model corresponding to Figure 3.1 with one activity level. The model actually used in the calculations involve difference equations with a one–month time step. Here it is shown that the stability threshold for the differential equations model also works for the difference–equations model.

The difference equations for the one activity level model are

$$Y_0^{n+1} = Y_0^n + (\delta + \mu)(N - Y_0^n) - \left[\sum_{j=1}^{m}\lambda_j Y_j^n\right]\left[Y_0^n\bigg/\sum_{k=0}^{m}Y_k^n\right]$$
$$Y_1^{n+1} = Y_1^n + \left[\sum_{j=1}^{m}\lambda_j Y_j^n\right]\left[Y_0^n\bigg/\sum_{k=0}^{m}Y_k^n\right] - (\delta + \mu + \gamma_1)Y_1^n \tag{4.14}$$
$$Y_k^{n+1} = Y_k^n + \gamma_{k-1}Y_{k-1}^n - (\delta + \mu + \gamma_k)Y_k^n \text{ for } 2 \leq k \leq m+1 .$$

As in Section 4.1, let $I_j^n = Y_j^n/N$ be the fraction of the population in stage j so the model (4.14) becomes

$$I_1^{n+1} = I_1^n + g(I^n)I_0^n - \zeta_1 I_1^n$$
$$I_k^{n+1} = I_k^n + \gamma_{k-1}I_{k-1}^n - \zeta_k I_k^n \text{ for } 2 \leq k \leq m+1 \tag{4.15}$$

where $g(I^n) = (\sum_{j=1}^{m}\lambda_j I_j^n)/(1-I_{m+1}^n)$, $\zeta_k = (\delta + \mu + \gamma_k)$, $\gamma_{m+1} = 0$, and $I_0^n = 1 - \sum_{j=1}^{m+1}I_j^n$.

The equilibria for the difference–equations model (4.15) are precisely the same as those for the differential–equations model (4.2). The disease–free equilibrium (DFE) is the origin and the endemic equilibrium (EE) is given by (4.4) and (4.6). Lemma 4.1 shows that the EE is a distinct equilibrium if $\sigma > 1$, where σ is the contact number given by (4.7). Let V^n be the vector of I_k for $1 \leq k \leq m+1$ and $V^{n+1} = F(V^n)$ be the nonlinear difference equations (4.14). The linearization of (4.15) at the DFE is

$$\mathbf{V}^{n+1} = T\mathbf{V}^n = (E + A)\mathbf{V}^n \tag{4.16}$$

where E is the identity matrix and A is the matrix in (4.9).

The matrix T is irreducible and nonnegative if $\zeta_k < 1$ for $1 \leq k \leq m+1$. This condition that the mean waiting times $1/\zeta_k$ are greater than one month is always satisfied for our application of the model for HIV/AIDS. The Perron–Frobenius theory applies to the matrix T so that T has a real simple eigenvalue equal to its stability modulus $s(T)$ and equal to its spectral radius $\rho(T)$, the corresponding eigenvector ω is positive, and any nonnegative eigenvector is a positive multiple of ω. Since $\rho(T) = s(T) = s(A+E) = s(A)+1$, the condition $s(A) < 0$ is equivalent to $\rho(T) < 1$. In Section 4.2 the condition $s(A) < 0$ is shown to be equivalent to $\sigma < 1$ where the contact number σ is given by (4.6). Recall that an equilibrium for a difference equation is locally stable iff the spectral radius of the linearization is less than 1. Thus we have proved the following Theorem, which is analogous to Theorem 4.5.

Theorem 4.8. _If $\sigma < 1$, then the DFE for the model (4.15) is locally asymptotically stable. If $\sigma > 1$, the DFE is unstable._

Although the analog of Theorem 4.6 is probably true for the difference–equations model (4.15) so that the endemic equilibrium (EE) is locally asymptotically stable for $\sigma > 1$, the obvious proof method does not quite work. The Jacobian at the EE is $V = E + B$, where B is given by (4.13), and $s(V) = s(E + B) = 1 + s(B)$. From Theorem 4.7 $s(B) < 0$ if $\sigma > 1$, so $s(V) \leq 1$ if $\sigma > 1$. But $V = E + B$ is not nonnegative since $\tau_{m+1} = -(1 - 1/\sigma)g(I) < 0$, so that the Perron–Frobenius theory does not guarantee that $\rho(V) = s(V)$. Thus this approach does not quite prove that $\rho(V) < 1$, which is needed for local stability.

4.5 Stability for the Difference–Equations Model with Two Sexual Activity Levels

The stability analyses of the difference–equations model and the differential–equations model corresponding to Figure 3.1 with very active and active groups are analytically intractable. Here the linearization at the DFE is found for the difference–equations model so the spectral radius can be evaluated numerically. This is the model which is used in later chapters in this monograph. Since the spectral radius (the largest absolute value of an eigenvalue) is often used as a measure of the contact number or intrinsic reproduction number [Hethcote and Van Ark, 1987; Diekmann et al., 1988], its size indicates how far above or below the threshold value of one the current parameters for the infectious disease process are.

The difference equations for the very active and active risk groups in the model corresponding to Figure 3.1 are:

$$X_0^{n+1} = X_0^n + (\delta + \mu)[fN - X_0^n] - g_1 X_0^n - \phi X_0^n + \theta Y_0^n$$

$$X_1^{n+1} = X_1^n + g_1 X_0^n - \xi_1 X_1^n - \phi X_1^n + \theta Y_1^n$$

$$X_k^{n+1} = X_k^n + \gamma_{k-1} X_{k-1}^n - \xi_k X_k^n - \phi X_k^n + \theta Y_k^n \quad \text{for } 2 \leq k \leq m+1.$$

$$Y_0^{n+1} = Y_0^n + (\delta + \mu)[(1-f)N - Y_0^n] - g_2 Y_0^n + \phi X_0^n - \theta Y_0^n \qquad (4.17)$$

$$Y_1^{n+1} = Y_1^n + g_2 Y_0^n - \xi_1 Y_1^n + \phi X_1^n - \theta Y_1^n$$

$$Y_k^{n+1} = Y_k^n + \gamma_{k-1} Y_{k-1}^n - \xi_k Y_k^n + \phi X_k^n - \theta Y_k^n \quad \text{for } 2 \leq k \leq m+1.$$

where $\sum\limits_{j=0}^{m+1} X_j^n = fN$, $\sum\limits_{k=0}^{m+1} Y_k^n = (1-f)N$, $\theta = f\phi/(1-f)$, $\xi_k = (\delta+\mu+\gamma_k)$ for $2 \leq k \leq m+1$, $\gamma_{m+1} = 0$,

$$g_1 = (1-\eta)\sum_{j=1}^{m} R\lambda_j X_j^n/[fN-X_{m+1}^n] + \eta\sum_{j=1}^{m} R\lambda_j(R\, X_j^n + Y_j^n)/[R(fN-X_{m+1}^n)+(1-f)N-Y_{m+1}^n],$$

$$g_2 = (1-\eta)\sum_{j=1}^{m} \lambda_j Y_j^n/[(1-f)N-Y_{m+1}^n] + \eta\sum_{j=1}^{m} \lambda_j(R\, X_j^n + Y_j^n)/[R(fN-X_{m+1}^n)+(1-f)N-Y_{m+1}^n],$$

and $\lambda_k = \rho_k \times PH \times \omega_k \times QH$.

This system of nonlinear difference equations could be converted to a system for the fractions in each class as in Section 4.4, but this is not necessary here since the eigenvalues and spectral radius will be found numerically. Since there is some redundancy in the system above, the subsystem for X_k^n and Y_k^n with $1 \leq k \leq m+1$ is considered, where $X_0^n = fN - \sum\limits_{j=1}^{m+1} X_j^n$ and $Y_0^n = (1-f)N - \sum\limits_{k=1}^{m+1} Y_k^n$. The disease–free equilibrium (DFE) for this subsystem is the origin and the matrix for the linearization around this DFE is given by:

$$T = \begin{bmatrix} T_{11} & T_{12} \\ \hline T_{21} & T_{22} \end{bmatrix},$$

where

$$T_{11} = \begin{bmatrix} 1-\xi_1-\phi+\tau_1 & \tau_2 & \tau_3 & \cdots & \tau_m & 0 \\ \gamma_1 & 1-\xi_2-\phi & 0 & & & 0 \\ 0 & \gamma_2 & 1-\xi_3-\phi & & & \\ \vdots & & & & & \vdots \\ & & & & & 0 \\ 0 & & 0 & \cdots & \gamma_m & 1-\xi_{m+1}-\phi \end{bmatrix},$$

$$T_{22} = \begin{bmatrix} 1-\xi_1-\theta+\omega_1 & \omega_2 & \omega_3 & \cdots & \omega_m & 0 \\ \gamma_1 & 1-\xi_2-\theta & 0 & & & 0 \\ 0 & \gamma_2 & 1-\xi_3-\theta & & & \\ \vdots & & & & & \vdots \\ & & & & & 0 \\ 0 & & 0 & \cdots & \gamma_m & 1-\xi_{m+1}-\theta \end{bmatrix},$$

$$T_{12} = \begin{bmatrix} \chi_1+\theta & \chi_2 & \chi_3 & \cdots & \chi_m & 0 \\ 0 & \theta & 0 & \cdots & & 0 \\ 0 & & \theta & & & \\ \vdots & & & & & \vdots \\ & & & & & 0 \\ 0 & 0 & \cdots & & 0 & \theta \end{bmatrix},$$

$$T_{21} = \begin{bmatrix} \nu_1+\phi & \nu_2 & \nu_3 & \cdots & \nu_m & 0 \\ 0 & \phi & 0 & \cdots & & 0 \\ 0 & & \phi & & & \\ \vdots & & & & & \vdots \\ & & & & & 0 \\ 0 & 0 & \cdots & & 0 & \phi \end{bmatrix},$$

$$\tau_k = \left[\frac{(1-\eta)R\lambda_k}{fN} + \frac{\eta R\lambda_k R}{RfN+(1-f)N} \right] fN,$$

$$\chi_k = \left[\frac{\eta R\lambda_k fN}{RfN+(1-f)N} \right],$$

$$\nu_k = \left[\frac{\eta\lambda_k(1-f)N}{RfN+(1-f)N} \right],$$

$$\omega_k = \left[\frac{(1-\eta)\lambda_k}{(1-f)N} + \frac{\eta\lambda_k R}{RfN+(1-f)N} \right](1-f)N.$$

The eigenvalues of T above are found numerically for the parameter sets in later Chapters. If the spectral radius satisfies $\rho(T) < 1$, then the DFE is stable. If $\rho(T) > 1$, the DFE is unstable, and solutions approach the endemic equilibrium.

CHAPTER 5

HOMOSEXUAL MEN IN SAN FRANCISCO:
ESTIMATION OF PARAMETERS AND INCIDENCES

San Francisco (SF) has been chosen as the site for modeling HIV transmission in homosexual men because very good data are available there. The large open community of homosexual men in SF has been the source of numerous sexual behavior surveys. Additionally, data are available in SF for AIDS incidence each year and for HIV incidence as early as 1978. In this application of the simulation model, men who have sex with men (homosexual and bisexual men) are called homosexual men. Since most (85%) of the reported AIDS cases in SF have occurred in homosexual men, the modeling here does not include transmission between homosexual/bisexual men and others such as their heterosexual partners or homosexual intravenous drug users.

5.1 Estimation of Parameters Related to the Stages

The model and parameter values in Section 2.1 for staged progression to AIDS based on clinical phases is used here.

5.1.1 Probabilities of Transmission in the Stages

Recall that ω_k ⋅ QH is the probability of transmission by people in stage k where $\omega_k = 1$ for an asymptomatic stage. Persons in the pre–antibody stage, symptomatic stages and AIDS stage seem to be more infectious than asymptomatic persons (Goedert et al., 1987, 1989; May, 1988; De Gruttola and Mayer, 1987; Padian et al., 1987; Osmund et al., 1988; Burke et al, 1989). Longini et al. (1990), using data on partnerships with HIV–infected persons, have estimated that the transmission rate of AIDS patients is 7.5 times that of symptomatic patients. In the model the factors ω_k are 2 for the pre–antibody stage, 1 for the asymptomatic stages, 2 for the symptomatic stages, and 15 for the AIDS stage.

5.1.2 Behavioral Changes in the Stages

Recall that ρ_k ⋅ PA is the average number of new sexual partners per month in stage k, where $\rho_k = 1$ for asymptomatics. Homosexual men might reduce their (unprotected) sexual activity either because they do not feel well in the symptomatic and AIDS phases or because they know that they have an HIV infection and do not want to infect others. Data presented by Coates et al. (1987) showed that in homosexual men in SF knowledge of HIV positive status resulted in a decrease in unprotected sexual activity from 18% to 12% between 1984 and 1986. Cates and Handsfield (1988) summarized studies showing that counseling and testing for HIV lead to reductions in high–risk behavior and that HIV positive individuals change their behavior more than HIV negative individuals. Thus the values chosen are $\rho_k = 1$ for stages in the pre–antibody or asymptomatic phases, $\rho_k = 0.75$ for stages in the symptomatic phase, and $\rho_k = 0.5$ for the

AIDS stage. There is significant uncertainty in the data leading to the parameter estimates for the $\omega_k \times \rho_k$ values of $(2, 1, 1.5, 7.5)$ in the four phases so the sensitivity analysis in Section 6.4 considers $(1, 1, 1, 1)$ and $(10, 1, 1, 1)$.

5.2 Estimation of Population Sizes and Turnover Rate Constants

The SF Department of Public Health (Lemp et al., 1990) estimated that there were 55,816 homosexual males in the city of San Francisco in 1984. A similar estimate was obtained by Pickering et al. (1986). The size of the homosexual male population probably increased during the 1970s due to the popularity of SF with homosexual men and may have decreased in recent years. However, because precise information is not available, the male homosexual population size in SF is assumed to be constant at 56,000 in the model during the HIV epidemic. The sensitivity analysis considers sizes of 40,000 and 80,000.

A survey by Communications Technologies (Bye, 1987) found that 26% of the homosexual men in SF had lived there for five years or less. The immigration and emigration rates are therefore assumed to be 5% per year, so that $\delta = 0.05/12$ per month. Although the migration rate of 5% per year seems to be a reasonably good estimate, the sensitivity analysis considers migration rates of 0%, 3%, and 8%. Using mortality data (US Bureau of the Census, 1987) for men between 18 and 54, the death rate for homosexual men in the model is $\mu = 0.000532$ deaths per person per month.

The San Francisco City Clinic Cohort (SFCCC) consists of approximately 6700 homosexual men recruited between 1978 and 1980 from a clinic for sexually transmitted diseases to participate in a hepatitis B study. Because of the selection procedures, these men were probably more sexually active than most homosexual men in SF. In the SFCCC, 166 (2.4%) were reported to have AIDS by December 1984; 147 of these men still lived in SF, and 19 had moved to ten other U.S. cities. AIDS cases in the SFCCC were 38.5% of all AIDS cases in SF in the last half of 1981 and 16.4% of the cumulative AIDS cases in SF in December 1984 (Jaffe et al., 1985). Subsets of the SFCCC have been used to examine factors associated with HIV infection (Darrow et al., 1987) and progression to AIDS (Hessol et al., 1989). Data from the SFCCC are used here and in the next section.

The sexually very active fraction (F) and the sexual activity ratio (R) can be estimated by using the data from the SFCCC (Darrow, 1989). The choice of $F = 0.1$ is consistent with the data showing that there is a small percentage of sexually very active men. For 751 SFCCC men, the 10, 25, 50, 75, 90 and 95 percentiles for the average number of nonsteady sexual partners per year from the time of enrollment to the first followup (reinterview of diagnosis of AIDS) were 0, 12, 36, 84, 204 and 329 which make the median numbers of partners per year about 36 for the least active 90% and 329 for the most active 10%. For 500 SFCCC men interviewed between 1978 and 1984–85 the analogous percentiles for the number of partners per month were 0, 1, 3, 8, 18 and 28 so that the median numbers of partners per month were about 3 for the least active 90% and 28 for the most active 10%. For 413 SFCCC men interviewed between 1984–85 and 1986–87, the analogous data were 0, 0, 1, 4, 11, 18 so that the median numbers of partners per month were about 1 for the least active 90% and 18 for the most active 10%. These data suggest that 10% of the homosexual men in SF are approximately ten times more sexually active than the others so that $F = 0.1$ and $R = 10$ are reasonable estimates. The sensitivity analysis considers combinations where F and R are halved and doubled.

Although the information on the distributions of numbers of sex partners of homosexual men in SF is less complete in three other articles (Darrow et al., 1987; Winkelstein, Lyman et al., 1987; Winkelstein, Samuel et al., 1987) the data are consistent with 10% being ten times as active. The Gay Report (Jay and Young, 1979) was a survey of 4212 homosexual men in the U.S. carried out by gay organizations. In this sample, the lifetime median number of sexual partners was 49.5, with 12.5% reporting over 500 sex partners. This suggests that 12.5% were at least 10 times as sexually active as the other homosexual men. Note that data between 1979 and 1989 suggests that $F = 0.1$ and $R = 10$ are reasonable parameter values. Brauer et al. (1992) consider an HIV/AIDS model in which the fraction in the very active (core) group changes as a function of incidence–driven changes in behavior.

The rate constant (ϕ) for moving from the very active to active compartments is chosen to correspond to a 5% inflow and a 5% outflow per year so that $\phi = 0.05/12$ per month. The sensitivity to this choice is examined in Section 6.4.

5.3 Sexual Behavior Parameter Estimates

In the fitting of the simulations the most reliable parameter values are fixed and the six least reliable parameter values are varied to fit the simulation model to the HIV and AIDS incidence data. These six parameters are the epidemic starting date, the four parameters in Chapter 3 defining the average number of new sexual partners per month and the external mixing fraction. The *a priori* estimates or ranges for these six parameter values obtained in this section serve as initial guesses for the fitting iterations and as checks on the best–fitting parameter estimations.

5.3.1 Probability of Transmission Per Partner

Grant et al. (1987) found that the mean probability of infection through unprotected receptive anal intercourse was 0.102 per sex partner for the homosexual contacts of the 672 homosexual men studied. Since asymptomatic individuals in our model have relative infectivity $\omega_k = 1$ and the people in the other stages have higher degrees of infectiousness, the average relative infectivity of the infected persons contacted by the 672 men is assumed to be 2. Thus $2QH = 0.1$ so that the probability of homosexual transmission of HIV to sex partners of active asymptomatic infected persons is $QH = 0.05$. The value of QH based on receptive anal intercourse may be too large since homosexual partnerships can involve many other types of sexual contacts. Since QH and the average number PA of different partners per month always appear as a product in the model, QH is held fixed while PA is varied.

5.3.2 New Partners Per Month

Surveys by Johnson (1988) and Becker and Joseph (1988) cite studies showing that HIV seropositivity in homosexual men is associated with receptive anal intercourse and the number of sexual partners. Like QH above, the number of new sexual partners per month, PA, is really a simplified average over a variety of types of partnerships. Recall that PA is defined in Chapter 3 in terms of the four parameters PAS, STR, STP, and RDN given in Table 3.1.

Subsets of men from stratified random samples of the SFCCC (see Section 5.2) were interviewed in 1978, 1984, 1985, and 1987 (CDC: 1985e; 1985f; 1987d; Doll et al., 1987; Doll, 1988). The mean numbers of nonsteady partners (defined as individuals with whom the participant had sexual contact just once or twice) during a four–month period were 29.3 per person (median = 16) in 1978, 14.5 (median = 3) in 1984 and 5.5 (median = 1) in 1985. The medians yield a yearly reduction factor of $0.67 = (1/16)^{1/7}$. In these studies, the risk index of a sexual activity is the product of the percentage of time the participant engaged in this type of activity and the number of nonsteady male partners during the same period. The risk index for receptive anal intercourse with ejaculation with nonsteady partners was 10.9 in 1978, 3.3 in 1984, 0.4 in 1985 and 0.09 in 1987. These data yield a yearly reduction factor of $0.59 = (0.09/10.9)^{1/9}$. The risk index for insertive anal intercourse with nonsteady partners was 12.9 in 1978, 3.5 in 1984, 1.0 in 1985, and 0.35 in 1987 so the yearly reduction factor was $0.67 = (0.35/12.9)^{1/9}$.

In the SFCCC, of the 25% who were negative for hepatitis B, 359 took part in hepatitis B vaccine trial. Of these men, 313 agreed to participate in a HIV study (Hessol et al., 1989). Although the SFCCC men were probably more sexually active than other homosexual men in SF, those in the vaccine trial cohort were probably less active than others in the SFCCC, since they were negative for hepatitis B. Hessol et al. (1989) suggest that these vaccine trial men might be typical of SF homosexual men, since the decrease in HIV seroconversion in this cohort parallels a decrease in their high–risk sexual behavior and a city–wide decrease in gonococcal proctitis. In this vaccine trial cohort, the estimated average number of partners with whom the index cases engaged in receptive anal intercourse was approximately constant at about 17 per year (1.4 per month) through 1981, and then decreased to about 0.1 in 1987. This suggests a yearly reduction factor of $0.43 = (0.1/17)^{1/6}$ in high–risk sexual behavior.

The San Francisco Men's Health Study (SFMHS) was started in June 1984 to study the epidemiology of AIDS in a six square kilometers area (19 census tracts), in which the early AIDS incidence had been highest. It was estimated that there were approximately 18,000 homosexual men living in this area. The initial cohort in the SFMHS consisted of 1034 single men aged 25 to 55 recruited by area probability sampling (Winkelstein, Lyman et al., 1987). In a sample from the SFMHS the average lifetime number of sex partners was 200 so that there may have been about 20 partners per year or about 1.7 per month (Winkelstein, Samuel et al., 1987). Winkelstein, Wiley et al. (1988) report behavior changes in the SFMHS participants. Among HIV–positive men, insertive anal intercourse with 2 or more partners in 6 months declined from 40% in early 1984 to 15% in early 1985, was approximately constant through late 1986, and then declined to 5% in early 1987. Among HIV—negative men, receptive anal intercourse with 2 or more partners in 6 months decreased from 15% in early 1984 to 5% in late 1984 and remained low, with a value of 3% in early 1987. These data suggest large decreases in high–risk sexual behavior in 1984, and smaller decreases since 1985.

The decreases in high–risk sexual activity reported above are consistent with observed decreases in gonococcal proctitis cases per year in SF (Pickering et al., 1986; Hessol et al., 1989; Kohn, 1990). As shown in Figure 3.2, cases were approximately level from 1978 to 1981, decreased rapidly between 1982 and 1987, and then decreased slowly in 1988 and 1989. Since gonorrhea incidence responds rapidly to changes in behavior (Hethcote and Yorke, 1984), the changes in gonorrhea incidence are a good indication of behavior changes. Decreases in high–risk sexual activity starting in 1982 are consistent with the increasing awareness of AIDS among homosexual men in SF at about that time (Darrow et al., 1987; CDC: 1985f; 1987d).

A simplified version of the model in Chapter 3 can be used for gonorrhea transmission in homosexual men in SF. This gonorrhea model has only one infectious phase with an average infectious period of one year, after which the recovered men are susceptible again. Figure 3.3 shows the monthly gonococcal proctitis incidence in the simulation model when the average contact rate decreases by a factor of 0.70 each year from January 1982 to December 1984. The similarity of the simulation incidences to the observed gonorrhea incidences suggest that decreases in the average number of sexual partners started in about 1982 and occurred for several years.

Although the four parameters defining the average number PA of different partners per month are varied to satisfy the fit criteria, initial estimates and reasonable ranges are necessary. In the paragraphs above, the yearly reduction factors in sex partners per month are 0.59, 0.67, 0.43, and 0.70, which makes 0.4 to 0.7 a reasonable range for the yearly reduction factor RDN in the HIV simulations. The data above indicate that a good estimate for the reduction starting date STR would be January 1982, but other dates in 1981 or 1982 are also considered acceptable in the simulations. Reductions in high–risk sexual behavior may be continuing in recent years, but they are probably smaller than in previous years. The initial guess for the reduction stopping date STP is December 1984, but other stopping dates are also acceptable.

Values for the average number of partners per month in the paragraphs above are $29.3/4 = 7.3$ (median $= 4$) in 1978 for the SFCCC, 1.4 before 1981 for the SFCCC vaccine trial sample, and 1.7 before 1984 for the SFMHS. Thus a reasonable initial guess for PAS, the average number of partners per month before STR, is 2. This corresponds to an average number of partners per month of 1.05 for active individuals, and 10.5 for very active individuals when 10% are ten times as active.

5.3.3 Other Parameters

The blood samples in the SFCCC indicate that some men were HIV positive in 1978 so that the HIV epidemic probably started several years earlier. Hence the epidemic starting date STD might be in 1974, 1975 or 1976. In the model for heterosexual transmission of gonorrhea which had sexually active and very active subpopulations (Hethcote and Yorke, 1984), the external mixing fraction was 0.8, so that the *a priori* estimate of the external mixing fraction η in this model is $\eta = 0.8$.

5.4 Estimation of HIV and AIDS Incidences

5.4.1 HIV Incidence in San Francisco

More information is available on HIV seroconversions in SF than in any other location. Because blood samples were saved for participants in a hepatitis B vaccine trial starting in 1978 (Hessol et al., 1990), SF is the only place where data on HIV incidence is available before 1984. Two other sources of HIV incidence data are the SF Men's Health Study (Winkelstein, Lyman et al., 1987) and the SF General Hospital Cohort (Moss et al., 1988). Using three data sets, Bacchetti and Moss (1989) estimated the HIV seroincidence for homosexual men in SF from 1978 to 1989. Bacchetti (1990) refined this approach and obtained monthly HIV seroincidence estimates. His HIV seroincidences were found by scaling up a seroincidence curve estimated from the cohort studies so that the cumulative HIV seroconversions through September 1984 matched his city–wide estimate of 20,060. Since HIV infection occurs approximately 2 months before HIV seroconversion, the HIV incidence estimates before 1985 in Figure 5.1 are obtained by shifting the Bacchetti seroincidence estimates back 2 months.

Because Bacchetti's HIV seroconversion estimates in 1985 to 1988 were based on closed cohorts of aging men, they may not reflect the higher HIV incidence occurring in younger men. Based on the low seroincidence in the SF City Clinic Cohort (SFCCC) and the SF Men's Health Study, Lemp et al. (1990) assumed that 0.8% of the susceptible homosexual men would become HIV–infected each year from 1988 to 1993. In the Multicenter AIDS Cohort Study consisting of 3095 initially seronegative homosexual men recruited in mid–1984, the overall annual HIV infection rate over 5 years was 1.4%, but the seroconversion rate in the younger men was significantly higher (Kingsley et al., 1990). Thus the HIV seroconversion rate of about 1% per year may be correct for older homosexual men in these closed cohorts, but seroconversion rates are higher in younger homosexual men.

Among homosexual men visiting STD clinics in SF, Kellogg et al. (1990) found 40.7% HIV seroprevalence in 59 men ages 20–24 and 60.7% seroprevalence in 125 men ages 25–29. They suggested that previously uninfected young men may have seroconverted since 1983 when the annual incidence of new infections began to decline in SF. Clearly, the HIV seroconversion rates in these younger homosexual men (one third of the sample survey) must have been much higher than 1% per year in recent years in order to reach the observed HIV seroprevalence levels of 40.7% and 60.7%. If the annual HIV seroconversion rates in recent years were 4% for the susceptible homosexual men in SF under 30 and 1% for those over 30, then the average seroconversion rate in recent years for all homosexual men in SF would be $(1/3)4\% + (2/3)1\% = 2\%$. These estimates are consistent with other estimates (Hessol et al., 1990; Winkelstein, Wiley et al., 1988). The HIV seroprevalence is approximately 20,000 out of about 56,000 homosexual men in SF (Bacchetti, 1990), so that the annual number of seroconversions may have been about 2% of 36,000 susceptibles, or 720 per year. This 720 HIV seroincidence per year is plausible

Table 5.1. Estimates of yearly HIV and AIDS incidences for homosexual men in SF

		AIDS Incidence			
			Consistent Cases		
year	HIV incidence	all cases adjusted for reporting delays	cases adjusted for reporting delays	modified non–consistent cases	total adjusted cases
1978	439	0	0	0	0
1979	1963	0	0	0	0
1980	4390	2	2	0	2
1981	5721	22	22	0	22
1982	4337	86	86	0	86
1983	2362	228	228	0	228
1984	1269	443	442	0	442
1985	762	681	678	0	678
1986	720	1029	1009	1	1010
1987	720	1320	1272	3	1275
1988	720	1354	1276	9	1285
1989	720	1449	1321	17	1338
1990	720	1635	1522	29	1551

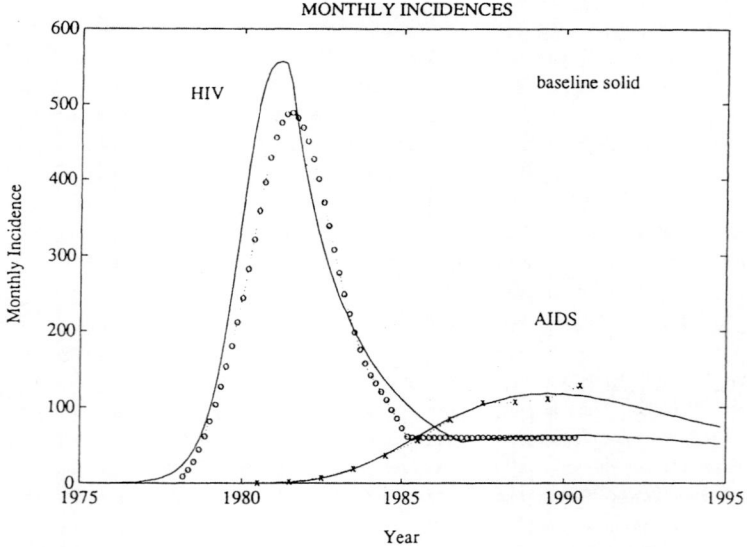

Figure 5.1. The HIV incidence curve (circles) and the AIDS incidence curve (x symbols) correspond to the estimates in Table 5.1. Baseline simulations for HIV and AIDS incidences corresponding to Tables 6.1 and 6.2 from Chapter 6.

since it is about one–fourth of the estimated 2800 (5% of our 56,000 estimate) homosexual men immigrating to SF each year. Thus the best approximation of HIV incidence in homosexual men in SF seems to be the Bacchetti's HIV incidence curve in Figure 5.1 until May 1986, and then about 60 per month between 1986 and 1990. The yearly estimated HIV incidences are given in Table 5.1.

5.4.2 AIDS Incidence in San Francisco

In the United States, AIDS cases meeting a surveillance definition (CDC: 1982, 1985c, 1987j) are reported locally and then forwarded to the Centers for Disease Control (CDC). The reported AIDS incidence in SF has been obtained from these case reports sent to CDC through May 1991. (Note that the data used throughout this chapter is for the city of SF, not the SF Metropolitan Statistical Area.) Lindan et al. (1989) found that the reporting delay pattern did not change from 1985 through 1988; consequently, methodical adjustments are possible. Cases diagnosed after March 1985 have been adjusted for reporting delays after grouping cases by quarters of diagnosis (Karon et al., 1988, 1989). The resulting estimates are shown in Table 5.1.

The AIDS surveillance definition was expanded in September 1987 (CDC: 1987j). The expansion allowed patients with a positive HIV antibody test to be reported if they had presumptive (instead of definitive) diagnoses of certain diseases in the previous definition, or if they had certain other diseases indicating severe morbidity associated with HIV infection. Patients satisfying what is called the consistent case definition (Karon et al., 1988) are those with a diagnosis (definitive or presumptive) of a disease in the pre–1987 case definition. The expansion of the surveillance definition increased the number of patients reported with AIDS by adding some patients who die before satisfying the consistent definition and allowing others to be reported earlier in the course of the disease. For homosexual men in SF, 3%, 4%, 8%, and 7% of the cases diagnosed in the years 1987–1990 respectively, were not consistent with the pre–1987 surveillance definition.

The effect of the 1987 change in the AIDS surveillance definition has been estimated (Lemp, 1991). There were 477 persons diagnosed with AIDS in SF between September 1, 1987, and December 31, 1989, based on diseases not consistent with the pre–1987 definition. In seven of these persons, the AIDS diagnosis was not made before the date of death. Of the remaining 470 patients, about half died before developing a disease consistent with the pre–1987 definition, and 130 (28%) had developed such a disease by December 31, 1990. The Kaplan–Meier procedure estimates the median time for progression to the consistent case definition to be 27 months. Of those who reach the consistent case definition before death, the estimates are that 21, 29, 38, 47, and 58% would develop a disease in the consistent case definition at 6, 12, 18, 25, and 31 months, respectively.

The total consistent case estimates in Table 5.1 of annual AIDS incidence are obtained as follows. Monthly incidences (cases diagnosed through December 1990) are adjusted for estimated reporting delays based on cases reported through March 1991 (Karon et al., 1989), both for cases consistent with the pre–1987 definition and for cases not consistent with that definition that did not die during the month of diagnosis. Based on the progression data from SF, the non—consistent cases are modified by assuming that 10% would satisfy the consistent definition six months after the month of diagnosis, and that 5% more would satisfy the consistent definition at the end of each of the following six—month intervals up to three years (i.e., after 12, 18, 24, 30, and 36 months.) For example, the estimate that 10% would satisfy the consistent definition six months later is based on half of the persons with non—consistent diagnoses dying before meeting the consistent definition, and 20% of the remaining persons satisfying the consistent definition within six months. The estimates in Table 5.1 of the total consistent AIDS incidences are obtained as the sums of the consistent and modified non—consistent cases.

One study (Lindan et al., 1989) found that approximately 10% of the total cases in homosexual men in SF from 1985 through 1988 were not reported. A previous study (Rauch et al., 1989) found that at least 98% of the AIDS cases diagnosed in SF before 1987 were reported. Since the extent of underreporting is unclear, the adjusted consistent AIDS cases in Table 5.1 are not further adjusted for underreporting. Thus the HIV and AIDS incidences found by fitting the simulation model to this data need to be scaled up by a factor to account for underreporting.

CHAPTER 6

HOMOSEXUAL MEN IN SAN FRANCISCO: SIMULATIONS AND SENSITIVITY ANALYSIS

Since homosexual men in San Francisco (SF) are probably the most studied AIDS
population in the world, it is useful to demonstrate that one can simulate HIV and AIDS in this
population in a manner consistent with all available information. The analysis in Chapter 5 and
this chapter is important not only for a better understanding of HIV and AIDS in homosexual
men in SF but also as a foundation for further work. It provides a basis for simulation modeling
in later chapters of other geographic locations and other risk groups.

Chapter 3 contains the formulation of a simulation model for HIV transmission and the
development of AIDS in homosexual men in SF. Here the term "homosexual men" includes
bisexual men but excludes homosexual intravenous drug users. In this dynamic simulation model,
the population is divided into sexually active and very active subpopulations, and the HIV
incidence is proportional to the infectivity of the infected persons during their staged progression
to AIDS and death. In Chapter 5 many data sources are used to estimate values or ranges of
values for all parameters in the model.

Recently there has been speculation about the effects on AIDS incidence of zidovudine
(ZDV), aerosol pentamidine and other forms of therapy or health care. The model is modified in
Section 6.3 to include therapy for some symptomatic and AIDS patients, and data on estimated
fractions of patients receiving therapy between 1987 and 1989 are presented. Parameter sets and
simulations consistent with therapy fractions are compared to the baseline parameter set and
simulations. Comparisons suggest the relative influences on AIDS incidences of saturation in the
high–risk group, changes in sexual behavior, and therapy.

The simulation modeling approach to the HIV epidemic in homosexual men in SF has been
used previously. Pickering et al. (1986) used a discrete time, nonlinear model for sexual
transmission of HIV with several possible courses of infection and used reported anal–rectal
gonorrhea data to estimate the changes in homosexual behavior. They analyzed and forecast
AIDS incidence in homosexual men in three cities including SF, but they concluded that there was
insufficient data before 1986 to choose between radically different forecasts. Ahlgren et al. (1990)
developed a dynamic transmission model and found parameter values which optimized the fit to
the seroconversion data from the SF Vaccine Trial Cohort and AIDS incidence in homosexual men
in SF for 1978 to 1986. Their modeling experiments suggested that the high infectivity of the
short–lived, antigen–bearing first stage of HIV infection may have caused the rapid rise in the
early epidemic in SF. Direct projections of AIDS incidence can be made by using an HIV
seroincidence curve and a distribution for the AIDS incubation period, but this method yields no
information on HIV transmission. This approach has been used in SF by Lemp et al. (1990).

The simulation modeling approach used here yields an HIV transmission dynamics model
with parameter estimates. The major emphasis in this analysis is to obtain a priori parameter
estimates from multiple sources and then to see if all of these parameter estimates are consistent
in a simulation model with estimated HIV and AIDS incidences. Thus the goal is not to provide

AIDS incidence forecasts but to provide a dynamic simulation model with parameter values which reconstructs what has occurred up to the present. The primary limitation of our modeling is that the model is only a simple approximation of reality; moreover, it is not possible in this model which simulates transmission dynamics to estimate the deviations of the model simulations from reality. When interpreting modeling results, one must be aware of the approximations involved in the formulation of the model. Further discussion of the purposes and limitations of epidemiologic modeling is given in Section 1.6.

6.1 The Fit Criteria

The first fit criterion for the simulations is that the parameter values must be close to the parameter estimates obtained in the Chapter 5. The second criterion is that the HIV and AIDS incidence in the simulations must be close to the estimated HIV and AIDS incidence values given in Table 5.1. The goodness of fit is measured by the chi−square (χ^2) statistic, i.e., the sum of the squares of the observed values minus the expected values of the incidences divided by the expected values. The quantity minimized in the fitting procedure is the sum of 0.02 times the χ^2 value for the HIV incidences and 0.98 times the χ^2 value for the AIDS incidences. These weights are chosen so that the two contributions to the minimized quantity are of the same magnitude.

In Table 6.1 the most reliable parameter values have been fixed at values equal to their listed *a priori* estimates. Values for the starting and stopping dates and initial estimates for the other three optimization parameters have been entered into a computer program that varies η, PAS and RDN in order to minimize the weighted sum of the χ^2 values. The six optimization parameters (see Table 6.1) whose values and simulation best satisfy the fit criteria have been found by comparing computer runs. The sensitivity to changes in the fixed and optimization parameters is considered in Section 6.4.

6.2 The Baseline Parameter Set

6.2.1 Simulation Results

The effects of changes in parameters have been explored by using a "baseline parameter set." Table 6.1 gives the baseline parameter set, and Table 6.2 and Figure 5.1 give the corresponding simulation results. In Table 6.1 the fixed parameter values are equal to their *a priori* estimates in Chapter 5. The optimization parameters which give the best fit in the sense of minimizing the weighted sum of the χ^2 values are consistent with the *a priori* estimates. The epidemic starting date is October 1975, and the external mixing fraction is 0.82. Decreases in homosexual partnership rates occur each month between August 1981 and December 1986 with a yearly reduction factor of 0.61. Note that these values are consistent with the *a priori* estimates that the reduction occurred for several years starting around 1982 with a yearly reduction factor in the interval (0.4, 0.7). The average number PAS of partners per month before reduction is 0.75, which is less than the *a priori* estimate of 2, but in the model PAS is multiplied by QH,

Table 6.1 Baseline parameter set

Fixed Parameters

Population size	Q	=	56,000
Natural mortality rate constant	μ	=	0.000532
Monthly migration percentage	δ	=	0.05/12
Monthly activity level change rate constant	ϕ	=	0.05/12
Probability of transmission	QH	=	0.05
Mean times in phases			2.2, 52.6, 62.9, and 18.0 months
Very active fraction	F	=	0.10
Activity level ratio	R	=	10
Relative weights $(\omega \times \rho)$ of transmission in 4 phases			2, 1, 1.5, and 7.5
Number of stages	m	=	7

Optimization Parameters

Starting date of the epidemic	STD	=	October 1975
Reduction starting date	STR	=	August 1981
Reduction stopping date	STP	=	December 1986
External mixing fraction	η	=	0.82
Average number of partners per month before STR	PAS	=	0.75
Yearly reduction factor	RDN	=	0.61

---

the probability of transmission per partner. If QH were changed from 0.05 to 0.019, then PAS would change from 0.75 to 2.0, the *a priori* estimate. In the baseline parameter set, the average time between new sex partners before reduction starts is 0.25 months for very active men and 2.5 months for active men. After reduction by a factor of about 0.07 through December 1986, the average time between new partners is 3.5 months for very active men and 35 months for active men.

Figure 5.1 and Table 6.2 show that the HIV incidences before 1985 in the simulation follow the general pattern of the estimated HIV incidences of Bacchetti (1990), but are usually above those estimates. Bacchetti obtained his estimates by using a scaling factor to match his HIV prevalence estimate of 20,060 in September 1984; if his scaling factor were increased by only 10%, then the HIV simulation curve would be closer to his estimates. As seen in Table 6.2, the HIV incidences after 1986 in the simulations are close to the estimates of 720 per year. The HIV prevalence of approximately 18,700 in 1984 is close to the cumulative HIV incidence of 20,060 by September 1984 obtained by Bacchetti (1990). The fit of the simulated AIDS incidence to the estimated AIDS incidence is quite good. Lang et al. (1991) estimated that there were 2381 living

Table 6.2 Simulation results for parameters in Table 6.1.

YEAR	YEARLY HIV INCIDENCE EST*	SIM+	HIV PREV	PREVALENCE+ FRACTIONAL ALL	V_A	PREV ACT	YEARLY AIDS RESULTS INCIDENCE EST*	SIM+	AIDS PREV+	AIDS DEATHS	AIDS OUTSIDE SF
1975	*****	1.	2.	.00	.00	.00	******	0.	0.	0.	0.
1976	*****	15.	17.	.00	.00	.00	******	0.	0.	0.	0.
1977	*****	84.	98.	.00	.01	.00	******	0.	0.	0.	0.
1978	439	469.	553.	.01	.06	.00	0	0.	0.	0.	0.
1979	1963	2162.	2642.	.05	.26	.02	0	1.	1.	0.	0.
1980	4390	5489.	7859.	.14	.66	.08	2	4.	4.	1.	0.
1981	5721	6284.	13538.	.24	.87	.17	22	21.	19.	6.	3.
1982	4337	4021.	16680.	.30	.90	.23	86	78.	72.	25.	11.
1983	2362	2562.	18178.	.32	.88	.26	228	213.	203.	81.	38.
1984	1269	1709.	18656.	.33	.85	.28	442	437.	441.	199.	94.
1985	762	1161.	18401.	.33	.79	.28	678	717.	774.	384.	185.
1986	720	788.	17583.	.31	.73	.27	1010	997.	1152.	619.	306.
1987	720	686.	16488.	.29	.66	.25	1275	1226.	1513.	865.	439.
1988	720	733.	15305.	.27	.60	.24	1285	1370.	1802.	1082.	565.
1989	720	758.	14073.	.25	.55	.22	1338	1424.	1986.	1240.	667.
1990	720	761.	12839.	.23	.50	.20	1551	1399.	2058.	1327.	735.
1991	*****	746.	11649.	.21	.46	.18	******	1316.	2031.	1343.	767.
1992	*****	718.	10541.	.19	.43	.16	******	1201.	1930.	1302.	766.
1993	*****	683.	9537.	.17	.40	.15	******	1074.	1784.	1221.	739.
1994	*****	644.	8646.	.15	.37	.13	******	950.	1617.	1117.	694.
1995	*****	606.	7868.	.14	.35	.12	******	838.	1448.	1007.	640.

*These are the estimated (EST) values in Table 5.1.
+These are the values from the simulation (SIM) model; V_A means very active, ACT means active, PREV means prevalence, and
OUTSIDE SF is the AIDS incidence outside San Francisco.

AIDS cases in SF in October 1989. Since 85% of AIDS cases in SF in 1989 were in homosexual/bisexual men, their estimate yields 2024 as the AIDS prevalence in homosexual men in 1989, which is close to the prevalence of 1986 in the simulation in Table 6.2. The weighted sum of the χ^2 values of the HIV incidences (594) and the AIDS incidences (35.4) is 46.6.

Certain patterns can be seen in Table 6.2 and Figure 5.1. The peak AIDS incidence in 1989 occurs 5 years after the peak in HIV prevalence in 1984 and 8 years after the peak HIV incidence in 1981. The peak in AIDS deaths occurs about 1 year after the peak in AIDS incidence. The eight–year delay between the peaks in HIV incidence and AIDS incidence is reasonable, since the median incubation period for the seven–stage progression model is 9.6 years. This reinforces the concept that a change in HIV incidence (such as a peak) can cause a similar change many years later in AIDS incidence.

Saturation in the very active group can be seen in Table 6.2. The fractional HIV prevalence in the very active group reaches a peak of 90% infected in 1982, about 1 year before the overall fractional prevalence peak of 33% and about 2 years before the peak prevalence of 28% in the active group. The increase in the HIV prevalence in the very active group between 1979 and 1981 is very dramatic. In the early years, nearly everyone with AIDS was in the very active group, but by 1988, the percentage of those with AIDS who were very active was 26% (value not given in Table 6.2). The large number of homosexual men who were infected with HIV while living in SF but developed AIDS after they left is shown in Table 6.2. Although the migration rate is only 5% per year in the simulation, the AIDS incidence in former SF residents is 53% of the AIDS incidence in SF residents in 1990.

6.2.2 Calculations of the Contact Number

It is interesting to calculate the *spectral radius* ρ of the matrix T given in Section 4.5 using parameter values corresponding to the baseline parameter set in Table 6.1. Recall from Chapter 4 that the spectral radius $\rho(T)$ is the contact number (reproduction number) for the difference equation model used here, so it determines whether the disease dies out $(\rho(T) \leq 1)$ or remains endemic $(\rho(T) > 1)$. In this model with the average number of new sexual partners per month given by PAS = 0.75, corresponding to the situation before any behavioral changes, the average number of new partners per month is 3.95 for people in the very active group and 0.395 for people in the active group. In this case, the spectral radius is found numerically using MATLAB to be $\rho(T) = 1.32$. This means that the average HIV–infected person has a contact sufficient for transmission with 1.32 persons during the average infectious period (about 10 years in length). It also means that at the endemic equilibrium, the HIV–infected fractional prevalence would be $1 - 1/\rho(T) = 0.24$ if the population were homogeneous. Of course, the population model is not homogeneous so the equilibrium HIV fractional prevalence is higher than 0.24 in the very active group and lower in the active group.

Using the yearly reduction factor RDN = 0.61 in Table 6.1 for the reduction time period of 5 years and 5 months reduces PAS from 0.75 to 0.0516, which changes $\rho(T)$ to 1.0091. Even though PAS has been reduced by a factor of 15, the disease persists since $\rho(T)$ is still above the threshold of 1. In order to get the spectral radius below 1, PAS must be below 0.03 so PAS must be reduced by another factor of about 1.7 in order to get below the threshold. Of course, if PAS is barely below 0.03, then $\rho(T)$ would be barely below 1 and HIV would die out very slowly. For example, if $\rho(T) = 0.99$, then it would take 69 ten—year intervals for the number of cases to decrease by half. It is important to realize that the modeling results are insensitive to the reduction stopping date, so the fit to the HIV and AIDS incidence data is almost as good if the yearly reduction with RDN = 0.61 did not stop in December 1986, but continued through 1990. In this case PAS would now be below 0.03 and the spectral radius $\rho(T)$ would be below 1 so that the HIV epidemic would be dying out. The significant conclusion is that we cannot determine from the modeling or the data whether $\rho(T)$ is now above or below the threshold, i.e., whether the HIV epidemic is now persisting or is slowly dying out.

It is surprising that a reduction in PAS, the average number of new partners per month, by a factor of 15 only decreases the spectral radius by a factor of about 1.3 from 1.32 to 1.0091. Moreover, PAS must be reduced by a factor of about 25 from 0.75 to 0.03 in order to get the spectral radius $\rho(T)$ reduced from 1.32 to 1.0. It seems plausible that the low responsiveness of the spectral radius to changes in the partnership rate PAS is due to factors such as the very long infectious period for HIV infecteds or the ability of HIV to persist in the "core" population of very active homosexual men.

6.3 Modeling Zidovudine Therapy

Recently there has been great interest in the possible effects on AIDS incidence of the treatment of some patients with zidovudine (ZDV) and the use of PCP prophylaxis (usually aerosol pentamidine) (Gail et al., 1990). The simulation model has been modified to include therapy; here therapy primarily refers to ZDV treatments, but it also includes aerosol pentamidine, other drugs, and other recent improvements in health care. Estimates of the fractions of HIV—positive homosexual men in SF receiving therapy are given for recent years, and simulations which satisfy the fit criteria and fit the therapy data are found.

6.3.1 Modification of the Simulation Model to Include Therapy

The simulation model is modified to include therapy by creating a separate track for treated people in the final symptomatic stage and in the AIDS stage, with longer mean residence times in these treated compartments. The final symptomatic stage (stage 6 if $m = 7$) with mean residence time of 1.7 years corresponds closely to a symptomatic stage with CD4 cell count below 200 cells/ml, which has a mean residence time of 1.6 years (see Chapter 2). The new parameters in the model are: 1) the monthly rate constants TF6 and TFA for moving stage 6 and AIDS patients into the treated track, 2) the starting dates ST6 and STA for the treatment of stage 6 and AIDS patients and 3) the multiplying factor TP of the transfer rate constants for the treated stages. Thus, TP = 0.5 means that the transfer rate constant is halved for the treated patients, so that the mean time in the stages is doubled for treated patients.

6.3.2 Estimates of the Therapy Percentages and Effects

Using data from the SF Men's Health Study and the SF General Hospital Cohort, Lang et al. (1991) have estimated that the percentages of homosexual men with AIDS in SF receiving ZDV were 36% in 1987, 54% in 1988, and 58% in 1989. They also estimated that the percentages of HIV–positive homosexual men in SF with CD4 count below 200 (but without AIDS) receiving treatment were 24% in 1987, 55% in 1988, and 52% in 1989. For HIV positive homosexual men in SF with CD4 count between 200 and 499, the percentages receiving ZDV were estimated to be 1% in 1987, 10% in 1988, and 16% in 1989. Andrews et al. (1990) report that ZDV was primarily available to AIDS patients after it had been officially approved on March 24, 1987, and became broadly available on September 15, 1987. Thus initial estimates for the starting dates for ZDV therapy are STA = April 1987 and ST6 = October 1987.

Zidovudine therapy lengthens the survival time of AIDS patients and slows progression to AIDS for HIV–positive symptomatic individuals. Gail et al. (1990) used relative risk factors of 0.5 or 0.33, which correspond to doubling or tripling the mean progression and survival times. Lemp (1990) recently surveyed reports on the effects of therapy on AIDS survival, and although there are many different measures of the effectiveness of ZDV therapies, they seem to be roughly consistent with doubling the mean time in the AIDS stage or in stage 6, which corresponds to a transfer rate multiplying factor of TP = 0.5.

6.3.3 Simulations Including Therapy

The therapy information above imposes two additional fit criteria. The first is that the percentages of AIDS patients treated in the simulation are close to the estimated 36%, 54%, and 58% in 1987, 1988, and 1989, respectively. The starting date STA and transfer rate constant TFA for treated AIDS patients are adjusted to achieve this. The second additional fit criterion is that the percentages of stage 6 men treated in the simulations are close to the estimated 24%, 55% and 52% in 1987, 1988 and 1989, respectively. In this case the starting date ST6 and transfer rate constant TF6 for therapy of stage 6 patients are adjusted. The small percentages of men with CD4 counts between 200 and 499 who received ZDV are ignored; they would have almost no influence on AIDS incidence through 1990. The transfer rate multiplying factor TP for stage 6 and the AIDS stage is equal to the *a priori* estimate of 0.5 which corresponds to doubling the mean residence times for treated patients.

The fixed parameters in Table 6.1 are used in the simulations with therapy. For TP = 0.5, STA = April 1987, and ST6 = October 1987, the transfer rate constant values TFA = 0.05 and TF6 = 0.05 give treatment percentages consistent with the *a priori* estimates. Transfer rate constants TFA = 0.025 and TF6 = 0.025 give treatment percentages which are about half of the *a priori* estimates. The simulation results for the best fit using these parameters is given in Table 6.3. Most of the parameter values corresponding to Table 6.3 are similar to those in Table 6.1. The epidemic starting date STD is July 1975 and the external mixing fraction η is 0.82. The average number PAS of partners before reduction is 0.71, the yearly reduction factor RDN is 0.57, reduction starts in April 1982 and ends in December 1986.

Table 6.3 Simulation results with therapy transfer constant of 0.025.

YEAR	YEARLY HIV INCIDENCE EST*	YEARLY HIV INCIDENCE SIM+	HIV PREV	YEARLY AIDS INCIDENCE EST*	YEARLY AIDS INCIDENCE SIM+	TREATMENT+ STAGE 6 TREATED	%	AIDS TREATED	TREATED %
1975	*****	3.	4.	*****	0.	0.	0.	0.	0.
1976	*****	19.	22.	*****	0.	0.	0.	0.	0.
1977	*****	101.	121.	*****	0.	0.	0.	0.	0.
1978	439	512.	616.	0	0.	0.	0.	0.	0.
1979	1963	2143.	2683.	0	1.	0.	0.	0.	0.
1980	4390	5146.	7561.	2	5.	0.	0.	0.	0.
1981	5721	6227.	13208.	22	22.	0.	0.	0.	0.
1982	4337	5146.	17460.	86	79.	0.	0.	0.	0.
1983	2362	3084.	19423.	228	210.	0.	0.	0.	0.
1984	1269	1936.	20054.	442	433.	0.	0.	0.	0.
1985	762	1246.	19806.	678	722.	0.	0.	0.	0.
1986	720	806.	18921.	1010	1023.	0.	0.	0.	0.
1987	720	689.	17758.	1275	1275.	173.	7.	249.	17.
1988	720	746.	16589.	1285	1352.	690.	25.	592.	32.
1989	720	783.	15448.	1338	1374.	1014.	34.	908.	44.
1990	720	805.	14347.	1551	1360.	1204.	40.	1164.	52.
1991	*****	813.	13299.	*****	1301.	1294.	45.	1349.	58.
1992	*****	808.	12317.	*****	1209.	1308.	48.	1462.	62.
1993	*****	793.	11414.	*****	1101.	1270.	51.	1509.	66.
1994	*****	771.	10596.	*****	991.	1200.	53.	1503.	69.
1995	*****	745.	9863.	*****	889.	1113.	54.	1457.	71.

*These are the estimated (EST) values in Table 5.1.
+These values are from the simulation (SIM) model.

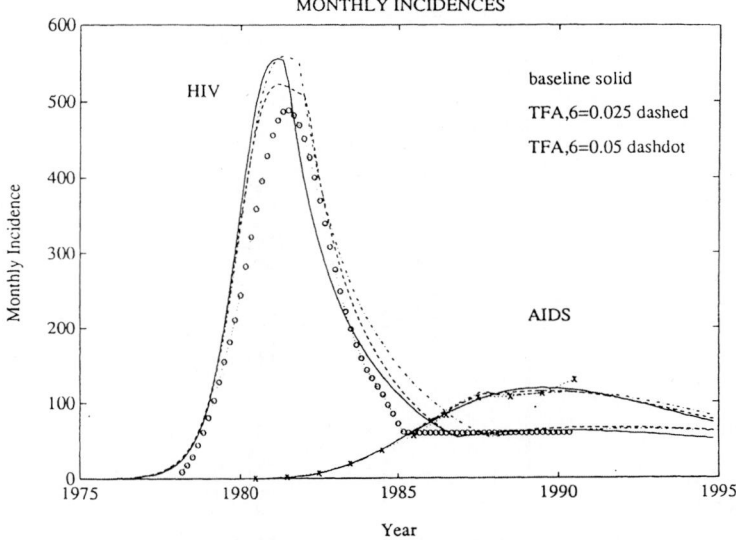

Figure 6.1 The best–fitting simulations with therapy are shown for therapy transfer constants of 0.025 and 0.05.

Figure 6.1 shows the simulation results for the best fits with the two sets of transfer rate constants. Although the two HIV incidence curves in Figure 6.1 are above the estimated curve, they give as good a fit to the estimated HIV incidence curve as the baseline parameters. The estimated AIDS incidence curve is best fit by the baseline parameter set (weighted $\chi^2 = 47$), adequately by the TFA = TF6 = 0.025 curves ($\chi^2 = 52$) and slightly worse by TFA = TF6 = 0.05 curves ($\chi^2 = 73$.) None of the three AIDS incidence curves match the 1990 AIDS incidence data. The better fits with half the estimated percentages treated suggest that the estimates of Lang et al. (1991) on the percentages in SF receiving ZDV therapy from 1987 to 1989 could be too large, possibly because the samples in the cohorts used for the estimates may not have been representative of all homosexual men in SF.

Thus the simulations with and without therapy all give adequate fits to the HIV and AIDS incidences. If the AIDS incidence in 1990 is ignored, then the models with therapy give a better fit, since they have a plateau in AIDS cases between 1987 and 1989 consistent with the data. Since all simulations with and without therapy give adequate fits, it is not possible to determine the importance of therapy from the model at this time.

Table 6.4. Sensitivity summary for parameters in Table 6.1

Parameter	Sensitivity
Q	relatively insensitive when Q is increased or decreased by 30–40%.
μ	imperceptible changes when μ is zero or doubled.
δ	somewhat sensitive to δ as seen in Figure 6.2.
ϕ	insensitive when ϕ is halved or doubled.
QH	sensitivity is the same as for PAS below.
γ_i	not very sensitive to scaling up or down by 10% as seen in Figure 6.4.
F & R	not very sensitive to halving or doubling F and R.
$\omega_i \rho_i$	fits with a wide variety of weights of transmission are possible.
m	somewhat sensitive to m as seen in Figure 6.3.
STD	insensitive to 6 month changes.
STR	insensitive to 3 month changes.
STP	insensitive to 6 month changes.
η	not sensitive for $0.50 \leq \eta \leq 1$, but sensitive for small η.
PAS	somewhat sensitive to 10% changes.
RDN	relatively insensitive to 10% changes.

6.4 Sensitivity Analysis

A dynamic model is said to be sensitive to a parameter if small changes in the parameter value have a big effect on the outcome, and insensitive to a parameter if small changes in the parameter value have little effect. In this section, all parameters are assumed to be equal to those in the baseline parameter set in Table 6.1 unless otherwise specified. Table 6.4 summarizes the sensitivity results described below.

6.4.1 Population Structure and Dynamics

When the best–fitting simulations have been found for a population size Q of 40,000, the HIV incidence curve is wider and lower than for the baseline parameter set, but the AIDS incidence curve is very similar. When the population size Q is changed to 80,000, both the HIV and AIDS incidence curves for the best–fitting simulation are similar to those for the baseline parameter set. Thus the simulations are relatively insensitive to the population size Q. The simulations are also insensitive to the mortality rate constant μ since changes are imperceptible when μ is halved or doubled.

Changing the yearly migration rate δ from 5% of the population to other values such as 0%, 3%, and 8% does cause changes in the best–fitting simulations for both the HIV and AIDS incidence curves, as shown in Figure 6.2. The AIDS incidence in 1995 is 57% higher when δ is 0% than when δ is 8%. The explanation is that with the larger values of δ, many of those infected in SF emigrate before they are diagnosed with AIDS, so the number of SF residents diagnosed with AIDS in 1995 is lower.

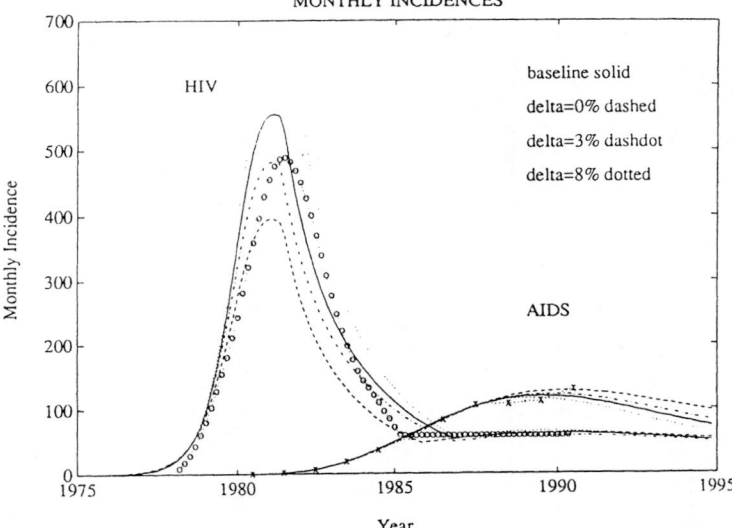

Figure 6.2. The best–fitting simulations are shown where the yearly migration rate δ is 5% (baseline), 0%, 3%, and 8%.

6.4.2 Epidemiological Structure and Mixing

The two parameters that define the activity structure are the very active fraction F and the activity level ratio R. The *a priori* baseline values for them are F = 0.1 and R = 10, so that 10% of the population is ten times as active. Halving or doubling F with R fixed at 10 leads to only minor changes in the best–fitting simulation. Halving or doubling R with F fixed at 0.1 also leads to minor changes. Doubling F to 0.2 and halving R to 5 leads to only minor changes. Changes in the activity level transfer rate constant ϕ away from the baseline value of 5% transfer per year cause imperceptible changes in the best–fitting simulations. Since the simulated HIV incidence curves are reasonably close to the estimated HIV curve and the simulated AIDS incidence curves are essentially the same for all of these changes in F, R, and ϕ, the simulation modeling is relatively insensitive to changes in these parameters.

Homogeneous mixing with no activity levels corresponds to R = 1. A best–fitting simulation with R = 1 has HIV and AIDS incidence curves which are similar to the estimated incidence curves. For R = 1 this best fit has STD = January 1976, STR = April 1979, STP = December 1986, PAS = 2.8, RDN = 0.61, and η = 1. All of these are consistent with the *a priori* estimates except the starting year STR for the reduction in the average number of partners per month, which is at least 2 years earlier than the *a priori* estimate. This best fitting simulation is not allowable since the STR value is unrealistic. The best fit with STR values in 1981 or 1982

76

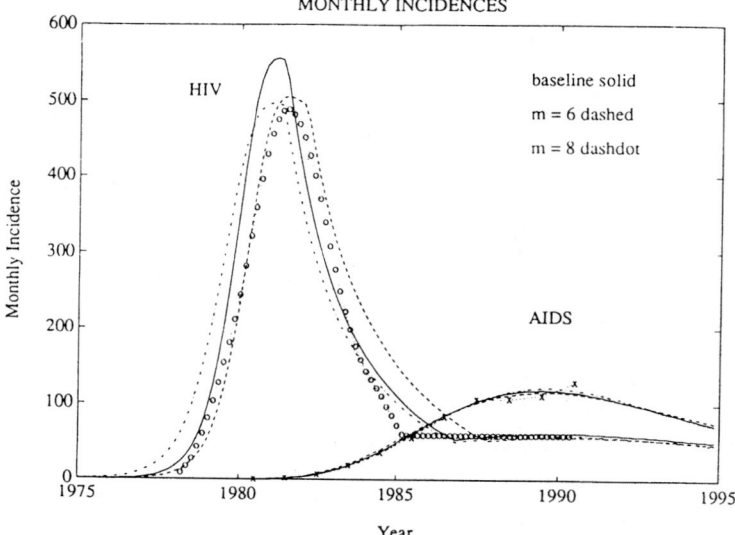

MONTHLY INCIDENCES

Figure 6.3 The best–fitting simulations are shown where the number m of infectious stages is 7 (baseline), 6, and 8.

does not give an adequate fit ($\chi^2 > 500$.) Thus homogeneous mixing with R = 1 is not adequate so that there must be two sexual activity levels.

The external mixing fraction η is 0.82 in the baseline parameter set in Table 6.1, which means that the mixing pattern between people in the activity levels is quite close to the standard proportionate mixing corresponding to $\eta = 1$. Changing η to 1, 0.9, or 0.75 and varying PAS and RDN to give the best fits yields simulations with HIV incidence curves similar to that of the baseline and AIDS incidence curves almost identical to that of the baseline. Thus the simulations are not very sensitive to η near 0.82, but they are sensitive to η when η is near zero, which corresponds to uncoupling the sexual activity levels. Choosing $\eta = 1$ reduces the number of parameters by one since this corresponds to assuming that the sexual partnership formation is governed by the proportionate mixing assumption as defined in Chapter 3.

The epidemic starting date STD is October 1975 in the baseline parameter set. If this starting date is shifted by six months earlier or later, the best–fitting simulations are only slightly different from the baseline simulations. Thus the simulation modeling is relatively insensitive to changes in the epidemic starting date.

6.4.3 Parameters Related to the Stages

The best–fitting simulation curves when the number m of infectious stages is 6, 7, or 8 are shown in Figure 6.3. Although the HIV incidence curves are somewhat different, the AIDS

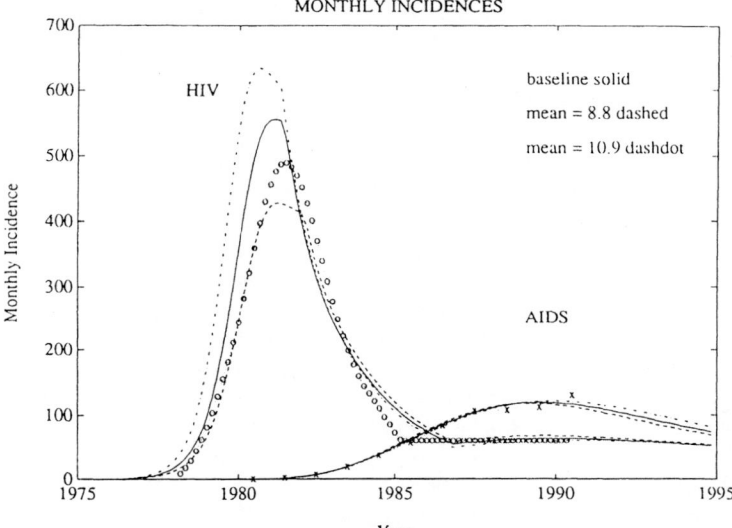

Year

Figure 6.4 The best–fitting simulations are shown where the mean AIDS incubation period is 9.8 years (baseline), 8.8 years, and 10.9 years.

incidence curves are very similar. The $m = 7$ curves correspond to the baseline parameter set. For $m = 6$, the optimization parameters are STD = January 1976, $\eta = 0.75$, PAS = 0.70, RDN = 0.63, STR = April 1982, and STP = December 1987; these are all consistent with the *a priori* estimates. For $m = 8$, the epidemic starting date of July 1974 is early but plausible; the other optimization parameters are consistent with the *a priori* estimates.

Best–fitting simulations have been found when the mean incubation period is 8.8 years = $(9/10) \times 9.8$ years, so that the baseline rate constants γ_i for progression between the stages are all multiplied by a $10/9$ factor. Best fits have also been found when the mean incubation period is 10.9 years = $(10/9) \times 9.8$ years so that the baseline γ_i values are all multiplied by $9/10$. As seen in Figure 6.4, the HIV incidence simulation curve corresponding to a mean of 8.8 years is close to the estimated HIV curve, but the simulation curve corresponding to a mean of 10.9 years is not as close. However, the HIV curves for means of 8.8, 9.8, and 10.9 years are all reasonable and the AIDS incidence curves are all similar. Hence the simulations are not very sensitive to changes in the mean incubation period.

Recall that the relative weights of transmission in the four phases are the products of the relative infectivities and the relative sexual activities (as compared to asymptomatic men) of the men in each of the phases. The baseline parameter set values assumed that asymptomatic men were less infectious than men in the other phases and that men with symptoms or AIDS were less sexually active. Changing the baseline relative weights of $(2,1,1.5,7.5)$ in the four phases to $(1,1,1,1)$ causes minor changes in the best–fitting simulation curves. Changing the baseline relative weights of (2,1,1.5,7.5) to (2,1,0,0), (2,0,1.5,7,5), (10,1,1,1) and (1,1,1,1) causes some small changes in the best—fitting simulation curves, but they all give acceptable fits and the parameter values which give these best fits are consistent with the *a priori* estimates. Thus it is not possible to exclude various possible relative weights of transmission from the fits obtained.

6.4.4 Sexual Behavior Parameters

Satisfying the fit criteria by using the simulation model is not possible if there is no reduction in partnership formation rates. If the simulation with no reductions fits the early AIDS incidence, then the AIDS incidence is too high in later years. This result is consistent with all of the SF surveys described in Chapter 3, which report some decreases in high—risk behavior during part of the time interval from 1982 to 1989.

The simulation results are relatively insensitive to changes in the starting date STR and stopping date STP for the reduction in the average partnership formation rate per month. Changes of these dates by 3 months in either direction lead to best—fitting simulation curves which are very similar to the baseline curves. Changes by 6 months lead to minor changes from the baseline curves.

Ten percent changes in the yearly reduction factor lead to relatively small changes in the simulation curves. When the baseline RDN value of 0.61 is changed to 0.56 or 0.66 and the other parameters are varied to give the best fit, the resulting simulation curves are similar to those for the baseline parameter set. When the average number PAS of new partners per month before reduction is changed by 10%, there are some changes in the best—fitting HIV incidence simulation curves, but the AIDS incidence curves are all close together. For example, when the baseline value of 0.75 for PAS is changed to 0.82, the HIV epidemic curve rises more steeply and falls more steeply; when PAS is changed to 0.67, the best—fitting simulation has a lower and wider HIV incidence curve. Although both simulations give adequate fits to the data curves, the simulations are somewhat sensitive to 10% changes in PAS.

6.5 Conclusions

The AIDS incidence in Table 5.1 increases steadily from 1980 to 1987 and then remains approximately level on a plateau from 1987 to 1989 before increasing again in 1990. As shown in Figure 1.5, this plateau in AIDS incidence in homosexual men also occurred in other cities such as New York City and Los Angeles (CDC, 1989b; Berkelman et al., 1989). An increase in AIDS incidence in homosexual men from 1989 to 1990 also occurred in the entire United States (CDC, 1991a). Thus these trends in AIDS cases in homosexual men are not unique to SF.

Various explanations for the plateau in 1987 − 89 of AIDS cases in homosexual men have been presented (Gail et al., 1990; CDC: 1990a). These include the effects of therapy, behavior change (and possibly saturation) resulting in decreased HIV incidence in the early 1980s, changes in reporting delays or practices, the 1987 change in the AIDS surveillance definition and evolution of attenuated HIV strains. Linden et al. (1989) found that the plateau could not be explained by late reporting or underreporting. It cannot be due to the 1987 definition change since adjustments for this are made in Table 5.1.

This temporary plateau in the yearly AIDS cases in homosexual men in SF makes forecasting very difficult. The simulations here which fit the data seem to smooth out AIDS incidences from 1987 to 1990. The best–fitting simulations are reasonably consistent since the AIDS incidences usually have a peak in about 1989 and then decrease slowly. This shape is a consequence of the estimated shape of the HIV incidence curve, which has a peak in early 1981 and then declines rapidly until it levels off in 1986 at 720 new infections per year. Thus the peak in the AIDS incidence curve in 1989 is due to the peak in the estimated HIV incidence curve in 1981. If the estimated HIV incidence curve is inaccurate, then the corresponding AIDS incidence curve would also be inaccurate. Our forecasts are based on fits to estimated HIV and AIDS curves; they do not reflect possible changes in sexual behavior after about 1987. Even in SF where good information is available, the fitting of the simulation model is not easy and the remaining uncertainty in the parameter values implies that forecasts from the simulations are also uncertain. Caution should be observed in using simulation modeling for forecasting in other risk groups and regions.

Other forecasts of AIDS incidences in homosexual men in SF have been given. Bacchetti and Moss (1989) gave a range of projections with peak AIDS incidences between 1989 and 1991. Ahlgren et al. (1990) found similar peaks in AIDS incidences using simulation modeling. Thus two other modeling groups have made forecasts similar to ours. Lemp et al. (1990) projected increasing total AIDS incidences (all risk groups) in SF through 1993.

A basic principle which has emerged from the simulations is that the AIDS incidence at a given time is primarily due to the HIV incidence about 6 to 10 years earlier and is less influenced by HIV incidence in the past 5 years and beyond 11 years earlier. This finding is consistent with the distribution curves for the AIDS incubation period in Chapter 2 in which less than 10% develop AIDS in the first five years after infection for $m = 7$. If the estimated HIV incidence were increased by 50% to 1080 per year from 1985 to 1989, then the best–fitting simulation still has a peak AIDS incidence in 1989, but the AIDS incidence decreases more slowly after 1989. Increases or decreases in recent years or in the future in high–risk sexual behavior of homosexual men in SF would affect future AIDS cases.

A group is said to be saturated by an infectious disease if the prevalence of infection is high enough so that transmission decreases significantly due to an insufficient density of susceptibles. A key question is whether the apparent decrease in HIV incidence around 1982 and the plateau in AIDS incidence in 1987 through 1989 in SF homosexual men are exclusively due to saturation in a high–risk group, to changes in sexual behavior, or to both. The results in Section 6.4.4 suggest that there must have been reductions in high–risk behavior, since, otherwise, the fit criteria cannot be satisfied. Because the fit criteria are not satisfied without separate activity level groups, the model must have a very active (high–risk) group. The prevalence in this group reaches 90%, so that there is saturation, with rapid and early spread of HIV infection in the very active (high–risk) group, followed by slower, later spread in the active (lower–risk) group (Table 6.2). Thus both saturation in a high–risk group and changes in sexual behavior are important in obtaining simulations which satisfy the fit criteria. Since the fit criteria are least satisfied when there are no changes in behavior, behavior modification is more important than saturation.

Fitting a simulation model to data on HIV and AIDS incidence can yield rough estimates of parameter values. For example, the starting dates of the epidemic in the simulations is consistently somewhere in 1975–1976 so it is plausible that the actual HIV epidemic started in SF in this time interval. The starting dates for reduction in the average number of partners per month are usually in 1981 or early 1982; these simulation estimates are consistent with estimates from sexual behavior surveys in SF. The yearly reduction in the average number of sexual partners of 0.61 in the baseline simulation is consistent with the estimates of 0.59, 0.67, 0.43, and 0.70 found from sexual behavior surveys. These and other consistencies between the simulation and *a priori* estimates increase our confidence in these parameter values.

The theoretical implications of a mixture of proportional mixing and internal mixing within each activity level for the development of an AIDS epidemic in populations with different activity levels have been analyzed by using simulations (Jacquez et al., 1988; Blythe and Anderson, 1988; Castillo–Chavez et al., 1989; Kaplan and Lee, 1990). If the sexual–activity–level groups have their sexual contacts distributed by proportional mixing, then the speed of development of the epidemic is similar to the speed for homogeneously mixing populations. However, if the mixing is very biased so that nearly all partners are within the same sexual–activity–level groups, then the overall speed of development is slower, since the disease seems to sweep through the highest sexual–activity–level group, then the second highest sexual–activity–level group, etc. For very weakly connected sexual–activity–level groups, the overall development of the epidemic is similar to the development when the groups are completely disconnected and each group starts with a few infected individuals. The baseline parameter set in Table 6.1 has the external (proportional) mixing fraction η equal to 0.82, but in Section 6.4.2 it has been found that the best–fitting simulations with $\eta = 1$ are almost as good. Thus for modeling the homosexual men in SF, the sexual–activity–level groups are strongly connected so that the simple proportional mixing assumption is adequate.

In Chapter 5 the *a priori* estimates are $PAS = 2$ for the average number of different sexual partners per month of homosexual men in SF before 1982 and $QH = 0.05$ for the probability of transmission to a partner by an infected asymptomatic man, so that the average number of partnerships per month of susceptibles which result in transmission is $PAS \times QH = 0.1$. The values for the baseline parameter set in Table 6.1 are $PAS = 0.75$ and $QH = 0.05$, so that their product is 0.0375, which is less than the *a priori* estimate by a factor of 2.7. This suggests that one or both of the *a priori* estimates were too high; for example, if the *a priori* estimate of $PAS = 2$ were correct, then a better estimate of QH would be 0.017. In Section 6.4.4 it has been found that the best–fitting simulation curves are sensitive to 10% changes in PAS, so they would also be sensitive to similar small changes in QH. Better estimates of these two parameters would be desirable, but it may be unrealistic to expect to obtain accurate estimates of these parameters from sexual behavior surveys.

In the sensitivity analysis in Section 6.4, the best–fitting HIV and AIDS incidence curves are sensitive to changes in values of some parameters. In Section 6.4.1, they have been found to be sensitive to changes in the yearly migration rate δ. The immigration and emigration rate estimate of 5% per year has been based on one sexual behavior survey (see Chapter 5). If the turnover rate is only 5% per year in the simulations, then the AIDS incidence in former SF residents is 53% of the AIDS incidence in current SF residents. Since this migration parameter is important in forecasting the long–range HIV and AIDS incidence in a risk group, it would be advantageous if questions to determine inflow and outflow rates in risk groups were included in future surveys. Although the simulations are sensitive to the yearly migration rate constant δ, they are not sensitive to the natural mortality rate constant μ or the monthly activity level change rate constants ϕ and θ so that the current estimates of those last three parameters are probably adequate.

The simulation model for the staged progression to AIDS has the advantage that it is consistent with the slow deterioration of the immune system and the decline in CD4 cells. In all of the simulations, the AIDS incidence peak occurs about 8 to 10 years after the HIV incidence peak. This observation is consistent with the median incubation period of 9.6 years for $m = 7$. When the progression to AIDS is slower or faster, the delay from the peak in HIV incidence to the peak in AIDS incidence is longer or shorter, as seen in Figure 6.4, but the overall patterns in the HIV and AIDS incidences are the same.

Although there is a large amount of information on HIV and AIDS in homosexual men in SF, the values of some parameters are still uncertain and the sensitivity analyses show that these uncertainties lead to variabilities in the fits to the estimated HIV and AIDS incidences. For example, very little information is available on the relative infectivity or the relative partnership formation rates of HIV–positive men in the stages leading to AIDS. The sensitivities to the relative weights of transmission, which are the products of the corresponding relative infectivities and relative sexual activities, are analyzed in Section 6.4.3. The fits are almost as good when the relative weights of transmission are $(10,1,1,1)$ for the four phases as when the weights are $(2,1,1.5,7.5)$; this agrees with the suggestion of Ahlgren et al. (1990) that the HIV incidence could be due to a high infectivity of infected people in the short pre–antibody phase. Adequate fits are also obtained when the relative weights of transmission are $(1,1,1,1)$ or $(2,1,0,0)$ or $(2,0,1.5,7.5)$ so that it is not possible on the basis of the fit to the data to exclude any possibilities regarding the relative infectivity and sexual activity of individuals in the various stages

Therapy with zidovudine delays the onset of AIDS and increases AIDS survival times, at least in some patients. In Section 6.3 the simulation model is modified to incorporate treatment of AIDS and final–stage symptomatic patients. Simulations using the estimated percentages treated (Lang et al., 1991) give marginally adequate fits to the data. Simulations with half as many treated and with no treatment give better fits. These simulations suggest that the percentages treated effectively with zidovudine may be lower than originally estimated by Lang et al. (1991). It is clear that more and better data are needed on the effects of therapy.

The dynamic simulation model formulated in Chapter 3 is designed to incorporate all features considered essential for modeling the sexual spread of HIV infections in homosexual men in SF and yet is also designed to be simple enough so that estimating the values of the parameters is possible. Most of the parameter values have been estimated from various data sources and the remaining few parameters have been adjusted to fit the estimates of HIV and AIDS incidence for homosexual men in SF. Thus the simulation modeling provides a conceptual and quantitative means of organizing, coalescing and cross–checking diverse information on homosexual men in SF. The simulation modeling has evaluated the relative roles of saturation and behavior modification, shown that there must be a high–risk very sexually active group, shown that the sexual–activity–level groups are strongly connected, estimated parameter values, and identified the most sensitive parameter values so that data can be collected to get improved estimates.

CHAPTER 7

THE HIV TRANSMISSION DYNAMICS MODEL FOR FIVE MAJOR RISK GROUPS

Chapters 2 and 3 have focused on modeling the transmission dynamics of HIV and the progression to AIDS for homosexual men. That model is now expanded in Section 7.1 to include five major risk groups: homosexual (and bisexual) men, homosexual (and bisexual) men who are intravenous drug users, intravenous drug users (IVDUs), heterosexual partners of IVDUs and neonates of female IVDUs and heterosexual partners. In this model the homosexual men have homosexual partnerships within their own group and also with homosexual–IVDUs. The IVDUs have needle–sharing partnerships with other IVDUs and also with homosexual–IVDUs. Obviously, the heterosexual partners of IVDUs have sexual partnerships with people who are IVDUs. Perinatal transmission occurs from the female IVDUs and the female heterosexual partners. Figure 7.1 summarizes the risk groups and possible routes of transmission of HIV infection. The fitting procedure for the five–group model is outlined in Section 7.2. This model with the first three risk groups is used for New York City in Chapter 8. The full model is used for regional comparisons in Chapter 10.

The five risk groups above are chosen since they account for 94% of the adult/adolescent cases and 78% of the perinatal pediatric cases with known source of infection reported through December, 1991 in the United States (CDC: 1992). See Tables 1.1 to 1.3. The model does not include other heterosexual contacts, hemophiliacs, blood transfusion recipients, and children with other perinatal transmission. It is not reasonable to include more risk groups in an initial model for a local population. Blood transfusion recipients (2% of AIDS cases) could be included, but blood banks are regional instead of local. Similarly, the incidence in hemophiliacs (1% of all AIDS cases) is quite uniform throughout the United States, so this is a nationwide phenomenon instead of a local phenomenon, particularly since the blood factor concentrate is prepared in a few places and distributed nationwide. It is probably not necessary to include a separate population of bisexual men since heterosexual contacts with bisexual men accounts for only 651 out of 206,392 AIDS cases in the United States through December 1992. It is not possible to include people or sexual partners born in pattern II countries since the immigration times and HIV status of these people is not known.

7.1 The General Model

Recall that the homosexual men are subdivided into active and very active subpopulations. In the modeling of homosexual men in San Francisco (SF), the 10% of the homosexual men in the very active class were ten times as sexually active as those in the active class (the parameter values are $F = 0.10$ and $R = 10$). Here the IVDU population is also subdivided into these two activity level classes based on their number of needle–sharing partners per month.

The needle–sharing contacts are modeled in a way analogous to the homosexual contacts in that there is an average number of new needle–sharing partners per month and there are probabilities of transmission per new needle–sharing partner that are dependent on the stage of

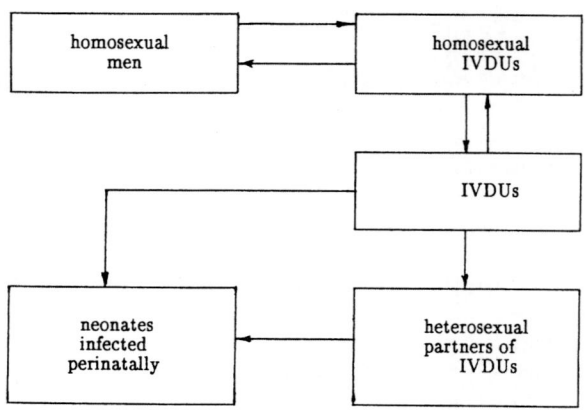

Figure 7.1 Risk groups and infection transmission connections.

infection of the partner just as for homosexual partners. As indicated previously the homosexual–IVDUs have both homosexual partners and needle–sharing partners.

The progression of HIV infecteds to AIDS has been developed carefully as a sequence of stages in Chapter 2 and the same progression is used for all adult risk groups in this general model. The progression for children has also been described in Chapter 2. The progression variables and parameters in Figure 3.1 and Table 3.1 now exist for all five risk groups: the homosexual men with suffix H, the homosexual–IVDUs with suffix B for both, the IVDU population with suffix D for drug user, the population of heterosexual partners of IVDU with suffix P for partners, and the neonates with suffix C for children. Thus the model consists of five sets of finite difference equations for the numbers in each compartment, which are similar to those in Figure 3.2. All populations except the heterosexual partners and children are subdivided into very active and active subgroups where the activity is either sexual or needle–sharing partnership formation. For example, the quantities for homosexual men are QVH, SVH, XH(1), $\cdots$, XH(8), QAH, SAH, YH(1), $\cdots$, YH(8), ZH(1), $\cdots$, ZH(6) and ZAIDSH.

The suffixes H, D, B, P and C are also used for other parameter values. For example, QHH, QHD, QHP and QHC are the probabilities of transmission of HIV infection by an infective in an asymptomatic stage during a homosexual partnership, needle–sharing partnership, heterosexual partnership, and childbirth, respectively. The quantities PAH, PAD and PAP are the average number of new homosexual, needle–sharing and heterosexual partnerships per month.

As in the model for homosexual men, the fraction η of new partnerships are distributed by proportionate mixing and the fraction $1-\eta$ of new partnerships occur internally to each group. The total incidences in the active and very active subpopulations are the sums of the internal incidences and the external proportionate mixing incidences. The incidences with suffixes H and

D on the variables and parameters are used for homosexual partners and needle–sharing partners, respectively. Thus the incidence for homosexual men is the sum of the internal and external (proportionate–mixing) homosexual incidences given in Section 3.2, where each parameter and variable now has the suffix H. For the IVDUs, the incidence is the sum of similar internal and external needle–sharing incidences, with suffix D. Thus the incidence in the active subpopulation of IVDUs is

$$\left[\sum_{i=1}^{m} (1\text{--ETAD}) \times \rho_i \times \text{PHD} \times \omega_i \times \text{QHD} \times \text{YD(i)} \right] \times \frac{\text{SAD}}{\text{QAD--YD(m+1)}}$$

$$+ \sum_{i=1}^{m} \text{ETAD} \times \rho_i \times \text{PHD} \times \omega_i \times \text{QHD} \times [\text{R} \times \text{XD(i)} + \text{YD(i)}] \times \frac{\text{PHD} \times \text{SAD}}{\text{CD}} \,,$$

where

$$\text{CD} = \text{PHD} \times (\text{QAD} - \text{YD(m+1)}) + \text{R} \times \text{PHD} \times (\text{QVD--XD(m+1)}) \,,$$

and the incidence in the very active subpopulation of IVDUs is

$$\left[\sum_{i=1}^{m} (1\text{--ETAD}) \times \rho_i \times \text{R} \times \text{PHD} \times \omega_i \times \text{QHD} \times \text{XD(i)} \right] \times \frac{\text{SVD}}{\text{QVD--XD(m+1)}}$$

$$+ \sum_{i=1}^{m} \text{ETAD} \times \rho_i \times \text{PHD} \times \omega_i \times \text{QHD} \times [\text{R} \times \text{XD(i)} + \text{YD(i)}] \times \frac{\text{R} \times \text{PHD} \times \text{SVD}}{\text{CD}} \,.$$

The homosexual–IVDUs are considered to have both homosexual partnerships and needle–sharing partnerships. The incidence in the homosexual–IVDUs with suffix B is the sum of both the homosexual and needle–sharing incidences.

The incidence for the heterosexual partners of IVDUs is not given by the incidences above, but is given by

$$\sum_{i=1}^{m} \rho_i \times \text{PAP} \times \omega_i \times \text{QHP} \times [\text{XD(I)} + \text{YD(I)}] \times \frac{\text{SAP}}{\text{QAP--YP(M+1)}}.$$

Note that the IVDUs do not have two activity levels in mixing with heterosexual partners and the heterosexual partners have only one activity level. This incidence term for the heterosexual partners of IVDUs is a very simple version of a complicated process. Although heterosexual partnerships with IVDUs are constantly being formed and dissolved, it is difficult to model this pairing process. The incidence term above assumes that people in the population of heterosexual partners of IVDUs are mixing with the IVDUs and forming partnerships. It is helpful to think that this population is a changing amalgamation consisting of those who have been or currently are or will become heterosexual partners of IVDUs. The incidence expression above seems to be the simplest way to model heterosexual partners of IVDUs.

The incidence of perinatal HIV infections is the product of the fecundity rate FC (children born per female per month), the probability QHC of transmission by an asymptomatic mother to a neonate and the weighted sum of infected females. The weighted sum of female IVDUs is the sum of the products of the relative weights of transmission, the fraction PIW of IVDUs who are women and the number of infected IVDUs. The weighted sum of female heterosexual partners is the sum of the relative weights of transmission, the fraction PHW of heterosexual partners who are females and the number of infected heterosexual partners. The sum of these two is the weighted sum of infected females. Thus the incidence of perinatal HIV infections is

$$FC \times QHC \times \left[\sum_{i=1}^{m} \rho_i \times \omega_i \times PIW \times [XD(I)+YD(I)] + \sum_{i=1}^{m} \rho_i \times \omega_i \times PHW \times YP(I) \right]$$

7.2 The Fitting Procedure

The fit criteria given in Section 6.1 for the model for homosexual men in San Francisco must be expanded for this more general model. As before, the first criterion for the simulations is that the parameter values must be consistent with the *a priori* parameter estimates obtained from data. Since estimates of HIV incidence are generally not available, the second criterion is now that the yearly AIDS incidences in the risk groups in the simulations must be close to the yearly AIDS incidence data supplied by the Centers for Disease Control (CDC).

Many of the parameter values in the model are fixed at their estimated values, but some are allowed to vary to give the best fit. For example, the population sizes of the homosexual men, IVDUs and heterosexual partners of IVDUs are all fixed, but the population size of the homosexual–IVDUs is varied in order to obtain the best fit to the AIDS incidence data in this population. The migration rates and natural mortality rates are fixed at the estimated values.

The parameters related to the progression through the stages (m and γ_i for i = 1,$\cdots$,7) are all fixed and equal to the values found in Chapter 2. Other fixed parameter values are the probabilities (or proportions) of transmission QHH, QHD and QHP per asymptomatic partner, the parameters ω_k which multiply these QH values to determine the probability of transmission by a stage k infective and the parameters ρ_k which are the fractions still active in stage k.

The predicted AIDS cases in the five risk groups in the NYC model must be close to the delay–adjusted AIDS incidence. The number of AIDS cases per year are not linearly independent so that a hypothesis of the chi–square goodness of fit test is not satisfied. Nevertheless the chi–square value of the sum of the squares of the observed minus the expected divided by the expected values is computed as a measure of the fit. Separate chi–square sums are also computed for each of the five risk groups.

The fit to the AIDS incidence data in the population of homosexual men is obtained by varying the initial average number PASH of partners per month, the year STRH in which reduction in partners starts and the yearly reduction factor RDNH. Similarly, the fit to the AIDS incidence data in the IVDU population is obtained by varying the analogous parameters

PASD, STRD and RDND. The fit to the AIDS incidence data in the homosexual–IVDU population is obtained by adjusting the population size NSIZEB.

The fitting procedure involves choosing parameter values sequentially with those subject to the most uncertainty chosen last or adjusted to fit the AIDS incidence data. Fixed values are used for many parameters such as population sizes, migration rates, natural mortality rates, number of stages, stage transition rates, probabilities of transmission by asymptomatic infectives, multiplying factors for probability of transmission and fractions still active in the stages, activity level fractions and ratios, and the transfer rate constants between the activity levels.

After the parameters above are fixed, the reduction starting years STRH and STRD are chosen and the size NSIZEB of the homosexual–IVDU population is chosen. Initial guesses are made for four parameters: the average numbers of partners per month (PASH and PASD), and the yearly reduction factors (RDNH and RDND). A Fortran computer program uses the IMSL subroutine BCONF to find the values of these four parameters which minimize the sum of the chi–square values for the homosexual men, homosexual–IVDUs and IVDUs. This program is similar to FIT10.FOR listed in the Appendix.

After the simulation model has been fit to the IVDUs, then the model is fit to the heterosexual partners of IVDUs by varying only one parameter, the average number PAP of new heterosexual partners per month. After both the IVDUs and their heterosexual partners have been fit, then the model is fit to the perinatal cases by varying only one parameter, the fecundity rate FC. This program is similar to IVDU10.FOR listed in the Appendix.

7.3 Discussion of the Model

Epidemiological modelers attempt to capture the essential features of an epidemiological process in a precisely stated model. Of course, the models are extreme simplifications of the complex human and biological processes that contribute to the spread of an infectious disease, but they can be very useful in attempting to understand the basic epidemiological mechanisms. The art of epidemiological modeling is to formulate a model so that it has enough complexity to be consistent with all observations, but is not more complicated than necessary to fit the data. Thus there is a balance between the goals of simplicity and realism.

The model formulated here for the spread of HIV in the five risk groups shown in Figure 7.1 attempts to capture the essential aspects in a relatively simple model. This model consists of five sets of nonlinear difference equations similar to those in Figure 3.2 for compartments similar to those in Figure 3.1. The model incorporates the major transmission mechanisms of homosexual and heterosexual intercourse, needle–sharing by IVDUs and perinatal infection.

Heterogeneity in sexual and needle–sharing behavior is reflected by the division of each population of homosexual men, homosexual IVDUs and IVDUs into two subgroups consisting of those who are active and those who are very active. The model includes migration into and out of the risk populations, normal, non–HIV related deaths, and changes in sexual (or needle–sharing) behavior by some individuals. Because there is no solid data on changes in the sizes of the risk groups over time, the modeling here assumes that the population sizes remain constant. The subdivision into only two sexual (or needle–sharing) activity levels is reasonably simple, but it is consistent with the survey data and it is adequate to fit the HIV and AIDS incidence data. Based on four surveys of homosexual behavior, it is estimated in Section 5.2 that for two sexual activity levels, ten percent of the population has ten times as many new sexual partnerships per month. The corresponding needle–sharing parameters are estimated in Section 8.2.4.

Heterogeneity in behavior is an important factor in the transmission of sexually transmitted diseases. Hethcote and Yorke (1984) explored the effects of heterogeneity in the transmission of gonorrhea and found that a "core" group of sexually very active, highly–efficient transmitters were central to the transmission and persistence of gonorrhea. One of the major barriers to a better understanding of the HIV transmission process is the lack of information on the social, sexual and needle–sharing mixing which occurs between subgroups of the risk groups. Many authors have used a modeling approach to explore the effects on HIV transmission and AIDS of behavioral heterogeneity and different mixing structures. Attempts have been made to estimate the entries in contact or mixing matrices from survey data. Papers exploring sexual mixing and heterogeneity include: Ahlgren et al. (1990), Anderson (1988a, 1988b), Anderson and May (1991), Blythe and Anderson (1988), Blythe and Castillo–Chavez (1989), Busenberg and Castillo–Chavez (1991), Cardell and Kanouse (1989), Castillo–Chavez et al. (1989), Hyman and Stanley (1988, 1989), Jacquez et al. (1988, 1989), Knox (1986), Koopman et al. (1989), Pickering (1986), Sattenspiel and Simon (1988) and Simon and Jacquez (1992). Papers modeling HIV transmission in IVDUs include Blower et al. (1991) and Kaplan et al. (1989, 1990).

Staged progression has become the standard way to model the long infectious period leading to AIDS. Here the progression from HIV infection to AIDS is modeled by a sequence of seven infectious stages with AIDS as the seventh stage and death due to AIDS as the eighth stage. The mean times in each stage are given in Chapter 2 for both clinical staging and T4–cell count staging. The infectivity and amount of sexual activity vary with the stage of infection. The relative infectivity and relative sexual activity compared to those in the asymptomatic stage are estimated in Sections 5.1.1 and 5.1.2.

The HIV incidence terms are all based on the principle of mass action; i.e., the incidence is directly proportional to the product of the number of susceptibles and the number of infectives in the stages. The simplest formulation for the interactions between subgroups of a risk group is based on the assumption of proportionate mixing. In this case the activity levels are specified for each subgroup and then the new partnerships of a person are distributed in proportion to the activity levels and population sizes of the subgroups (Hethcote and Yorke, 1984). Thus a person is more likely to have a new partner from a more active subgroup than from a less active subgroup. This assumption of proportionate mixing has the immense advantage that the n^2 entries in the $n \times n$ contact matrix can be estimated from n pieces of information (Hethcote and Van Ark, 1987). Unfortunately, this proportionate mixing assumption does not seem to be realistic since very active people seem to be much more likely to form new partnerships with other very active people. The next simplest formulation for subgroup interactions seems to be a convex combination of proportionate mixing and internal mixing (in which people mix only with their own subgroup). This formulation, which was used in modeling gonorrhea (Hethcote and Yorke, 1984, p. 83), is now often called preferred mixing (e.g., Jacquez et al., 1988, 1989). In the modeling here, the incidences are formulated with preferred mixing and the convex combination parameter η is adjusted to fit the data.

As indicated in Section 7.1, the incidence terms for HIV transmission between needle–sharing IVDUs are also formulated with preferred mixing. It may seem strange to use the same form for the incidence terms for homosexual men and for IVDUs; however, this same form is based on the following similarities. People in both groups do form partnerships that consist of one or more contacts (homosexual or needle–sharing). Bath houses or gay bars might be analogous to shooting galleries as places where multiple partnerships occur. The number of contacts and duration of partnerships vary greatly in both populations so that the very active and active categories are a simplification for both populations. People in both populations can have multiple simultaneous partnerships and the incidence terms account for this somewhat since this behavior could correspond to frequent partner change. Thus the incidence term above is a simplification for both populations, but is reasonable for both populations.

There are data from sexual behavior surveys which show that the average partnership rate of homosexual men in some cities has changed over time (see Section 5.3.2). There are also some indications that the needle–sharing behavior of IVDUs may have decreased over time (see Section 8.2.4). Here changes in behavior are modeled by specifying the initial average number of new partners per month, the starting and stopping dates for changes in the partnership rate and the yearly reduction factor.

Modeling HIV transmission and AIDS in heterosexual partners of IVDUs is handled with the simplest possible formulation. The HIV incidence for these heterosexual partners is proportional to the number of new partnerships per month of heterosexuals with IVDUs; consequently, the only parameter to be adjusted in the fitting process is the average number of IVDU partners per month of heterosexuals. Although there is some evidence that the probability of heterosexual transmission is different depending on whether the infected person is male or female (Padian et al., 1991), this possible asymmetry is not included in our model. If this asymmetry were included, then the model would need separate classes for male and female IVDUs and for male and female heterosexual partners of IVDUs. This more complicated model would have more parameter values to be estimated, and this might be difficult since the yearly AIDS incidence is often small and erratic in the risk groups of female IVDUs and their male heterosexual partners. The simple model used here works well in fitting the AIDS incidence data for heterosexual partners.

The modeling of perinatal transmission from HIV–infected mothers to their newborn children before, during or just after birth is also modeled in the simplest way possible. The perinatal HIV incidence involves only the fecundity rate (birth rate), the probability of transmission during birth and the number of HIV–infectious females. The progression of perinatally–infected children to AIDS is modeled using the two–track staging system given in Section 2.3. For further clarification of the incidence terms or other aspects of the model, see the sample computer programs in the Appendix.

CHAPTER 8

WEAK LINKAGE BETWEEN HIV EPIDEMICS IN HOMOSEXUAL MEN
AND INTRAVENOUS DRUG USERS IN NEW YORK CITY

The largest number of AIDS cases in the United States have occurred in homosexual men and intravenous drug users (IVDUs). The transmission mechanisms for HIV in these groups are needle–sharing between IVDUs and homosexual intercourse. Since homosexual men who are also IVDUs have both possible transmission mechanisms and interact with both homosexual men and IVDUs, they could be an important transmission link between these two groups. It is conceivable that a primary HIV epidemic in one of these groups could sustain a secondary HIV epidemic in the other group through the linkage provided by the homosexual IVDUs. The goal of this chapter is to evaluate the relative importance of HIV transmissions by homosexual IVDUs and to decide if they form an essential linkage between the HIV epidemics in homosexual men and IVDUs.

A geographic analysis of where HIV epidemics in homosexual men and IVDUs are occurring together and separately suggests that these epidemics are not strongly connected. Major HIV epidemics in homosexual men are occurring throughout the United States, but major epidemics in IVDUs are focused in the Northeast region of the U.S. (NE region). If epidemics in homosexual men generally sustained epidemics in IVDUs, then there would be major epidemics in IVDUs throughout the U.S., and this has not occurred. If HIV epidemics in IVDUs generally sustained HIV epidemics in homosexual men, then the minor epidemics in IVDUs outside the NE region would probably cause only minor HIV epidemics in homosexual men in these areas, and this has not occurred since there are major HIV epidemics in homosexual men in many places outside the NE region. Thus it does not appear likely that HIV epidemics in either homosexual men or IVDUs are supporting HIV epidemics in the other. It is possible that the reason why major HIV epidemics in IVDUs are occurring in the NE region but not elsewhere is that the needle–sharing and other IVDU behaviors are different in the NE region. Thus it seems desirable to investigate possible connections between epidemics in homosexual men and IVDUs more thoroughly in the NE region. The most AIDS cases in the NE region occur in New York City (NYC), so it seems appropriate to use NYC to test the theory that the epidemics are essentially independent and separate.

During the early phase of the HIV epidemic in homosexual men and IVDUs, the HIV transmission process was probably like a random or stochastic process. In this early phase the homosexual IVDUs may have been involved in the seeding of HIV in the populations of homosexual men and IVDUs (Battjes, Dickens and Amsel, 1989). The stochastic nature of the beginning of the HIV epidemic is not of interest here. The main concern is the role of homosexual IVDUs when the epidemics are established and growing. Although many simplifying assumptions are necessary in order to use a deterministic model for an HIV epidemic, this type of model is well–suited as a quantitative descriptor of an epidemiological process. A deterministic HIV epidemiological model has been developed for one population in Chapter 3 and applied to homosexual men in San Francisco in Chapters 5 and 6. This model has been generalized in

Chapter 7 to five risk groups including homosexual men, homosexual IVDUs, and IVDUs. This model is available to explore the importance of homosexual–IVDUs in connecting the HIV epidemics in homosexual men and IVDUs.

How can one test the hypothesis that the HIV epidemics in homosexual men and IVDUs are not crucially linked by homosexual IVDUs and are essentially separate epidemics? The approach used here is to first fit one risk group models to the AIDS incidence data in NYC for homosexual men and IVDUs separately; then the three risk group model for homosexual men, homosexual IVDUs, and IVDUs is fit to the AIDS incidence data. If the parameter values obtained in the simultaneous fitting of the three risk groups are quite similar to those obtained in the separate fits, then the homosexual IVDUs are not a crucial link between the other two groups, and their HIV epidemics can be treated separately.

Information on HIV and AIDS in NYC is given in Section 8.1, and parameter values are estimated in Section 8.2. A modified fit criterion which accounts for HIV–related deaths is presented in Section 8.3. Fits of the one group model to the NYC populations of homosexual men and IVDUs are found in Sections 8.4 and 8.5. Section 8.6 presents the simultaneous fitting to the AIDS incidence data for the three risk groups. A key conclusion in Section 8.7 is that the HIV epidemics in homosexual men and IVDUs are not strongly connected by the homosexual IVDUs. Thus the HIV epidemics in homosexual men and IVDUs can be modeled separately. This separation of the HIV epidemics in homosexual men and IVDUs is assumed to also hold in other subregions and in racial/ethnic groups.

8.1. Data on HIV and AIDS in New York City

The incidences of AIDS in NYC and SF given in Table 8.1 have been adjusted for reporting delays and for the 1987 change in definition in the AIDS surveillance definition. The delay–adjusted incidence data, as reported by October 1, 1991, were supplied by John Karon and Debra Hansen in the Division of HIV/AIDS, Center for Infectious Diseases, Centers for Disease Control (CDC). Patients are said to satisfy the consistent case definition of AIDS if they have a diagnosis (definitive or presumptive) of a disease in the pre–1987 case definition. Based on a study of homosexual men in SF, a procedure in Section 5.4.2 was developed for estimating when the nonconsistent cases would later meet the consistent case definition. This procedure has been used to obtain the total adjusted consistent cases in Table 8.1 as the sums of the consistent and the modified nonconsistent cases. The data have not been adjusted for underreporting.

Note that the pattern of yearly AIDS incidence for homosexual men in NYC is similar to the patterns in homosexual men in SF for the first five years in the sense that the ratios of incidences in succeeding years are similar. After the first five years, the AIDS incidence in homosexual men in NYC seems to grow faster than in SF. The AIDS incidence in homosexual men in SF is approximately equal to that in NYC about one year earlier so the NYC epidemic undoubtedly started earlier. The data in Table 8.1 are consistent with the observations of Karon and Berkelman (1991) that AIDS incidences in homosexual men in NYC was roughly constant from mid–1986 to 1990. The simulation modeling in Chapter 6 suggests that the AIDS incidence

Table 8.1. The AIDS incidence by categories in New York City is adjusted for
reporting—delays and the 1987 AIDS definition change. The adjusted AIDS incidence in
homosexual men in San Francisco is included for comparison.

Year	homosexual men	homosexual IVDUs	IVDUs	homosexual men — SF
1979	5	1	0	0
1980	23	3	5	2
1981	95	9	21	22
1982	272	45	115	86
1983	577	73	276	228
1984	1017	82	503	442
1985	1463	142	871	678
1986	2068	167	1314	1010
1987	2321	206	1754	1275
1988	2489	174	2326	1285
1989	2451	180	2542	1338
1990	2378	158	2895	1551

in homosexual men in SF reached a plateau in about 1989 and may decline in the future.

The pattern for about the first five years for AIDS incidence in IVDUs in NYC is similar to
that for homosexual men in NYC one year earlier, but after five years the incidence in IVDUs
continues to grow instead of leveling off or reaching a peak. Indeed, the AIDS incidence in IVDUs
jumps significantly in 1988 and then increases slowly. The AIDS incidence in homosexual—IVDUs
in NYC is roughly 7 to 9% of that in homosexual men with larger differences in a few years.
Thus the AIDS incidence pattern in homosexual men in NYC who are also IVDUs is similar to
that for homosexual men in NYC.

In modeling the HIV prevalence in IVDUs it is significant that some HIV positive IVDUs
are dying from HIV—related causes that do not meet the AIDS definition. These causes include
pneumonia, endocarditis and tuberculosis. Stoneburner et al. (1988) estimated these HIV—related
deaths by comparing observed narcotics—related deaths in 1982 to 1986 with those that would be
expected without the AIDS epidemic and those reported as AIDS—related deaths. The number of
IVDUs was assumed to be constant from 1979 to 1986 and AIDS—related cases were subtracted so
that the average annual narcotics—related deaths for 1979 to 1981 was 488 deaths per year. Thus
2440 narcotics—related deaths would be expected for 1982 to 1986. Hence of the actual 6157
narcotics—related deaths in 1982 to 1986, 2440 were expected and 1197 were AIDS—related deaths,
so that the excess deaths were 2520. Stoneburner at al. (1988) provide evidence that these 2520
excess deaths are HIV—related, but they occur in people who do not have AIDS.

In February 1989, the NYC Department of Health (NYCDOH, 1989) gave revised
estimates of the number of NYC residents in various risk groups who were HIV—positive. Their
estimated ranges were 33,015 to 75,998 for men who have sex with men (MSM), 60,000 to 90,000
male IVDUs, 20,000 to 30,000 female IVDUs, 10,000 to 15,000 other men, 1,000 to 20,000 other
women and 1600 to 4400 children. Their estimated range for MSM were obtained in three ways.
Assuming 15% underreporting, they compared white and other categories of MSM in NYC with
MSM in San Francisco. Using back—calculation, they obtained the estimate of 33,015. By direct

calculation with 30% to 50% positivity and a risk population estimate of about 150,000, they obtained a range of 42,406 to 75,998 for HIV prevalence in MSM. The IVDU estimates are based on 40% to 60% prevalence in a population of 200,000 IVDUs where one quarter of them are women. They note that there is some evidence for a leveling off of HIV prevalence in IVDUs beginning in 1985 (Des Jarlais et al., 1988).

8.2. Parameter Estimates for New York City

The linkage between the HIV epidemics in homosexual men and IVDUs in NYC is analyzed in later sections. The simulation modeling needs *a priori* estimates and initial estimates for parameter values for the three group model consisting of homosexual men, homosexual IVDUs, and IVDUs. These estimates are used in fitting the model or as initial estimates of parameters that are adjusted in the fitting process.

8.2.1 Estimates of Population Sizes and Turnover

Estimates of the population size of the homosexual men in NYC have ranged up to 500,000, but the estimate in 1988 was reduced to about 100,000 (Lambert, 1988). A recent estimate of the NYC Department of Health of this population size is about 150,000 (NYC DOH, 1989). In the NYC model the size of the population of homosexual men is taken to be 100,000. The migration rate with equal immigration and emigration is taken to be 5% per year as it was in the SF model in Section 5.2.

Friedland and Klein (1987) note that ninety percent of the IVDUs are heterosexual, implying that 10% are homosexual. If there are about 200,000 IVDUs in NYC, then there would be about 20,000 homosexual–IVDUs in NYC, but this estimate is very crude. In a study of homosexual men (Darrow et al., 1987), 20% said that they had injected drugs and 60% of the drug users said that they had shared hypodermic needles. Since 12% of these homosexuals were needle–sharing IVDUs, roughly 12,000 of the 100,000 would be homosexual–IVDUs who share needles. Due to the uncertainty of the size of the homosexual–IVDU population, this size is taken as a variable in the NYC model which is to be determined to fit the homosexual–IVDU AIDS data.

Many papers (e.g., Friedland and Klein, 1987; Selwyn et al., 1987; Drucker, 1986) have given 200,000 as the approximate size of the IVDU population in NYC; however, it is not clear if these are independent estimates or are all based on one original source. Dolan et al. (1987) found that 59% of 193 in a drug abuse treatment program (1983–1985) reported that they had shared needles. Other studies of IVDUs in treatment programs found that 66% (Mulleady and Green, 1985) and 68% (Black et al., 1986) reported needle–sharing. Of course, these percentages may be unrealistically low since they are based on self–reporting of people in treatment programs. Darrow (personal communication, 1988) states that nearly all IVDUs share needles. Schuster (1988) reports that 70% to 90% of IVDUs are needle–sharers. If 20,000 (10% of 200,000 IVDUs) are homosexuals, and 30,000 (17% of the remaining 180,000 IVDUs) do not share needles, then the size of the non-homosexual needle–sharing IVDU population in NYC would be 150,000. In the rest of this chapter IVDU will mean non–homosexual needle–sharing IVDUs, and the size of this population in the NYC model is taken to be 150,000.

It is not clear whether the size of the needle–sharing population has changed with time. Kozel and Adams (1986) reported that the number of heroin users seems to have remained reasonably stable, but the number of people injecting forms of cocaine has increased. Others found that needle–sharing among drug users has decreased. Des Jarlais et al. (1987, 1988) found that 54% of 59 IVDUs in a treatment program in 1985 reported some risk reduction in needle–sharing; 75% in 1986 and 85% in 1987 reported some AIDS reduction behavior. Of course, self–reported changes of these IVDUs may be biased. In the model the number of needle–sharing IVDUs is fixed at 150,000, but it would be possible to change this size with time if more information becomes available.

Since three–fourths of all IVDUs in the United States are male (Des Jarlais et al., 1988) it is assumed that this fraction is also true for needle–sharers in NYC. This means that there are about 37,500 female IVDUs and 112,500 male IVDUs in NYC. Friedland and Klein (1987) state that 30% to 50% of the IVDU women have engaged in prostitution.

The migration or turnover rates in homosexual men and in IVDUs in NYC are difficult to estimate. One study found an annual inactivation rate of 13–25% for IVDUs who died, relocated outside of NYC, or ceased all intravenous use (Drucker and Vermund, 1989). Another study (Des Jarlais et al., 1989) of a 1987 subject group found that 11% had begun injecting illicit drugs after 1980 and 4% had begun after 1984; thus the entry rate was about 2% per year. The high exit rate is not consistent with the low entry rate. As a compromise, the migration rate is chosen as 5% per year, which is the same as for homosexual men.

The transfer rates between the very active and active classes is estimated to be 5% per year as in the SF model in Section 5.2. The natural mortality rate in all four risk groups is taken to be $\mu = 0.000532$, which is the value used in the SF model for homosexual men. This corresponds to the death rate of men aged 45–54. Although not all people in the risk groups are men or are in this age bracket, this slightly higher death rate is suitable for people in these groups with a somewhat risky lifestyle.

8.2.2 Estimates of Parameters Related to the Stages

Very little information seems to be available for the progression of IVDUs from HIV infection to AIDS. Thus it is assumed that all adults who become infected progress through the T4–cell count stages to AIDS in the same way as that found for homosexual men in Section 2.2. The probabilities w_k of transmission by a person in stage k and relative sexual or needle–sharing activity ρ_k of a stage k individual are assumed to be the same as those estimated in Section 5.1 for the baseline parameter set in Section 6.1. The fixed parameters in Table 6.1 are based on many data sources and sexual behavior surveys; the optimization parameters are those values which give the best fit to the HIV and AIDS incidence estimates for SF.

8.2.3. Sexual Behavior Parameter Estimates

The AIDS incidence pattern for homosexual men in NYC in Table 8.1 is similar to that of homosexual men in SF about 1 year later. Thus the *a priori* estimates for homosexual men are the baseline parameter values in Table 6.1 except that the NYC population size is 100,000 and the epidemic starting date is one year earlier.

8.2.4. Needle–Sharing Behavior Parameter Estimates

Needle–sharing seems to occur primarily within a particular group. In a study of IVDUs in NYC, Selwyn et al. (1987) found that about half of those sharing needles gave as reasons the need to inject drugs with no clean needle being available and needle–sharing was done only with a close friend or relative. Thus a needle that is shared is most likely to have been used by someone in the same group. Since the pattern of development of the AIDS epidemic in IVDUs is similar initially to the pattern for homosexual men in NYC and SF, it is assumed that the distribution of the number of needle–sharing partners is similar to that for homosexual men. Thus, it is assumed that 5% or 10% are in the very active class and that they have ten times as many needle–sharing partners as those in the active class. The sensitivity of the results to these parameter choices is checked.

IVDUs may inject several times a day, but usually share needles less often. Although some needle–sharing occurs in shooting galleries with many people, it usually occurs with a few acquaintances. Although partnerships formed with unknown individuals in shooting galleries are of short duration and involve one needle–sharing, the partnerships with acquaintances can be of long duration and involve many needle sharings. No estimates have been found for the probability of transmission per needle–sharing partnership; however, the probability of transmission from one needle–sharing partner is likely to be higher than the probability of transmission from one homosexual partner. In the NYC model it is assumed that the probability of transmission QHD per new needle–sharing partner is 0.05.

It is not clear whether the needle–sharing partnership rate has changed with time. Selwyn et al. (1987) found that some IVDUs reported that they had either stopped needle-sharing or ceased being an IVDU. Des Jarlais et al. (1987, 1988, 1989) found in a drug treatment center that 54% of IVDUs in 1985, 75% in 1986 and 85% in 1987 reported some reduction in behavior that could lead to AIDS, but this reporting could be biased. Thus in the NYC model, the reduction factor per year in the average number of needle-sharing partners is expected to be near 1 in contrast to the expected range of 0.4 to 0.7 for homosexual men. Since the AIDS incidence of homosexual men in NYC is about a year ahead of the incidence in SF, the starting date of the epidemic in homosexual men should be at least a year earlier than the starting date of July 1976 in SF. It is likely that the epidemic started in the IVDUs and in homosexual men at about the same time.

8.3 Modified Fit Criteria for the New York City Model.

Because of the significant number of HIV–related deaths described in Section 8.1, the fitting criteria for the NYC model are changed slightly from that described in Section 7.2. The parameter ALP is the rate constant for HIV–related deaths in stages 4, 5, and 6 for IVDUs and is adjusted so that these deaths in 1982 to 1986 are close to the observed value of 2520 given in Section 8.1. The initial guesses for the IVDU parameters are that PASD is about half of PASH and RDND is one. If the 42 HIV–related deaths per month (2520 in 5 years) occurred in a population of 10,000 pre–AIDS IVDUs, then the death rate would be 0.0042 so that this is taken as an initial estimate for ALP. The fit to the AIDS incidence data in the homosexual–IVDU population is obtained by adjusting the population size NSIZEB which is initially assumed to be 10,000. The HIV–related death rate constant ALP now joins the list of optimization parameters. The expression to be minimized in the fitting procedure is now changed to

$$\text{CHISQH} + \text{CHISQB} + \text{CHISQD} + 0.01(\text{DTH26--2520})^2$$

which is the sum of the chi–square values for the homosexual men, homosexual–IVDUs and IVDUs plus a measure of how close the HIV–related deaths in IVDUs in later HIV stages are to the observed value of 2520. The coefficient 0.01 has been found by trial and error to give a reasonable balance between the last term and the chi–square terms.

8.4. Fitting in the New York City Population of Homosexual Men

The model for homosexual men in Chapter 3 is also used for NYC. Indeed, since the AIDS epidemic in NYC homosexual men is about the same, but one year earlier in NYC than in San Francisco, one would expect the pattern in NYC to be similar to that in SF.

The best fit for the NYC homosexual men is shown in Table 8.2. The parameter values are quite similar to those for the best fit in SF except that the population size in Table 8.2 is 100,000 instead of 56,000 in SF and the starting date in the NYC epidemic is May 1974 instead of October 1975 in SF. In Table 8.2 the average number of partners per month is 0.49 before July 1982 and the yearly reduction factor is 0.41 until December 1984. In the best fitting parameter set for the SF homosexual men, the average number of sexual partners per month was 0.75 before August 1981 and the yearly reductions factor was 0.61. The external mixing fraction η in the simulation of the epidemic in NYC homosexual men is 0.58, while η was 0.82 for the baseline simulation in SF. Some other parameter sets also give reasonable fits, so it is not possible to conclude much about the partners per month and changes in sexual behavior other than the general conclusion that the average number of partners per month was approximately constant until around mid–1982 and then it decreased rapidly. Note that it was not possible to get an adequate fit using a parameter set without any change in sexual behavior. For all parameter sets which satisfy the fit criteria, the pattern is similar to the pattern in Table 8.2. Namely, the yearly HIV incidence peaks in about 1980, the HIV prevalence peaks at in about 1983, the AIDS incidence peaks in 1988 or 1989 and the AIDS deaths peak in about 1989 or 1990. Note that the

Table 8.2 Simulation results for the best fit to the AIDS incidence data for NYC homosexual men.

```
THE POPULATION SIZE IS        100000, THE VERY ACTIVE FRACTION IS
1.000000E-01 AND THE ACTIVITY RATIO IS        10.000000
THE NATURAL MORTALITY RATE XMU IS     5.320000E-04
THE INTERCHANGE RATE   FROM THE VERY ACTIVE CLASS TO THE ACTIVE CLASS IS
  4.166667E-03  AND THE TURNOVER RATE IS DLT =      4.166667E-03
THE NUMBER OF INFECTIOUS STAGES IS  M =            7
THE G PARAMETERS FOR THE TRANSFER BETWEEN STAGES ARE      7.355444E-02
  6.433708E-02     4.867545E-02     4.199281E-02     3.997889E-02
  5.152515E-02     5.398798E-02
THE WEIGHTS OF TRANSMISSION PER INFECTIOUS PARTNER TIMES THE FRACTION STILL
SEXUALLY ACTIVE FOR THE STAGES ARE WRH(I) =          2.000000         1.000000
  1.000000        1.500000        1.500000        1.500000
  7.500000
THE PROBABILITY OF TRANSMISSION IS QH =       5.000000E-02
THE EXTERNAL MIXING FRACTION IS ETA =     5.750000E-01
THE AVERAGE NUMBER OF PARTNERS PER MONTH IS      4.923000E-01 BEFORE        1982
          7, THEN IT IS REDUCED EACH YEAR BY A FACTOR OF      4.088000E-01UNTIL
DEC,       1984
THE STARTING YEAR AND MONTH ARE          1974           5
THE STARTING NUMBER OF VERY ACTIVE INFECTIVES IS        1.000000

     **********************************************
```

YEAR	HIV INC SIM	HIV PREV	FRACTNAL PREV ALL V_A ACT			YR AIDS DATA	INC SIM	AIDS(SIMULATION) PREV DTHS OUTSF		
1974	4.	4.	.00	.00	.00	*****	0.	0.	0.	0.
1975	24.	28.	.00	.00	.00	*****	0.	0.	0.	0.
1976	132.	156.	.00	.01	.00	*****	0.	0.	0.	0.
1977	709.	843.	.01	.06	.00	*****	0.	0.	0.	0.
1978	3148.	3883.	.04	.26	.01	*****	1.	1.	0.	0.
1979	7699.	11189.	.11	.65	.05	5.	5.	4.	1.	1.
1980	8612.	18956.	.19	.87	.11	23.	24.	22.	7.	3.
1981	7745.	25432.	.25	.93	.18	95.	93.	85.	29.	14.
1982	6788.	30544.	.31	.93	.24	272.	265.	252.	98.	49.
1983	3277.	31809.	.32	.88	.26	572.	578.	577.	253.	126.
1984	1489.	31023.	.31	.82	.25	1017.	1018.	1076.	518.	263.
1985	1100.	29564.	.30	.75	.25	1463.	1520.	1708.	888.	459.
1986	1232.	27921.	.28	.68	.23	2068.	1987.	2376.	1319.	693.
1987	1336.	26091.	.26	.62	.22	2321.	2328.	2965.	1738.	930.
1988	1399.	24123.	.24	.57	.20	2489.	2494.	3383.	2076.	1133.
1989	1417.	22102.	.22	.52	.19	2451.	2490.	3587.	2286.	1273.
1990	1398.	20121.	.20	.49	.17	2378.	2355.	3586.	2356.	1340.

CHISQ =   7.490914

peak AIDS incidence occurs about 8 or 9 years after the peak HIV incidence and about 5 years after the peak HIV prevalence.

Note in Table 8.2 that in the very active class the HIV prevalence rises rapidly until 93% are infected in 1981–82, and then the HIV prevalence decreases as infected very–active people either die from AIDS, migrate out of NYC, or move into the active class. The prevalence in the active class rises more slowly and reaches a peak of 26% infected in 1983 and then declines slowly. Note that the HIV prevalence peaks in the very active class in 1981–82 and peaks in the total population and in the active class in 1983. Since very sexually active men have more partnerships and hence are more likely to be infected, it is reasonable that the HIV fractional

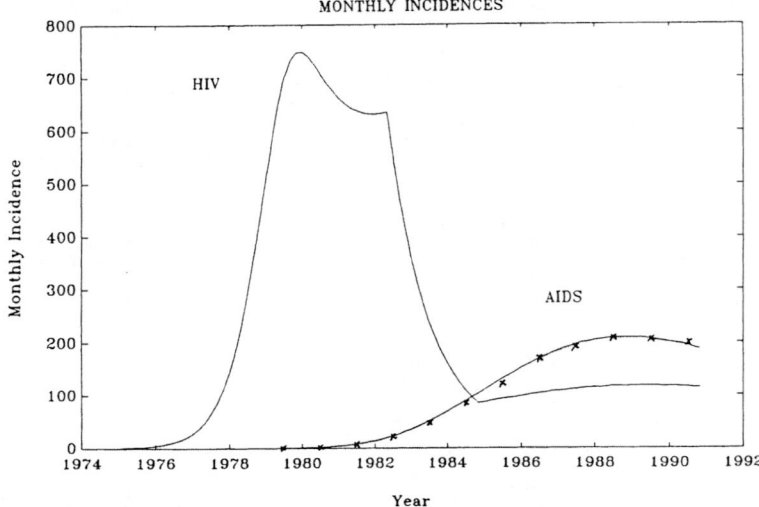

MONTHLY INCIDENCES

Figure 8.1. The best—fitting simulations for HIV and AIDS incidences for NYC homosexual men corresponding to Table 8.2. The AIDS incidence data (x symbols) correspond to the data in Table 8.1.

prevalence should have a peak in the very active class before the peak in the active class. As expected, nearly everyone with AIDS in the early years is in the very active class, but only 25% are in the very active class when the AIDS incidence peaks in 1988–89. Graphs of the HIV prevalence and yearly AIDS incidences are given in Figure 8.1.

A sensitivity analysis for the simulation for homosexual men in SF has been presented in Section 6.4. The relative sensitivities to the parameters found there would also apply here to the simulations for homosexual men in NYC. The peak HIV prevalence of about 32,000 in homosexual men in NYC is not too surprising since the AIDS incidence in homosexual men in NYC is similar to that in SF and the peak HIV prevalence there was about 20,000. If the AIDS incidence is uniformly underreported by 10% or 20%, then the HIV prevalence would increase by approximately these percentages. If all AIDS incidences in homosexual men were scaled up by 15% as done in the NYC Department of Health calculations, then the peak HIV prevalence in our model would be approximately 37,000. The HIV prevalence in this model is at the bottom of the range of 33,015 to 75,998 estimated for homosexual men in NYC in the NYC Department of Health report (NYCDOH, 1989). Note that the estimate in the dynamic model here is closest to their back—calculation procedure which yielded the estimate of 33,015 (see Section 8.1). Unless people develop AIDS more slowly than the current data indicates, the HIV prevalence cannot be higher and still lead to the given AIDS incidence data.

Table 8.3 Simulation results for the best fit to the AIDS incidence data for NYC IVDUs

```
THE IVDU POPULATION SIZE IS      150000
THE VERY ACTIVE FRACTION IS      1.000000E-01
THE ACTIVITY RATIO IS           10.000000
THE NATURAL MORTALITY RATE XMU IS    5.320000E-04
THE INTERCHANGE RATE  FROM THE VERY ACTIVE CLASS TO THE ACTIVE CLASS IS
    4.166667E-03  AND THE TURNOVER RATE IS DLT =    4.166667E-03
THE HIV-RELATED DEATH RATE CONSTANT IS    4.865000E-03
THE NUMBER OF INFECTIOUS STAGES IS  M =         7
THE G PARAMETERS FOR THE TRANSFER BETWEEN ADULT STAGES ARE    7.355444E-02
    6.433708E-02   4.867545E-02   4.199281E-02   3.997889E-02
    5.152515E-02   5.398798E-02
THE WEIGHTS OF TRANSMISSION PER INFECTIOUS PARTNER TIMES THE FRACTION STILL
SEXUALLY ACTIVE FOR THE STAGES ARE WRH(I) =         2.000000         1.000000
    1.000000      1.500000      1.500000      1.500000
    7.500000
THE PROBABILITY OF TRANSMISSION IS QH =      5.000000E-02
THE EXTERNAL MIXING FRACTION IS ETA =     4.734000E-01
THE AVERAGE NUMBER OF NEEDLE-SHARING PARTNERS PER MONTH IS    3.753000E-01
BEFORE      2000        1, THEN IT IS REDUCED EACH YEAR BY A FACTOR OF
    1.000000 UNTIL DEC,     2000
THE STARTING YEAR AND MONTH ARE        1974        1
THE STARTING NUMBER OF VERY ACTIVE INFECTIVES IS         1.000000
****************************************************
```

YEAR	HIV INC	HIV PREV	HIV DTHS	FRACTNAL_PREV ALL	V_A	ACT	YR AIDS DATA	INC SIM	AIDS(SIMULATION) PREV	DTHS	OUTSF
1974	5.	5.	0.	.00	.00	.00	****	0.	0.	0.	0.
1975	18.	22.	0.	.00	.00	.00	****	0.	0.	0.	0.
1976	68.	87.	0.	.00	.00	.00	****	0.	0.	0.	0.
1977	258.	335.	0.	.00	.02	.00	****	0.	0.	0.	0.
1978	949.	1245.	1.	.01	.06	.00	0.	1.	1.	0.	0.
1979	3062.	4170.	5.	.03	.20	.01	0.	2.	2.	1.	0.
1980	6972.	10733.	18.	.07	.48	.03	5.	9.	8.	3.	1.
1981	9179.	19022.	59.	.13	.74	.06	21.	31.	29.	10.	5.
1982	8546.	26121.	151.	.17	.86	.10	115.	97.	92.	34.	17.
1983	7997.	32088.	304.	.21	.88	.14	276.	250.	243.	99.	48.
1984	8078.	37493.	495.	.25	.88	.18	503.	521.	527.	236.	116.
1985	8432.	42539.	694.	.28	.85	.22	871.	900.	960.	467.	232.
1986	8815.	47205.	877.	.31	.83	.26	1314.	1343.	1514.	789.	396.
1987	9104.	51389.	1035.	.34	.79	.29	1754.	1795.	2134.	1174.	597.
1988	9254.	54986.	1168.	.37	.75	.32	2326.	2216.	2765.	1586.	816.
1989	9263.	57922.	1279.	.39	.72	.35	2542.	2586.	3361.	1990.	1034.
1990	9155.	60168.	1370.	.40	.68	.37	2895.	2901.	3898.	2363.	1241.

```
CHISQ =      22.860970
DTH26 =    2520.323000
```

8.5. Fitting in the New York City Population of IVDUs

Here the AIDS incidence data for the IVDU population is fit using the submodel obtained by ignoring the homosexual and homosexual–IVDU populations. In Section 8.6, all three risk groups are fit simultaneously. The best fitting simulation is given in Table 8.3 and shown in Figure 8.2. Note that 10% of the population of 150,000 is ten times as active and the external mixing fraction is 0.47. In Table 8.3 the epidemic starts in January of 1974 and the average number of needle–sharing partners is 0.38. Note that this best–fitting parameter set does not

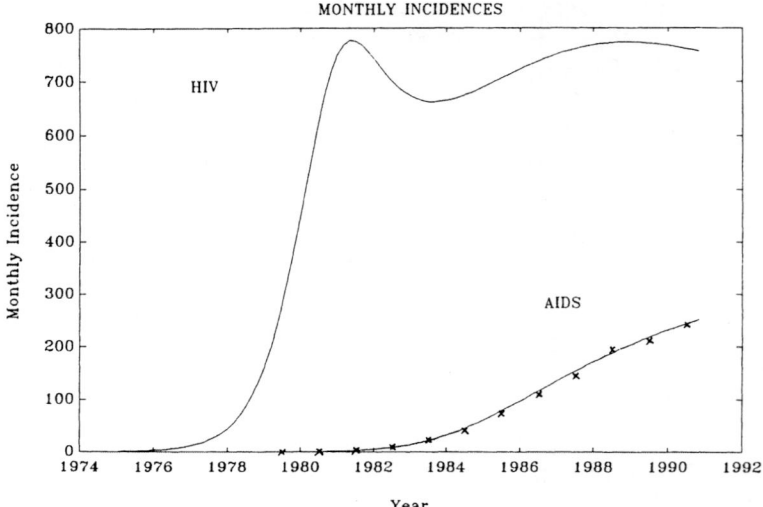

Figure 8.2 The best fitting simulations for HIV and AIDS incidences in NYC IVDUs corresponding to Table 8.3. The AIDS incidence data (x symbols) correspond to the data in Table 8.1.

have any reduction in the needle–sharing partnership rate. This is significantly different from the best fit in Section 8.4 for homosexual men.

The pattern in Table 8.3 is that the HIV incidence is approximately level after 1981, but both the HIV prevalence and AIDS incidence increase steadily. The HIV incidence of approximately 9000 per year is consistent with the HIV incidence of 10,000 cases per annum used in Pagano et al. (1991). The HIV–related deaths in the simulation match the estimated deaths of 2520 in the years 1982 to 1986. In the simulation, the HIV–related deaths are about 1000 to 1400 per year in 1987 to 1990. The simulation in Table 8.3 and Figure 8.2 is not intended to be used for forecasting; however, it does show that good fits to the AIDS data through 1990 are obtained without any reduction in needle–sharing partnership rates. There may have been changes in the needle–sharing behavior of IVDUs in NYC in recent years, since these changes would have almost no influence on the fit to the AIDS data through 1990.

The report (NYCDOH, 1989) of the Department of Health in NYC estimated that the HIV prevalence in IVDUs is 60,000 to 90,000 men and 20,000 to 30,000 women for a total of 80,000 to 120,000 (40% to 60%) out of their estimated IVDU population of 200,000. Their estimates of 40% to 60% HIV positivity are based on IVDUs in treatment centers in Manhattan and may be too high for NYC since the percentages are probably lower in the other boroughs. In Table 8.3 the predicted value is about 43,000 HIV positive IVDUs (non–homosexual) in 1988. This is lower than their estimated range and is 29% of the 150,000 needle–sharing IVDUs in the

NYC model. In Table 8.3 the simulated HIV prevalence increases up to about 60,000 in 1990, which is 40% of the NYC needle–sharing IVDUs.

8.6. Fitting in the Three New York City Risk Groups

In the previous sections the best fits were found for the populations of homosexual men and IVDUs. Here three risk groups are fit simultaneously by using the modified fitting procedure outlined in Section 8.3, which is the sum of the chi–squares and the weighted square of the deviation from the 2520 HIV–related deaths in 1982–86. Table 8.4 gives the parameter set an the computer simulation output which satisfies the modified fit criteria. Graphs of the monthly HIV and AIDS incidences for the three risk groups are given in Figure 8.3.

Table 8.4 Simulation results for the best fit to the AIDS incidence data for NYC homosexual men, homosexual IVDUs and IVDUs.

```
THE SIZE OF THE HOMO POPULATION IS        100000
THE SIZE OF THE HOMO-IVDU POPULATION IS        6500
THE SIZE OF THE IVDU POPULATION IS        150000
THE VERY ACTIVE FRACTIONS ARE     1.000000E-01 FOR HOMOSEXUALS
, AND     1.000000E-01 FOR IVDUs, AND THE ACTIVITY RATIO IS        10.000000
THE HIV-RELATED DEATH RATE CONSTANT FOR IVDUs IS     4.887000E-03
THE STARTING YEARS AND MONTHS ARE     1974             5
FOR HOMOSEXUALS, AND          1974          1 FOR IVDUs.
THE NATURAL MORTALITY RATE XMU IS     5.320000E-04
THE INTERCHANGE RATE   FROM THE VERY ACTIVE CLASS TO THE ACTIVE CLASS IS
    4.166667E-03   AND THE TURNOVER RATE IS DLT =      4.166667E-03
THE WEIGHTS OF TRANSMISSION PER INFECTIOUS PARTNER TIMES THE FRACTION STILL
SEXUALLY ACTIVE FOR THE STAGES ARE WRH(I) =       2.000000          1.000000
        1.000000        1.500000         1.500000        1.500000
        7.500000
THE PROBABILITY OF TRANSMISSION IS QH =      5.000000E-02
THE EXTERNAL MIXING FRACTIONS ARE ETAH, ETAD =      5.419000E-01     5.171000E-01
THE AVERAGE NUMBER OF HOMOSEXUAL PARTNERSHIPS PER MONTH IS     4.865000E-01 BEFO
RE       1982          7 AND IS REDUCED EACH YEAR BY A FACTOR OF
    4.191000E-01 UNTIL DEC,      1984
THE AVERAGE NUMBER OF NEEDLE-SHARING PARTNERS PER MONTH IS      3.445000E-01
BEFORE         2000          1, THEN IT IS REDUCED EACH YEAR BY A FACTOR OF
       1.000000 UNTIL DEC,     2000
***************************************************
```

CLASS	HIV INC	HIV PREV	HIV DTHS	FRACTNAL_PREV ALL	V_A	ACT	YR AIDS DATA	INC SIM	AIDS(SIMULATION) PREV	DTHS	OUTSF
--1970--											
HOMO	0.	0.	0.	.00	.00	.00	****	0.	0.	0.	0.
HMDU	0.	0.	0.	.00	.00	.00	****	0.	0.	0.	0.
IVDU	0.	0.	0.	.00	.00	.00	****	0.	0.	0.	0.
--1971--											
HOMO	0.	0.	0.	.00	.00	.00	****	0.	0.	0.	0.
HMDU	0.	0.	0.	.00	.00	.00	****	0.	0.	0.	0.
IVDU	0.	0.	0.	.00	.00	.00	****	0.	0.	0.	0.
--1972--											
HOMO	0.	0.	0.	.00	.00	.00	****	0.	0.	0.	0.
HMDU	0.	0.	0.	.00	.00	.00	****	0.	0.	0.	0.
IVDU	0.	0.	0.	.00	.00	.00	****	0.	0.	0.	0.
--1973--											
HOMO	0.	0.	0.	.00	.00	.00	****	0.	0.	0.	0.
HMDU	0.	0.	0.	.00	.00	.00	****	0.	0.	0.	0.
IVDU	0.	0.	0.	.00	.00	.00	****	0.	0.	0.	0.
--1974--											
HOMO	4.	4.	0.	.00	.00	.00	****	0.	0.	0.	0.
HMDU	0.	0.	0.	.00	.00	.00	****	0.	0.	0.	0.
IVDU	4.	5.	0.	.00	.00	.00	****	0.	0.	0.	0.

```
--1975--
HOMO    25.      29.      0.    .00   .00   .00   ****    0.     0.     0.     0.
HMDU     2.       3.      0.    .00   .00   .00   ****    0.     0.     0.     0.
IVDU    14.      18.      0.    .00   .00   .00   ****    0.     0.     0.     0.
--1976--
HOMO   146.     171.      0.    .00   .01   .00   ****    0.     0.     0.     0.
HMDU    12.      14.      0.    .00   .02   .00   ****    0.     0.     0.     0.
IVDU    55.      71.      0.    .00   .00   .00   ****    0.     0.     0.     0.
--1977--
HOMO   807.     954.      0.    .01   .07   .00   ****    0.     0.     0.     0.
HMDU    62.      74.      0.    .01   .08   .00   ****    0.     0.     0.     0.
IVDU   231.     293.      0.    .00   .01   .00   ****    0.     0.     0.     0.
--1978--
HOMO  3545.    4377.      0.    .04   .29   .02    0.     1.     1.     0.     0.
HMDU   262.     327.      0.    .05   .34   .02    0.     0.     0.     0.     0.
IVDU   977.    1234.      1.    .01   .06   .00    0.     0.     0.     0.     0.
--1979--
HOMO  7928.   11874.      0.    .12   .69   .06    5.     5.     5.     1.     1.
HMDU   571.     866.      0.    .13   .75   .06    1.     0.     0.     0.     0.
IVDU  3310.    4402.      5.    .03   .20   .01    0.     2.     2.     1.     0.
--1980--
HOMO  8202.   19202.      0.    .19   .89   .11   23.    27.    24.     7.     4.
HMDU   615.    1417.      0.    .22   .93   .14    3.     2.     2.     1.     0.
IVDU  6957.   10935.     18.    .07   .47   .03    5.     8.     7.     2.     1.
--1981--
HOMO  7398.   25324.      0.    .25   .93   .18   95.   102.    94.    33.    16.
HMDU   614.    1935.      0.    .30   .96   .22    9.     8.     7.     2.     1.
IVDU  8808.   18850.     61.    .13   .71   .06   21.    31.    28.    10.     5.
--1982--
HOMO  6605.   30255.      0.    .30   .93   .23  272.   285.   272.   107.    53.
HMDU   588.    2393.      0.    .37   .95   .30   45.    21.    20.     8.     4.
IVDU  8433.   25846.    155.    .17   .83   .10  115.    99.    93.    34.    17.
--1983--
HOMO  3291.   31535.      0.    .32   .88   .25  572.   605.   608.   269.   135.
HMDU   405.    2637.      0.    .41   .93   .35   73.    45.    45.    20.    10.
IVDU  7971.   31798.    307.    .21   .87   .14  276.   254.   247.   101.    49.
--1984--
HOMO  1545.   30798.      0.    .31   .82   .25 1017.  1044.  1112.   540.   275.
HMDU   324.    2770.      0.    .43   .90   .37   82.    78.    83.    40.    20.
IVDU  7983.   37124.    495.    .25   .87   .18  503.   525.   532.   239.   118.
--1985--
HOMO  1161.   29392.      0.    .29   .75   .24 1463.  1537.  1738.   911.   471.
HMDU   320.    2866.      0.    .44   .87   .39  142.   117.   132.    68.    35.
IVDU  8255.   42017.    691.    .28   .85   .22  871.   899.   962.   470.   233.
--1986--
HOMO  1303.   27814.      0.    .28   .68   .23 2068.  1990.  2393.  1335.   702.
HMDU   337.    2943.      0.    .45   .84   .41  167.   156.   185.   102.    54.
IVDU  8574.   46483.    872.    .31   .82   .25 1314.  1335.  1509.   788.   396.
--1987--
HOMO  1414.   26061.      0.    .26   .63   .22 2321.  2317.  2965.  1744.   935.
HMDU   348.    2995.      0.    .46   .80   .42  206.   188.   237.   137.    73.
IVDU  8817.   50439.   1028.    .34   .79   .29 1754.  1779.  2120.  1168.   594.
--1988--
HOMO  1482.   24181.      0.    .24   .58   .20 2489.  2475.  3368.  2072.  1132.
HMDU   354.    3021.      0.    .46   .76   .43  174.   212.   280.   168.    91.
IVDU  8935.   53800.   1157.    .36   .75   .32 2326.  2192.  2739.  1573.   809.
--1989--
HOMO  1505.   22254.      0.    .22   .53   .19 2451.  2468.  3562.  2273.  1268.
HMDU   354.    3023.      0.    .47   .73   .44  180.   225.   312.   193.   107.
IVDU  8925.   56506.   1263.    .38   .71   .34 2542.  2553.  3322.  1969.  1024.
--1990--
HOMO  1491.   20371.      0.    .20   .50   .17 2378.  2336.  3559.  2339.  1332.
HMDU   350.    3007.      0.    .46   .69   .44  158.   231.   332.   211.   118.
IVDU  8810.   58541.   1350.    .39   .68   .36 2895.  2856.  3845.  2334.  1225.
CHISQH =     12.757770
CHISQB =     93.055450
CHISQD =     22.162120
DTH26  =   2520.463000
```

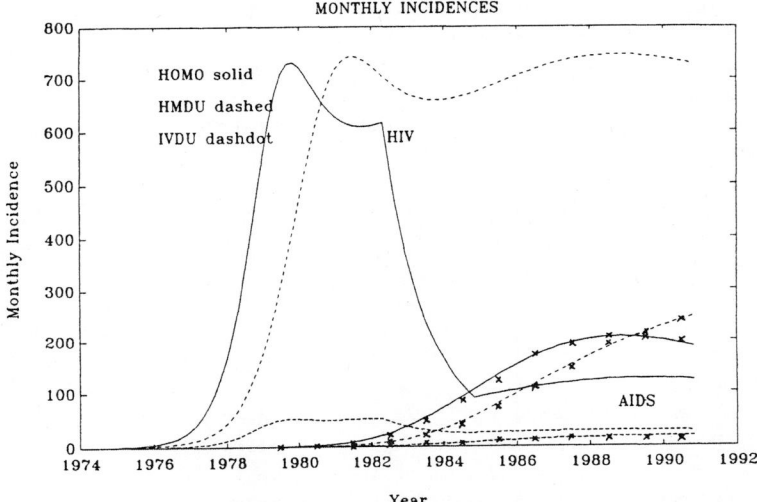

Figure 8.3 The best fitting simulations for HIV and AIDS incidences for homosexual men, homosexual IVDUs and IVDUs in NYC corresponding to Table 8.4. The AIDS incidences (x symbols) correspond to the data in Table 8.1.

The fits of the model simulations to the AIDS incidence data are quite good as shown in Figure 8.3 or as measured by the chi–square values at the bottom of Table 8.4. The largest chi–square value occurs for the homosexual–IVDUs and this is primarily because the 1988–90 AIDS incidence values are very low compared to a trend curve through the previous years. For the other risk groups the largest deviations also occur in 1988.

For the homosexual men the peak HIV incidence in Table 8.4 occurs in 1980, the peak HIV prevalence occurs in 1983, and the peak AIDS incidence occurs in 1988–89. This pattern is essentially the same as that in Table 8.2 where the population of homosexual men is fit separately. Essentially the same means that the peaks are within 5% of the previous peaks and they occur in the same year or within one year of the previous peaks. The starting date of the epidemic in Table 8.4 is May 1974 which is the same as in Table 8.2. The activity structure of 5% being ten times as active is like that in Table 8.2. The average number of homosexual partners per month before reduction and the external mixing fraction are slightly lower in Table 8.4, while the yearly reduction factor is slightly higher. The sexual activity reduction starting and stopping dates are the same in Tables 8.2 and 8.4. Thus the homosexual men part of the simultaneous fit in Table 8.4 is very similar to the separate fit for homosexual men.

For the IVDU population in Table 8.4 , the HIV incidence is approximately level after 1981, but both the HIV prevalence and the AIDS incidence increase steadily. This pattern for the IVDUs in the simultaneous fitting in Table 8.4 is very close to the pattern in Table 8.3 where the IVDUs were fit separately. In Table 8.4 compared to Table 8.3, the average number of new needle–sharing partnerships per month is slightly lower, the yearly reduction factor is still one (no reduction), and the external mixing factor is slightly higher. The decrease in the initial average number of needle–sharing partnerships per month is not surprising, since the IVDUs now also have some needle–sharing partnerships with homosexual–IVDUs. The dates for the start of the IVDU epidemic and the starting and stopping of reduction in partnerships per month are the same in Tables 8.3 and 8.4. Thus the IVDU part of the simultaneous fit in Table 8.4 is also very similar to the separate fit of the IVDUs in Table 8.3.

For the homosexual–IVDU population in Table 8.4 , the HIV incidence peaks in 1980–81, and then decreases before it levels off at about half the peak value. The HIV prevalence increases up to 1983 and then is approximately level. These behaviors are roughly between the corresponding behaviors for homosexual men and IVDUs. This is expected since the homosexual–IVDUs are linked to the HIV epidemics in both the other groups. The population size of 6500 homosexual–IVDUs is only 6.5% of the population size of 100,000 for homosexual men and only 4.3% of the population size of 150,000 for IVDUs. Thus the homosexual–IVDUs seem to be small in number compared to the other two groups. Although the homosexual–IVDUs do have some influence on the other two risk groups, this influence does not appear to be a crucial connection between the HIV epidemics in the two other risk groups.

From the simultaneous fitting of the three risk groups and the separate fittings of the homosexual men and IVDUs, one observes that the essential patterns are the same. Thus for these two groups the simultaneous fitting does not really change their patterns and the HIV epidemics in these two groups seem to be proceeding almost independently. This near independence is used in subsequent modeling.

8.7. Discussion of the Separate–Epidemic Theory

In both the separate fitting of the AIDS incidence in homosexual men in Section 8.4 and the simultaneous fitting in Section 8.6, the peak HIV incidence in homosexual men occurs in 1980, the peak HIV prevalence at about 32% occurs in 1983 and the peak AIDS incidence occurs in 1988–89. In Tables 8.2 and 8.4 the fractional HIV prevalence peaks at 93% in 1981–82 in the very active class and peaks at 25–26% in 1983 in the active class. Thus the general patterns of HIV and AIDS incidences and prevalences are the same for the separate fitting of homosexual men in Table 8.2 and the simultaneous fitting of the three risk groups in Table 8.4. In Table 8.4, the average number PASH of sexual encounters per month, the yearly reduction RDNH in sexual partners and the external mixing fraction ETAH are very close to those in Table 8.2. The dates for the start of the epidemic and the starting and stopping of partnership reduction are chosen to be the same in Table 8.4 as in Table 8.2. Thus the parameter values in the simultaneous fitting are close to the separate fitting of homosexual men. The patterns described above occur for a variety of parameter sets which satisfy the fit criteria. For example, they persist when the population size is doubled.

The pattern for the best–fitting parameter sets for IVDUs in Tables 8.3 and 8.4 is that the HIV incidence levels off around 1981, but both the HIV prevalence and the AIDS incidence are increasing. Thus the general patterns of HIV and AIDS incidences and prevalences are the same whether IVDUs are fit separately or simultaneously with homosexual men and homosexual–IVDUs. Moreover, the parameter values for the IVDU fit in Table 8.3 are the same as or similar to those in Table 8.4. Hence it seems that the simultaneous fitting of the three risk groups does not have much effect on the IVDU pattern and parameter values. This observation is consistent with the theory that the linkage provided by the homosexual–IVDUs is weak enough to be considered negligible.

In the fit of the data for the homosexual–IVDUs in Section 8.6, it is interesting to note that the best population size is 6500 which is 6.5% of the size of the non–IVDU homosexual men. It is plausible that a homosexual–IVDU population which is 6.5% of the population of homosexual men could have an AIDS incidence which is 7–9% of the AIDS incidence in homosexual men since homosexual–IVDUs can also be infected through needle–sharing. The pattern in the homosexual–IVDUs is that the HIV prevalence rises rapidly until it is about half of the population size and then remains approximately level. The fractional prevalence is high (near 50%) in homosexual–IVDUs since they are infected by both homosexual and needle–sharing partnerships. The early rise in HIV prevalence in homosexual–IVDUs seems to be due to infections from the homosexual men and then the HIV prevalence is maintained by infections from the IVDUs. Thus the pattern in homosexual–IVDUs is that their HIV epidemic follows and is sustained by the HIV epidemics in homosexual men and IVDUs. The HIV epidemic in homosexual–IVDUs does not seem to be a mechanism by which one of the HIV epidemics in homosexual men or in IVDUs supports or sustains the other.

Another argument supports the concept that the HIV epidemics in homosexual men and IVDUs are essentially independent. If one HIV epidemic were feeding another HIV epidemic, then there would be a delay of 4 to 6 years between the start (or peak) in the feeder epidemic and the start (or peak) in the sustained epidemic. In simulations of HIV epidemics in IVDUs and their heterosexual partners, delays of about 5 years are observed between the starts of the HIV epidemics, the peaks of the HIV epidemics, the starts of the AIDS incidences, and the peaks of the AIDS incidences (see Chapter 10). Similar delays are also observed for female IVDUs and perinatal cases in their children and for female heterosexual partners and perinatal cases in their children. A simplified explanation is that the delays of approximately 5 years occurs because the average time of infecting someone is in the middle of the 10 year infectious period. Since these delays do not occur between the HIV epidemics or between the AIDS incidence curves for homosexual men and IVDUs in NYC, this strongly suggests that neither of these epidemics is sustaining the other.

Forecasting future yearly AIDS incidence is difficult. The AIDS incidence data for homosexual men peaked in 1988–89 and declined slightly in 1990. This data and the best fitting simulations to this data suggest that a possible forecast is that the yearly AIDS incidence in NYC homosexual men has leveled off and may decline in the future. However, this forecast may be incorrect if the model is not realistic or if the data is incorrect for any reason. Possible data problems are recent increases in underreporting or recent changes in reporting delay patterns or a temporary leveling off of AIDS cases due to effects of the treatment of some pre–AIDS people with zidovudine (AZT) and aerosol pentamidine.

It is interesting to compare the HIV/AIDS epidemics in homosexual men in NYC and SF. In SF homosexual men the AIDS incidence in Table 8.1 appeared to be leveling off in 1987–89 and then it jumped up again in 1990. Thus the AIDS incidence in 1990 would probably not be consistent with a forecast based on data up through 1989. Simulations in Section 6.3.3 of the HIV/AIDS epidemic in SF homosexual men suggest that therapy may not have had much effect on the AIDS incidence in homosexual men there. Although saturation in the very active homosexual men did occur in the simulations of homosexual men in SF in Section 6.2.1, a reduction in sexual partners per month was essential in fitting the data there.

The simulations in Table 8.3 for NYC IVDUs suggest that there may not have been significant changes in needle–sharing behavior in IVDUs in NYC. Thus the HIV incidence remains high in Figure 8.2 and AIDS incidence continues to increase. This forecast without any change in behavior may be a "worst case" prediction, but it is consistent with the AIDS data so far. Blower et al. (1991) also modeled IVDUs in NYC and also found that their simulation scenario was able to fit the AIDS incidence data in NYC IVDUs without any change in needle–sharing behavior.

CHAPTER 9

RACIAL/ETHNIC PATTERNS OF AIDS IN THE UNITED STATES

For many reasons it is important to consider differences and similarities in the racial/
ethnic (r/e) patterns of AIDS cases in the United States (U.S.). Although most AIDS cases in
the U.S. have occurred in white homosexual men, the *per capita* risk of AIDS is generally higher in
Blacks and Hispanics. Understanding AIDS case rates and growth rates in r/e subgroups of a
risk group can lead to more focused educational or prevention programs. Moreover,
cross—checking r/e distributions between related risk groups and between regions provides a
simple measure of the confidence which can be placed in the data. Time trends in r/e AIDS cases
are analyzed in Chapter 10.

A primary source of r/e data is the January 1992 issue of HIV/AIDS Surveillance Report
published by the Centers for Disease Control (CDC, 1992). The r/e distributions given by the
percentages in three r/e groups in Tables in this Chapter are calculated from AIDS case data
taken from these CDC Tables. Tables 1.1, 1.2 and 1.3 in Chapter 1 give the AIDS cases through
December 1991 by exposure category and race/ethnicity for male adults/adolescents, female
adults/adolescents and pediatric (< 13 years old) cases. The r/e distributions of AIDS cases are
very useful for cross—checking data in related risk groups, but a better measure of connection of
the r/e groups is the relative risk. Using the risk for whites as a basis, the relative risk in an r/e
group is the ratio of the AIDS incidence per hundred thousand in the r/e group to the AIDS
incidence per hundred thousand in whites. Relative risks in r/e groups in the U.S. were analyzed
earlier by Selik et al. (1988).

In Section 9.1, the r/e distributions of cumulative AIDS cases in risk groups are
compared with the r/e distribution of the U.S. population. In Section 9.2, the r/e distributions
of cumulative reported AIDS cases are compared for exposure categories which are related by
sexual contacts between males and females. The r/e distributions of AIDS cases in exposure
categories related by perinatal transmission are considered in Section 9.3. Possible explanations
for observed differences in the r/e distributions are presented. In Section 9.4 the r/e patterns of
cases in three subregions of the Northeast (NE) part of the U.S. are analyzed and compared with
those in the U.S. The discussion in Section 9.5 summarizes the r/e patterns in the U.S. and NE
subregions.

9.1 Racial/Ethnic Patterns of AIDS Cases and Relative Risks

The r/e distributions of cumulative AIDS cases in risk groups of men, women and
children can be compared with the r/e distribution of the population in the U.S. In 1985 in the
U.S. about 78% of the population was white (not Hispanic), about 12% was black (not Hispanic),
about 7% was Hispanic and about 3% was other (Asian/Pacific Islander or American
Indian/Alaskan Native) (U.S. Bureau of the Census, 1989). For convenience these categories are
referred to as white, black, Hispanic and other. In Table 9.1 57% of the cumulative AIDS cases

Table 9.1. AIDS cases and percentages by race/ethnicity, age group, and sex, reported through December 1991, in the United States.

Adults/Adolescents

Race/ethnicity	Males		Females		Children <13 years old		Total	
	No.	(%)	No.	(%)	No.	(%)	No.	(%)
White, not Hispanic	104,180	(57%)	5,466	(26%)	739	(21%)	110,385	(53%)
Black, not Hispanic	47,037	(26%)	11,156	(53%)	1844	(53%)	60,037	(29%)
Hispanic	28,624	(16%)	4,400	(21%)	854	(25%)	33,878	(16%)
Asian/Pacific Islander	1,153	(1%)	105	(0%)	17	(0%)	1,275	(1%)
American Indian/ Alaskan Native	269	(0%)	45	(0%)	8	(0%)	322	(0%)
Total	181,696	(100%)	21,225	(100%)	3,471	(100%)	206,392	(100%)

in adult/adolescent males are white, 26% are black, 16% are Hispanic and 1% are other. Note that the r/e distribution of AIDS cases in males is much different from the r/e distribution of the population. A more detailed analysis of this difference and possible explanations for it are given below by examining risk groups of males.

For adult/adolescent females in Table 9.1, about 26% of cumulative AIDS cases are white, 53% are black, 21% are Hispanic and less than 1% are other. Comparing these percentages with the U.S. population percentages, it is clear that AIDS is much more likely for black and Hispanic females than for females in the white or other groups. R/e differences in AIDS in females in exposure categories are examined below and in Section 9.3. The r/e group of "other" is not usually considered in later analyses since the number of AIDS cases in this group is small. Cumulative AIDS cases in children less than 13 years old are about 21% white, 53% black and 25% Hispanic so that, as in females, AIDS is much more likely for black and Hispanic children than for white children. More details on pediatric AIDS cases in exposure categories are given below and in Section 9.3.

Overall annual case rates per 100,000 people are different among the r/e groups. Table 9.2 gives the AIDS cases and annual rates by r/e groups reported in 1991 in the U.S. (CDC, 1992). Among males the relative risk of AIDS is 3.4 for blacks, 2.5 for Hispanics, 1.0 for whites, 0.3 for Asians/Pacific Islanders and 0.3 for American Indian/Alaskan natives. Among females the relative risk of AIDS is 14.5 for blacks, 7.4 for Hispanics, 1.0 for whites, 0.5 for Asians/Pacific Islanders, and 0.9 for American Indian/Alaskan natives. Among children less than 13 years old, the relative risk of AIDS is 18 for black children, 5 for Hispanic children, 1 for white and Asian/Pacific Islander children, and 1.5 for American Indian/Alaskan native children. Racial/ethnic percentage distributions of AIDS cases are compared for sexually–related exposure categories of males and females in Section 9.2 and for perinatally–related exposure categories in Section 9.3.

Table 9.2. AIDS cases and annual rates per 100,000 population by race/ethnicity, age group, and sex, reported in the United States in 1991.

Adults/Adolescents

Race/ethnicity	Males		Females		Children <13 years old		Total	
	No.	Rate	No.	Rate	No.	Rate	No.	Rate
White, not Hispanic	20,716	27.8	1,358	1.7	142	0.4	22,216	11.7
Black, not Hispanic	11,059	95.3	3,102	24.6	400	7.4	14,561	49.2
Hispanic	6,850	69.9	1,213	12.6	133	2.0	8,196	31.4
Asian/Pacific Islander	247	8.5	24	0.8	4	0.3	275	3.7
American Indian/ Alaskan Native	65	9.2	12	1.6	2	0.6	79	4.4
Total	39,093	39.3	5,730	5.4	683	1.4	45,506	17.8

It is useful to compare the r/e distributions of cumulative AIDS cases in risk groups of men, women and children with the r/e distributions of the population which is about 78% white, 12% black and 7% Hispanic. Table 9.3 is constructed from data in Tables 1.1 and 1.2 in Chapter 1. In Table 9.3 the r/e distribution of cumulative AIDS cases in homosexual/bisexual males is 70% white, 17% black and 11% Hispanic so the relative risk is 1.6 for black males and 1.7 for Hispanic males and 1.0 for white males. Possible explanations are that black and Hispanic males are more likely to be homosexual/bisexual than white males, that black and Hispanic homosexual males are more likely to engage in risky behavior, or that black and Hispanic homosexual males are more likely to get HIV infection than white homosexual males.

The r/e distributions of AIDS cases in Table 9.3 for homosexual male IVDUs is 57% white, 27% black and 15% Hispanic so that the relative risk is 3.1 for black males, 2.9 for Hispanic males and 1.0 for white homosexual male IVDUs. Possible explanations are that black and Hispanic males are more likely to be homosexual IVDUs who share needles or that black and Hispanic male homosexuals are more likely to get an HIV infection than their white counterparts. The r/e distribution for AIDS cases for male IVDUs is 20% white, 48% black and 32% Hispanic so that the relative risk is 16 for black, 18 for Hispanic, and 1.0 for white IVDU males. Possible explanations are that black and Hispanic males are much more likely to be needle–sharing IVDUs than white males, or that they are more likely to get HIV infection than white males.

The r/e distribution of cumulative AIDS cases in Table 9.3 for female IVDUs is 21% white, 58% black and 20% Hispanic. Thus the relative risk is 18 for black female IVDUs, 11 for Hispanic female IVDUs, and 1.0 for white female IVDUs. Note that the relative risks for black male and female IVDUs are similar, but that the relative risks for Hispanic IVDUs are somewhat different. It is possible that black and Hispanic females are significantly more likely to be IVDUs than white females, or that they are more likely to get HIV infection than white females.

Table 9.3. AIDS cases by exposure category and race/ethnicity, reported through December 1991, in the United States.

male/female exposure category	White, not Hispanic		Black, not Hispanic		Hispanic		Total
	No.	(%)	No.	(%)	No.	(%)	No.
male homosexual/bisexual contact	83,205	(70%)	20,540	(17%)	13,240	(11%)	118,362
female–sex with bisexual male	343	(53%)	216	(33%)	78	(12%)	651
male homosexual IV drug user	7,547	(57%)	3,578	(27%)	1,925	(15%)	13,135
male (heterosexual) IV drug user	7,017	(20%)	16,798	(48%)	11,083	(32%)	35,048
female–sex with IV drug user	859	(19%)	2,244	(50%)	1,343	(30%)	4,484
male–sex with IV drug user	483	(26%)	1,077	(57%)	313	(17%)	1,882
female IV drug user	2,268	(21%)	6,185	(58%)	2,191	(20%)	10,705
male–hemophilia/ coagulation disorder	1,373	(82%)	127	(8%)	137	(8%)	1,671
female–sex with person with hemophilia	78	(83%)	10	(11%)	4	(4%)	94
male–sex with person with hemophilia	7	(70%)	1	(10%)	2	(20%)	10
female–hemophilia/ coagulation disorder	29	(69%)	10	(24%)	3	(7%)	42
male born in Pattern II country	8	(0%)	1,779	(99%)	11	(1%)	1,805
female–sex with person born in Pattern II country	10	(13%)	63	(83%)	2	(3%)	76
male–sex with person born in Pattern II country	40	(41%)	48	(49%)	9	(9%)	98
female–born in Pattern II country	5	(1%)	709	(99%)	3	(9%)	718
male–receipt of blood transfusion blood components or tissue	1,938	(72%)	418	(16%)	259	(10%)	2,679
female–sex with transfusion recipient with HIV infection	102	(63%)	28	(17%)	28	(17%)	161
male–sex with transfusion recipient with HIV infection	43	(54%)	19	(24%)	16	(20%)	79
female–receipt of blood transfusion, blood components or tissue	1,055	(63%)	349	(21%)	220	(13%)	1,668
male–other/undetermined	2,287	(37%)	2,269	(37%)	1,432	(23%)	6,114
female–sex with HIV–infected person, risk not specified	303	(28%)	514	(48%)	236	(22%)	1,065
male–sex with HIV–infected person, risk not specified	232	(29%)	383	(47%)	197	(24%)	813
female–other/undetermined	414	(27%)	828	(53%)	292	(19%)	1,561

The r/e distribution of AIDS cases in people with hemophilia/coagulation disorder cannot be simply compared to the r/e distribution of the population since some r/e groups in this category are more likely to have had other risk factors and some are more likely to have received single donor blood products (Stehr—Green et al., 1988). The r/e patterns of AIDS cases in people born in Pattern II countries clearly implies that nearly all of them are black.

In Table 9.3 the r/e distribution of AIDS cases in males who received blood transfusions, blood components or tissue is 72% white, 16% black and 10% white which is reasonably close to the r/e distribution of the population. For females who received blood transfusions, etc., the r/e distribution is 63% white, 21% black and 13% Hispanic so that the per capita AIDS case rate in these black and Hispanic females is about twice that in whites. This could be due to more frequent blood transfusions in black and Hispanic women.

In Table 9.3 the r/e distribution of cumulative AIDS cases in males in the other/ undetermined category is 37% white, 37% black and 23% Hispanic. Comparing this with the r/e distribution of all male AIDS cases in Table 9.1 shows that black and Hispanic males with AIDS are about twice as likely to be in the other/undetermined category as white males with AIDS. For females in the other/undetermined category, the r/e distribution of AIDS cases is 27% white, 53% black and 19% Hispanic which is close to the r/e distribution for all females with AIDS in Table 9.1. Thus white, black and Hispanic women with AIDS are all about equally likely to be in the other/undetermined category.

In Table 1.3 it is clear that most AIDS cases in children are perinatal from mothers who have or are at risk for HIV infection; these exposure categories are analyzed in Section 9.3. For children with hemophilia/coagulation disorder in Table 1.3, the r/e distribution is 69% white, 13% black and 16% Hispanic. Compare this to the r/e distribution of the population which is 78% white, 12% black and 7% Hispanic. It is possible that Hispanic children are more likely to be hemophilic or that Hispanic hemophilic children are more likely to get AIDS, but these explanations are probably too simplistic since the treatment received is not uniform for the r/e groups (Stehr—Green et al., 1988). For children who received blood transfusions, blood components or tissue, the r/e distribution of AIDS cases in Table 1.3 is 53% white, 22% black and 23% Hispanic. This r/e distribution does not match that of the U.S. population. As in females it is possible that blood transfusions are more common for Hispanic and black children.

9.2 Exposure Categories Related by Sexual Contacts

Racial/ethnic distributions of cumulative AIDS cases are compared for male and female exposure categories which are connected by sexual contacts between individuals in the categories. Table 9.3 contains the cumulative numbers of reported AIDS cases and percentages in three r/e groups for many exposure categories. Because the number of cases are usually small in the r/e groups of Asian/Pacific Islander and American Indian/Alaskan native, these r/e groups are not considered in this section.

9.2.1 Relating Exposure Categories

Many of the comparisons in this section assume that sexual pairing occurs primarily within the racial/ethnic groups so that the r/e percentages should match for exposure categories connected by sexual pairing. Of course, there is some pairing across r/e boundaries; however, the assumption above is reasonable if the pairing between people in different r/e groups is relatively infrequent and the cross pairings between men in a first group and women in a second group are nearly balanced by cross pairings between women in the first group and men in the second group.

The comparisons of r/e distributions in related exposure groups in this and succeeding sections are based on various assumptions. A typical comparison in this section is between the exposure categories of male (heterosexual) intravenous drug users (IVDUs) and (non–IVDU) females who have had sex with a male IVDU. It seems that the r/e distributions between these two directly–connected exposure categories should match, but this involves some implicit assumptions. A possible connecting chain is that:

1. the cumulative reported AIDS cases in females who have had sex with IVDU males is related to
2. the cumulative AIDS cases in these females, which is related to
3. the history of HIV incidence of these females who have had sex with IVDU males, which is related to
4. the history of HIV prevalence of IVDU males, which is related to
5. the history of HIV incidence in IVDU males, which is related to
6. the cumulative AIDS cases in IVDU males, which is related to
7. the cumulative reported AIDS cases in IVDU males.

Before discussing the relationships between the 7 items above, it is important to note that the details of the relationships do not have to be understood; all that is necessary is that the relationships between the numbered items are approximately the same for all of the r/e groups so that the overall relationship between 1 and 7 is the same for all of the r/e groups. If the history of underreporting is the same for all r/e groups, then the relationships between 1 and 2 above and also between 7 and 6 are the same for all r/e groups. If the progression from HIV infections to AIDS is similar historically for all r/e groups, then the relationship between 2 and 3 is the same for all r/e groups. A similar assumption implies that the relationship between 5 and 6 is the same for all r/e groups. Note that the relationship of 2 to 3 is not the same as the relationship of 6 to 5 since the HIV epidemic in females who have had sex with IVDU males is at an earlier stage than the HIV epidemic in IVDU males; i.e., the HIV incidence curve for these females rises later than the HIV incidence curve for the males since the females get the HIV infections from the infected males.

Item 3 is related to item 4 since the HIV incidence in these females at a given time is approximately proportional to the HIV prevalence in their male partners and the susceptible fraction of the females; it is assumed that this relationship is approximately the same for all r/e groups. Item 4 is related to item 5 since the HIV prevalence in these males at a given time is related to the history of HIV incidence in these males and their progression to AIDS and death; it is assumed that this relationship is approximately the same for all of the r/e groups. Thus the expectation that the r/e distributions of cumulative reported AIDS cases should match between the two exposure categories is based on the assumption that sexual pairing occurs primarily within the r/e groups and that the overall relationship between the two exposure categories is the same for the r/e groups. When the r/e distributions do not match for two related exposure categories, there could be many possible explanations; for example, the relationships between some items in the connecting chain above could be different in different r/e groups. When the r/e distributions do not match in the comparisons below, some possible explanations are given.

9.2.2. Homosexual/Bisexual Males

It would be expected that the racial/ethnic distributions of AIDS cases should match for the female exposure category of sex with a bisexual male and the exposure category of bisexual male. The exposure category of bisexual male is not in Table 9.3, but the r/e percentage distribution for bisexual males is about 59% white, 28% black and 12% Hispanic (J. Karon, personal communication). This r/e distribution matches reasonably well to that of the exposure category of females who had sex with a bisexual male. Note that the r/e distributions of bisexual males and males with homosexual/bisexual contact do not match very well. A possible explanation is that bisexual behavior is more common among black men than among whites and Hispanics. This observation that black homosexual/bisexual men may be more likely to be bisexual is consistent with reports in the sociology literature (Darrow, personal communication). Chu et al. (1992) reported that among 65,389 men who had sex with men, 26% were bisexual. Bisexual behavior was reported by 41% of black men, 31% of Hispanic men and 21% of white men in those men who had sex with men.

In Table 9.3 the r/e distribution of AIDS cases in males with homosexual/bisexual contact and IV drug use is 57% white, 27% black and 15% Hispanic. For each r/e group these percentages are between those for males with homosexual/bisexual contact and males with IV drug use. Since the r/e distribution for homosexual/bisexual IVDU males is closer to that of homosexual/bisexual males, the males with homosexual contact and IV drug use may behave more like homosexual/bisexual males than like IVDUs and hence may be more likely to be infected through homosexual contacts then through needle—sharing contacts with IVDUs.

9.2.3. Intravenous Drug Users

Consider cumulative reported AIDS cases in the exposure categories of male (heterosexual) IVDUs and female IVDUs. Although about the same percentages (20% and 21%) are whites in these exposure categories, 58% of female IVDUs are black compared to 48% black for male (heterosexual) IVDUs and 20% of females are Hispanic compared to 32% Hispanics for male (heterosexual) IVDUs. For all (heterosexual) IVDUs about 23% of AIDS case occur in females and 77% in males; this seems to suggest that 23% of IVDUs are females and 77% are males. For (heterosexual) IVDUs, about 24% of AIDS cases occur in females among whites, about 27% occur in females among blacks and only about 17% occur in females among Hispanics. This does not mean Hispanic females are less likely to be IVDUs than white and black females. Recall the implications from Section 9.2 that black males and females may be about 16 to 18 times as likely to be IVDUs as white males and females, but that his likelihood ratio may be about 16 for Hispanic males and 11 for Hispanic females. Although a smaller percentage of Hispanic IVDUs are females, Hispanic females are much more likely to be IVDUs than white females but slightly less likely than black females.

Two exposure categories connected by sexual contacts are male (heterosexual) IVDUs and females who had sex with IVDUs. Indeed, these two categories are used as the typical example at the beginning of this section. The r/e percentages in Table 9.3 for these categories match remarkably well. This suggests that the relationship between the HIV and AIDS epidemics in these two exposure categories is about the same for the r/e groups and that reporting for these two categories may be reasonably accurate.

The exposure categories of female IVDUs and males (heterosexual) who had sex with female IVDUs are also connected through sexual contacts. However, Des Jarlais (personal communication) believes that the exposure category of (non–IVDU) male (heterosexual) who had sex with female IVDUs is often used for men who should be in another category; he believes that it is rare for a female IVDU to have a sexual partner who is not also an IVDU. Nevertheless, the r/e distributions in Table 9.3 for these two groups show some consistency with slightly more white males then would be expected and slightly fewer Hispanic males than expected.

Based on his knowledge of IVDUs in New York City, Des Jarlais (personal communication) estimated that about 2/3 of IVDU males have female sexual partners who are not IVDUs, about 1/4 have female sexual partners who are also IVDUs, and very few have no sexual partner. He also estimated that nearly all IVDU females have a male sexual partner who is also an IVDU, and very few have partners who are not IVDUs or no sexual partner. This would mean that the exposure category of males (heterosexual) who had sex with an IVDU woman would be nearly empty and, indeed, in the New York City data, this exposure category is nearly empty.

It is possible to check the consistency of the estimates above of Des Jarlais if it is assumed that the numbers of HIV infected persons in the exposure categories are proportional to the numbers of AIDS cases in the exposure categories. If 77% of IVDUs are male and 25% of all male (heterosexual) IVDUs have a female sexual partner who is also an IVDU and there is a one to one correspondence, then 84% of female IVDUs must have a male sexual partner who is also an IVDU since $0.25 \times 0.77 = 0.84 \times 0.23$. This calculated 84% is consistent with the estimate that nearly all female IVDUs have a male sexual partner who is also an IVDU; the remaining 16% of female IVDUs would have no sexual partner or a male sexual partner who is not an IVDU.

9.2.4. Other Sexually–Related Categories

In Table 9.3 the r/e percentage distributions of AIDS cases for people with hemophilia/coagulation disorder and their sexual partners should match. Although the number of AIDS cases in females who had sex with a person with hemophilia is small, the percentage distribution matches reasonably well to that for AIDS cases in males with hemophilia/coagulation disorder. The number of AIDS cases in males who had sex with a female with hemophilia is too small to compare r/e distributions.

Now consider people born in Pattern II countries and their sexual partners. Although in Table 9.3 the number of AIDS cases is small for females in the exposure category of sex with a person born in a Pattern II country, the r/e distribution for this category matches reasonably well with that of AIDS cases for males born in Pattern II countries. This is not surprising since nearly everyone in these exposure categories is black.

The r/e distribution in Table 9.3 for males in the exposure category of sex with a person born in a Pattern II country is very different from that for females born in a Pattern II country. One explanation of the difference could be that a significant number of white males had sex with black females born in Pattern II countries; indeed, the data suggest that for women born in Pattern II countries, about half of these sexual partners are white and half are black. Another possibility is that many white men in this exposure category of sex with a woman born in a Pattern II country are misclassified.

Although the number of AIDS cases in Table 9.3 in males and females who had sex with recipients of transfusions, blood components or tissue is relatively small, these r/e distributions match reasonably well with the distributions of AIDS cases for the female and male recipients, respectively. Since the population is 78% white, 12% black and 7% Hispanic, it might be expected that this distribution would also hold for AIDS cases in recipients of blood transfusions, blood components or tissue. This distribution matches reasonably well for males, but not as well for females. The data suggests that black and Hispanic females may receive blood transfusions, blood components or tissue relatively more frequently than white females.

For the exposure categories of other/undetermined which contain miscellaneous and leftover AIDS cases, one might not expect matching of the r/e distribution of the AIDS cases in these categories and AIDS cases in the corresponding sexual partner category. Surprisingly, the r/e distributions of AIDS cases in Table 9.3 do match reasonably well for both males and females in the other/undetermined categories and female and male AIDS cases in the category of sex with HIV—infected person, risk not specified.

9.2.5. Estimating HIV Transmission

It was recently estimated that there are approximately one million people in the United States who are infected with HIV (CDC, 1990b). The cumulative number of AIDS cases reported in the U.S. at the end of 1991 was 206,392 (CDC, 1992). Since cumulative actual AIDS cases are slightly greater than cumulative reported AIDS cases, the ratio K of cumulative HIV incidence to cumulative AIDS cases is now approximately between 4 and 5 for all people in the U.S. As cumulative AIDS cases increase in the future, the ratio K will decrease towards the value one. Of course, the ratio K not only changes with time, but is also different for different risk groups. If only a few AIDS cases have appeared in a risk group, then the value of K would be large; however, the value of K would decrease as the epidemic progresses and the cumulative AIDS incidence increases in the risk group. Since children progress more rapidly to AIDS than adults, values of K for risk groups of children would be lower than if a similar HIV epidemic were occurring in adults.

The AIDS case data in Table 9.3 can be used to obtain some information on HIV transmission between people in exposure categories related by sexual contacts. As a concrete example, consider the exposure categories of male (heterosexual) IVDUs and (non–IVDU) female sexual partners of male IVDUs. For the ratio K defined in the previous paragraph, let K_1 be the current value for male (heterosexual) IVDUs and K_2 be the current value for female sexual partners of male IVDUs. Then the average number D of female sexual partners of male IVDUs infected per new HIV case in male (heterosexual) IVDUs who have female sexual partners is

$$D = \frac{\text{cumulative HIV incidence in female sexual partners of male IVDUs}}{\text{cumulative HIV incidence in male IVDUs who have female sexual partners}}$$

$$= \frac{K_2(\text{cumulative AIDS cases in female sexual partners of male IVDUs})}{K_1(\text{cumulative AIDS cases in male IVDUs})(\text{fraction who have female sexual partners})}$$

If K_2 were equal to K_1 at the current time, then they would cancel out in the last quotient above and the result would be an estimate of D. However, early in an HIV epidemic there are fewer AIDS cases per HIV case than later and the HIV infections in the female sexual partners occur later than the HIV infections in the male IVDUs, so that K_2 is probably somewhat greater than K_1. Thus

$$D \geq \frac{\text{cumulative AIDS cases in female sexual partners of male IVDUs}}{(\text{cumulative AIDS cases in male IVDUs})(\text{fraction who have female sexual partners})}$$

so that the right side is a lower bound on D for female sexual partners of male IVDUs. If reporting delays are similar for these females and males, then cumulative reported AIDS cases can be used in the numerator and denominator of the quotient above. Analogous quotients apply for other exposure categories related by sexual transmission.

Table 9.4 contains data from Table 9.3 on the cumulative reported AIDS cases for exposure categories and the categories related by sexual transmission. In Table 9.4 the fractions of male and female IVDUs with non–IVDU sexual partners are those estimated in a paragraph above. Since 72% of males over age 20 are married (World Almanac, 1988), this 72% is a reasonable estimate for the percent of adult males who have a female sexual partner. Since 44% of blood transfusion recipients are age 65 or older and 58% of transfusion recipients are women (NHLBI, 1985), many female transfusion recipients do not have a sexual partner so that the fraction 0.50 is used in Table 9.4. The last column in Table 9.4 contains the estimates of the quotient above, which are obtained using the values in the first three columns. These are estimates of lower bounds on the average number D of sexual partners infected per HIV case.

Table 9.4. Estimates of lower bounds on the average number D of sexual partners
infected per HIV case.

exposure category	AIDS cases	fraction with sexual partners	AIDS cases in sexual partners	lower bound on D
male (heterosexual) IVDUs	35,048	0.67	4,484	0.19
female IVDUs	10,705	0.08	1,882	2.20
males—hemophilia/coagulation disorder	1,671	0.72	94	0.08
males—born in Pattern II country	1,805	0.72	76	0.06
females—born in Pattern II country	718	0.72	98	0.19
males—blood transfusion recipients	2,679	0.72	161	0.08
females—blood transfusion recipients	1,668	0.50	79	0.09
males—other/undetermined	6,114	0.72	1,065	0.24
females—other/undetermined	1,561	0.72	813	0.72

The value 2.20 for (non—IVDU) male sexual partners of female IVDUs appears to be
unrealistically large; it would still be too large if the fraction of female IVDUs with (non—IVDU!)
male sexual partners were as large as 0.16. Thus this calculation reinforces the previous
suggestion that many males in this exposure category may be misclassified. The value of 0.72 for
male sexual partners of females in the other/undetermined category also seems too high, but this
is not surprising due to the miscellaneous nature of this category.

The remaining seven estimates for lower bounds for values in Table 9.4 range from 0.06
to 0.24 so that this range seems plausible. The lower bound 0.19 for D occurs for
(non—IVDU) female sexual partners of male IVDUs and for male sexual partners of females born
in Pattern II countries. For hemophiliacs and blood transfusion recipients, there have been almost
no new HIV infections since early 1985 when the testing of blood for HIV was started. Since HIV
incidence does not increase, but AIDS cases continue to occur in these groups, the ratio K would
be smaller for these groups than for their sexual partners where new HIV cases are still occurring.
Hence, K_2/K_1 would be larger than if the HIV epidemic had continued in hemophiliacs and
blood transfusion recipients. Thus it is not surprising that the quotient estimates for these groups
in Table 9.4 are lower. The range 0.08 to 0.09 for hemophiliacs and blood transfusion
recipients is enough lower that there may also be other factors involved. For example, the types
of sexual interactions might be safer or less likely to result in HIV transmission than the sexual
interactions occurring between male IVDUs and their sexual partners. It is not clear why the
estimated lower bound (0.06) is low for males born in Pattern II countries.

118

Table 9.5. AIDS cases by exposure category and race/ethnicity, reported through December 1991 in the United States.

female/pediatric exposure category[1]		White, not Hispanic		Black, not Hispanic		Hispanic		Total
		No.	(%)	No.	(%)	No.	(%)	No.
IV drug use	(female)	2,268	(21%)	6,185	(58%)	2,191	(20%)	10,705
	(pediatric)	224	(16%)	833	(58%)	365	(26%)	1,430
sex with IV drug user	(female)	859	(19%)	2,244	(50%)	1,343	(30%)	4,484
	(pediatric)	91	(15%)	269	(45%)	238	(39%)	603
sex with bisexual male	(female)	343	(53%)	216	(33%)	78	(12%)	651
	(pediatric)	22	(36%)	24	(39%)	14	(23%)	61
sex with person with hemophilia	(female)	78	(83%)	10	(11%)	4	(4%)	94
	(pediatric)	9	(69%)	3	(23%)	1	(8%)	13
born in Pattern II country	(female)	5	(1%)	709	(99%)	3	(0%)	718
	(pediatric)	1	(0%)	241	(99%)	2	(1%)	244
sex with person born in Pattern II country	(female)	10	(13%)	63	(83%)	2	(3%)	76
	(pediatric)	0		13	(93%)	0		14
sex with transfusion recipient with HIV infection	(female)	102	(63%)	28	(17%)	28	(17%)	161
	(pediatric)	4	(31%)	4	(31%)	4	(31%)	13
sex with HIV-infected person, risk not specified	(female)	303	(28%)	514	(48%)	236	(22%)	1,065
	(pediatric)	30	(21%)	70	(49%)	40	(28%)	144
receipt of blood transfusion, blood components or tissue	(female)	1,055	(63%)	349	(21%)	220	(13%)	1,668
	(pediatric)	22	(37%)	25	(42%)	13	(22%)	60
undetermined	(female)	414	(27%)	828	(53%)	292	(19%)	1,561
	(pediatric)	62	(18%)	222	(63%)	65	(18%)	354

[1]The pediatric exposure category describes the category of their mothers who are with or at risk for HIV infection.

9.3 Perinatally–Related Exposure Categories

Table 9.5 contains data on cumulative AIDS cases reported through 1991 for pediatric categories and corresponding exposure categories for females. The AIDS case data are taken directly from Tables 1.2 and 1.3 in Chapter 1. Racial/ethnic percentage distributions are compared for pediatric and female exposure categories connected by perinatal transmission.

A typical comparison of r/e distributions in this section is for AIDS cases for IVDU females and pediatric AIDS cases with a mother who was at risk due to IVDU. One assumed chain of connections in this case is that the cumulative reported pediatric AIDS cases with an IVDU mother is related to the cumulative number of AIDS cases in this group; which is related to the history of HIV incidence in these children, which is related to the history of HIV prevalence in female IVDUs, which is related to the history of HIV incidence in this group, which is related to the cumulative reported AIDS cases in female IVDUs. As in the previous section it is assumed that the relationships in this connecting chain are the same for all r/e groups so that the overall relationships are also the same. In particular, it is assumed that both the birthrates and the fractions infected by HIV infected mothers are constant and equal for the r/e groups.

For the category of IVDU in Table 9.5, the percentage distributions for females and pediatric cases do not match since there are fewer pediatric AIDS cases than expected in whites and more than expected in Hispanics. This same pattern also occurs in the four other exposure categories: sex with IVDU, sex with bisexual male, sex with HIV–infected person (risk not specified) and receipt of blood transfusions, blood components or tissue. What are possible explanations for the pattern observed in the five categories where there are fewer pediatric AIDS cases than expected in whites and more than expected in Hispanics?

Most of the mismatching above of the r/e distributions can be explained by the differences in birthrates in the r/e groups. In 1985 in the U.S. the births per 1000 women, aged 18 to 44 were 66.9, 76.4 and 107.3 for whites, blacks and Hispanics, respectively (World Almanac, 1988). Thus the birth rate for Hispanic females is 1.6 times as large as for white females and is 1.4 times as large as for black females. In Table 9.5 the ratios of pediatric AIDS cases to female AIDS cases for white, blacks and Hispanics, respectively are: 0.10, 0.13 and 0.17 for the IVDU category, 0.11, 0.12 and 0.18 for the sex with IVDU category and 0.06, 0.11 and 0.18 for the sex with bisexual male category. For these three categories the Hispanic ratios divided by the white ratios are 1.7, 1.6 and 3.0 and the Hispanic ratios divided by the black ratios are 1.3, 1.1 and 1.6; these quotients are roughly consistent with the birth rate quotients of 1.6 and 1.4 obtained above. Thus most of the mismatchings of r/e distributions between pediatric and female AIDS cases in perinatally related categories are explained by the higher birth rates for Hispanic women.

The birth rate for black women is between that for white and Hispanic women so that the matching of percentages for blacks in Table 9.5 is reasonably good. A category where the percentage match is not as good for blacks is the sex with bisexual male category, but the total pediatric AIDS cases (61) in this category is small so that misclassification of a few pediatric cases, particularly in black children , could greatly affect this r/e distribution of pediatric AIDS cases. On the other hand, the large percentage of black pediatric AIDS cases in this category reinforces the earlier suggestions that bisexual behavior may be more common among black homosexual/bisexual males than among white or Hispanic homosexual/bisexual males.

Some of the categories in Table 9.5 have so few pediatric cases that the r/e distributions between pediatric and female AIDS cases could not be expected to match; such categories are sex with person with hemophilia, sex with person born in Pattern II countries and sex with transfusion recipient with HIV. The r/e distributions of AIDS cases in females and children match well for the category of born in a Pattern II country, but they should match since nearly all AIDS cases here are black. For the category of blood transfusion recipients, the r/e distributions do not match well. This may be because the number of pediatric cases is small (60) or because the r/e distribution of pediatric cases depends on the r/e distribution of blood transfusions in women of child—bearing age; data in Section 9.2.4 suggest that blood transfusions are more common in black and Hispanic females. Despite the miscellaneous nature of the undetermined category, the r/e distribution of AIDS cases in females and children are reasonably close.

In a manner similar to the approach in Section 9.2, it is possible to obtain quantitative information about HIV transmission from HIV infected females to their offspring. At a given time the average number E of offspring infected per new HIV case in a female in a specified category is

$$E = \frac{\text{cumulative HIV incidence in offspring of these females}}{\text{cumulative HIV incidence in females in the category}}$$

$$= \frac{K_3(\text{cumulative AIDS incidence in offspring of these females})}{K_4(\text{cumulative AIDS incidence in females in the category})}$$

$$\approx \frac{\text{cumulative AIDS incidence in offspring of these females}}{\text{cumulative AIDS incidence in females in the category}}$$

The constant K_3 might be expected to be greater than the constant K_4 since the HIV epidemic is occurring later in the children, but K_3 would also be lower since children progress more rapidly to AIDS than adults. If these two factors balance out, then K_3 would be approximately equal to K_4 so that the last quotient may be a reasonable approximation to E. Table 9.6 contains cumulative AIDS case data taken from Table 9.5 and also contains the quotients above as estimates of E values.

For six of the ten exposure categories in Table 9.6, the estimates of E are between 0.13 and 0.23 so that they are fairly close together. This suggests that in most exposure categories, for every new HIV case in a female, one can expect approximately 0.18 HIV cases in a child. For females who have had sex with a bisexual male, the estimate of 0.10 for E is lower, but this was also a problem category because of r/e distribution mismatching in Tables 9.3 and 9.5. The low estimate in Table 9.6, together with the mismatching in Tables 9.3 and 9.5, suggest that there may be underreporting or misclassification of white females who were exposed through sex with bisexual males. For females born in Pattern II countries, the estimate of 0.34 for E is about

Table 9.6. Estimates of the average number E of offspring infected per HIV case in
females.

female exposure category	AIDS cases	AIDS cases in their offspring	estimates of E
IVDUs	10,705	1,430	0.13
sex with male IVDUs	4.484	603	0.13
sex with hemophilic males	651	61	0.09
born in Pattern II country	218	244	0.34
sex with male born in Pattern II country	76	14	0.18
sex with transfusion recipient with with HIV infection	161	13	0.08
sex with HIV–infected person, risk not specified	1,065	144	0.14
recipient of blood transfusion, blood components or tissue	1,668	60	0.04
undetermined	1,561	354	0.23

twice that for most of the other categories; it is possible that these black females are twice as
likely to have children as females in the other categories. For females infected through blood
transfusions, the estimate of 0.04 for E is very low, but this is easy to explain since many women
receiving blood transfusions are beyond child–bearing age. In blood transfusion recipients, only
0.34 of adult/adolescent AIDS cases are between 13 and 44 (CDC, 1992).

9.4 Racial/Ethnic Patterns of AIDS Cases in the Northeast Region

It is interesting to carry out these same r/e pattern analyses in the Northeast (NE) region
of the U.S. Comparisons of three subregions of the NE with each other and with the entire U.S.
yield some interesting results. Estimates of yearly AIDS incidences through 1990 in risk groups in
the U.S. and three subregions of the NE region of the U.S. have been obtained from the Centers of
Disease Control. The risk–undetermined AIDS cases have been redistributed and the data have
been adjusted for reporting delays using methods described in Karon et al. (1989). The total
consistent cases as described in Chapter 10 are used here. Graphs of these incidence data as a
function of time are given in Chapter 10.

The three subregions of the NE region are: region A consisting of New York City, region B
consisting of the rest of New York State, New Jersey (minus Philadelphia MSA), Connecticut and
Rhode Island, and region C consisting of Maine, New Hampshire, Vermont, Massachusetts,
Pennsylvania and the portion of Philadelphia MSA in New Jersey. Total consistent case data are
arranged by risk groups and r/e categories for the U.S. and NE regions A, B and C in Tables
9.7–9.9 and 9.12–9.13. These Tables also include r/e percentage distributions and cases per
100,000 population (in each r/e category). The population sizes and r/e percentage

distributions on July 1, 1985 (U.S. Bureau of the Census, 1989) are 185.0 million (78%) white, 28.8 million (12%) black, and 17.5 million (7%) Hispanic for the U.S. In subregion A, there are 7.9 million (65%) white, 2.2 million (18%) black, and 1.7 million (14%) Hispanic. In subregion B, there are 14.1 million (82%) white, 1.9 million (11%) black, and 1.0 million (6%) Hispanic. In subregion C, there are 18.5 million (82%) white, 1.4 million (7%) black, and 0.3 million (1.6%) Hispanic. These tables are useful for comparisons in the following subsections.

9.4.1. Racial/Ethnic Patterns of AIDS Cases in Risk Groups in NE Subregions

For homosexual/bisexual males the AIDS cases per 100,000 r/e population in Table 9.7 are higher for black and Hispanic males than for white males. In particular, the AIDS case rates for blacks and Hispanics are about 1.5 times those of whites in the U.S. and in region A, about 2 times in region B and about 3 times in region C. Note that the cumulative AIDS cases per 100,000 population in New York City are about 2 to 3 times higher than in the U.S. and in regions B and C. This is not surprising since New York City is usually thought to be a preferred place to live by many homosexual men.

From data on male homosexual IVDUs in Table 9.7, the AIDS case rates per 100,000 r/e population are much higher for blacks and Hispanics than for whites. Specifically, the case rates for blacks and Hispanics are about 2 to 3 times those for whites in the U.S., about 4 times in region A, about 6 times in region B and about 9 times in region C. Note for blacks and Hispanics, the cumulative AIDS case rates per 100,000 r/e population in regions B and C are almost as high as those in New York City (region A).

The patterns for male (heterosexual) IVDUs in Table 9.8 are interesting. The AIDS cases per 100,000 population in blacks and Hispanics are always at least 10 times those for whites in the U.S. and in regions A, B and C. For whites the AIDS cases per 100,000 population are about the same in the U.S. and region C and are about 4 times higher in region A (New York City) and region B. For black male (heterosexual) IVDUs the AIDS cases per 100,000 population are about the same in the U.S. and region C, and are about 4 times as high in regions A and B. For Hispanic male IVDUs, the AIDS cases per 100,000 population in regions A, B and C are about 3 to 5 times higher than those in the U.S. In summary, the higher AIDS cases per 100,000 population occur in blacks and Hispanics in regions A and B and in Hispanics in region C. The next highest rates occur in blacks in region C and then for whites in regions A and B. These results suggest that black and Hispanic males are much more likely to be needle–sharing IVDUs than white males or that they are more likely to get an HIV infection, and that the AIDS epidemic in IVDUs is focused in the NE part of the U.S.

The patterns of female IVDUs in Table 9.9 are similar to those for male IVDUs. Namely, the AIDS cases per 100,000 population for blacks and Hispanics are usually more than 10 times those for whites. For whites the AIDS case rates are about the same in the U.S. and region C and are about 3 to 5 times higher in regions A and B; this pattern for white female IVDUs is the same as for white male IVDUs. The pattern for black female IVDUs is similar since the AIDS cases per 100,000 population are similar in the U.S. and region C and are about 4 times higher in regions A and B. For Hispanic female IVDUs the AIDS case rate increases steadily from the U.S. to region

Table 9.7. Total consistent AIDS cases by exposure category and race/ethnicity, through December 1990, with percentages and cases per 100,000 population in the U.S. and the three NE subregions.

region	exposure category	White, not Hispanic		Black, not Hispanic		Hispanic		Total
		No. rate	(%)	No. rate	(%)	No. rate	(%)	No. rate
US	male homosexual/ bisexual contact	73.913 40.0	(71%)	17,878 62.1	(17%)	11,030 63.0	(11%)	104,020 45.0
	male homosexual IV drug user	6,572 3.6	(61%)	2,994 10.4	(28%)	1,151 6.6	(11%)	10,852 4.7
A	male homosexual/ bisexual contact	8,681 109.9	(57%)	3,371 153.2	(22%)	2,870 168.8	(19%)	15,154 128.4
	male homosexual IV drug user	393 5.0	(32%)	464 21.1	(37%)	370 21.8	(30%)	1,240 10.5
B	male homosexual/ bisexual contact	3,732 26.5	(69%)	1,105 58.2	(20%)	558 55.8	(10%)	5,431 31.9
	male homosexual IV drug user	312 2.2	(43%)	298 15.7	(41%)	98 9.8	(14%)	721 4.2
C	male homosexual/ bisexual contact	4,328 23.4	(75%)	1,212 86.6	(21%)	213 71.0	(4%)	5,778 28.6
	male homosexual IV drug user	279 1.5	(53%)	209 14.9	(40%)	37 12.3	(7%)	529 2.6

B to region C to region A with a 7 factor difference between the U.S. and region A. As for male IVDUs, the highest AIDS cases per 100,000 population occurred in blacks and Hispanics in regions A and B and in Hispanics in region C.

9.4.2 Exposure Categories Related by Sexual Contacts in NE Subregions

Two exposure categories linked by sexual contacts are male (heterosexual) IVDUs and females with male IVDU partners. In the U.S. the r/e percentage distributions from Table 9.8 are 22% white, 51% black and 26% Hispanic for male (heterosexual) IVDUs and 20% white, 54% black and 24% Hispanic for females with male IVDU sexual partners. Thus these r/e distributions match well. In region A (New York City) the r/e distributions from Table 9.8 are 15% white, 44% black and 41% Hispanic for male (heterosexual) IVDUs and 11% white, 44%

Table 9.8. Total consistent AIDS cases by exposure category and race/ethnicity, through December 1990, with percentages and case rates per 100,000 population in the U.S. and the three NE subregions.

region	exposure category	White, not Hispanic		Black, not Hispanic		Hispanic		Total
		No. rate	(%)	No. rate	(%)	No. rate	(%)	No. rate
US	male heterosexual IV drug user	5,6433 3.1	(22%)	13,308 46.2	(51%)	6,787 38.8	(26%)	25,918 11.2
	female–sex with IV drug user	735 0.4	(20%)	1,981 6.9	(54%)	868 4.7	(24%)	3,640 1.6
A	male (heterosexual) IV drug user	1,423 18.0	(15%)	4,208 191.3	(44%)	3,942 231.9	(41%)	9,633 81.6
	female–sex with IV drug user	146 1.8	(11%)	565 25.7	(44%)	546 32.1	(43%)	1,277 10.8
B	male (heterosexual) IV drug user	1,488 10.6	(24%)	3,341 175.8	(54%)	1,367 136.7	(22%)	6,222 36.6
	female–sex with IV drug user	166 1.2	(23%)	408 21.5	(58%)	133 13.3	(19%)	709 4.2
C	male (heterosexual) IV drug user	369 2.0	(27%)	553 39.5	(41%)	421 140.3	(31%)	1,354 6.7
	female–sex with IV drug user	59 0.3	(32%)	80 5.7	(43%)	47 15.7	(25%)	186 0.9

black and 43% Hispanic for females with male IVDU sexual partners. These r/e distributions in region A match reasonably well. In region B the r/e distributions from Table 9.8 are 24% white, 54% black and 22% Hispanic for male (heterosexual) IVDUs and 23% white, 58% black and 19% Hispanic for females with male IVDU partners. As in region A these r/e distributions match reasonably well. In region C the r/e distributions from Table 9.8 are 27% white, 41% black and 31% Hispanic for male (heterosexual) IVDUs and 32% white, 43% black and 25% Hispanic for females with male IVDU sexual partners. These r/e distributions in region C do not match as well as in those in regions A and B. The reasons for this mismatching are unknown, but the ratios in the left half of Table 9.10 suggest that there may be some misclassification in the white r/e category in region C. Either too many white females with AIDS are put in the sex with male IVDU category or too few white males with AIDS are put in the heterosexual IVDU

Table 9.9. Total consistent AIDS cases by exposure category and race/ethnicity, through December 1990, with percentages and case rates per 100,000 population in the U.S. and the three NE subregions.

region	exposure category	White, not Hispanic		Black, not Hispanic		Hispanic		Total
		No. rate	(%)	No. rate	(%)	No. rate	(%)	No. rate
US	female IV drug user	1,785 1.0	(22%)	4,885 17.0	(61%)	1,309 7.5	(16%)	8,052 3.5
	male–sex with IV drug user	409 0.2	(28%)	826 2.9	(56%)	193 1.1	(13%)	1,483 0.6
A	female IV drug user	444 5.6	(15%)	1,580 71.8	(53%)	943 55.5	(32%)	2,989 25.3
	male–sex with IV drug user	15 0.2	(20%)	35 1.6	(46%)	23 1.4	(30%)	76 0.6
B	female IV drug user	431 3.1	(24%)	1,199 63.1	(67%)	159 15.9	(9%)	1,796 10.6
	male–sex with IV drug user	71 0.5	(31%)	105 5.5	(45%)	45 4.5	(19%)	232 1.4
C	female IV drug user	150 0.8	(37%)	176 12.6	(44%)	68 22.7	(17%)	401 2.0
	male–sex with IV drug user	32 0.2	(41%)	34 2.4	(43%)	8 2.7	(10%)	79 0.4

category. Except for whites in region C the ratios of AIDS cases in female partners of male IVDUs and AIDS cases in male (heterosexual) IVDUs are all very similar in the left half of Table 9.10.

Two additional exposure categories linked by sexual contacts are female IVDUs and males who had sex with female IVDUs. In the U.S. the r/e distribution from Table 9.9 are 22% white, 61% black and 16% Hispanic for these females and 28% white, 56% black and 13% Hispanic for these males. Thus these r/e distributions do not match very well in the U.S. In region A the r/e distributions from Table 9.9 are 15% white, 53% black and 32% Hispanic for these females and 20% white, 46% black and 30% Hispanic for these males. Again, the r/e distributions do not match very well. In region B the r/e distributions from Table 9.9 are 24% white, 67% black and 9% Hispanic for these females and 31% white, 45% black and 19% Hispanic for these males. These r/e distribution do not match well. In region C the r/e distributions from Table 9.9 are 37% white, 44% black and 17% Hispanic for these females and 41% white, 43% black and 10% Hispanic for these males. The r/e distributions here also do not match well.

126

Table 9.10. Ratios of AIDS cases (from Tables 9.8 and 9.9) by race/ethnicity and region for exposure categories related by sexual contacts in the U.S. and the three NE subregions.

	AIDS cases in female partners / AIDS cases in male IVDUs			AIDS cases in male partners / AIDS cases in female IVDUs		
region	white	black	Hispanic	white	black	Hispanic
U.S.	0.13	0.15	0.13	0.23	0.17	0.15
A	0.10	0.13	0.14	0.03	0.02	0.02
B	0.11	0.12	0.10	0.16	0.09	0.28
C	0.16	0.14	0.11	0.21	0.19	0.12

The variability of the ratios in the right half of Table 9.10 compared to the left half is consistent with the observed mismatchings of r/e distributions. One pattern in the right half of Table 9.10 is that the ratios for region A (New York City) are much smaller than in the U.S. and regions B and C. This is consistent with the belief of Des Jarlais and others in New York City that very few men who are sexual partners of female IVDUs are not IVDUs. The erratic nature of the entries in the right half of Table 9.10 suggests that there may be many misclassifications in the exposure category of males who have a female IVDU sexual partner.

As in Section 9.2.5, it is possible for the NE subregions to estimate a lower bound on the average number D of sexual partners infected per new HIV case. The estimated lower bounds on D are shown in Table 9.11. For male (heterosexual) IVDUs these lower bounds generally agree in the U.S. and the NE subregions, but for female IVDUs and their sexual partners the lower bounds differ greatly. As in Section 9.2.5, these data suggest that some male AIDS cases may be misclassified as sexual partners of female IVDUs or that female IVDUs are highly efficient transmitters of HIV.

9.4.3 Perinatally–Related Exposure Categories in the NE Subregions

The r/e distributions can be compared for exposure categories connected by perinatal HIV transmission. First, consider the categories of pediatric AIDS cases with a mother who is an IVDU and female IVDUs in Table 9.12. In region A the r/e distributions are 9% white, 53% black and 37% Hispanic for these pediatric AIDS cases and 15% white, 53% black and 32% Hispanic for female IVDUs. These r/e distributions do not match very well; the r/e distributions for the U.S. and regions B and C are as bad or worse. Part of the mismatching can be explained as in Section 9.3 by the higher birth rate for Hispanics which is 1.6 times the birth rate for whites and 1.4 times that for blacks. Table 9.13 contains the r/e distribution for pediatric AIDS cases with a mother who is the sexual partner of an IVDU.

Table 9.11. Estimates of lower bounds on the average number D of sexual partners infected per HIV case in the U.S. and the three NE subregions.

region	exposure category	AIDS cases	fraction with sexual partners	AIDS cases in sexual partners	lower bound on D
US	male (heterosexual) IVDUs	25,918	0.67	3,640	0.21
A	male (heterosexual) IVDUs	9,633	0.67	1,277	0.20
B	male (heterosexual) IVDUs	6,222	0.67	709	0.17
C	male (heterosexual) IVDUs	1,354	0.67	186	0.21
US	female IVDUs	8,052	0.08	1,483	2.26
A	female IVDUs	2,989	0.08	76	0.32
B	female IVDUs	1,796	0.08	232	1.61
C	female IVDUs	401	0.08	79	2.46

Instead of looking at r/e percentage distributions it is better to look at the ratios of pediatric AIDS cases to female AIDS cases in the associated mother category; recall from Section 9.3 that this ratio is an estimate of the average number E of offspring infected per HIV case in females. These ratios as estimates of E are given in Table 9.14 of females who are IVDUs and females who have had male IVDU sexual partners. Note that the ratios in the r/e categories in the U.S. generally agree on the left and right sides of Table 9.14. This agreement reinforces the concept that most of the differences in these estimates of E can be explained by differences in birth rates in the r/e groups. In particular for female IVDUs the E estimates for Hispanics are 1.4 times that of blacks and 1.8 times that of whites; these are roughly consistent with the birth rate for Hispanics being 1.4 times that of blacks and 1.6 times that of whites (World Almanac, 1988).

In Table 9.14 the estimates of E in region A are somewhat like those in the U.S. in Table 9.6, but the estimates of E in regions B and C are more erratic. In the left half of Table 9.14 the low ratio for whites in region C suggests that there may be some underreporting of white pediatric AIDS cases with an IVDU mother or overreporting of female IVDUs. On both sides of Table 9.14 the estimates of E seem somewhat high for Hispanics in region C, which suggests overreporting in children or underreporting of AIDS cases in Hispanic females in region C (such underreporting could also explain why AIDS cases in female IVDUs are only 11% of all IVDU cases in region C). The large estimate of 0.26 for Hispanics in region B on the left side and the large estimate of 0.18 for blacks in region C on the right side do not have any obvious explanations.

Table 9.12. Total consistent AIDS cases by exposure category and race/ethnicity, through December 1990, with percentages and case rates per 100,000 population in the U.S. and the three NE subregions.

region	exposure category	White, not Hispanic		Black, not Hispanic		Hispanic		Total
		No. rate	(%)	No. rate	(%)	No. rate	(%)	No. rate
US	female IV drug user	1,785 1.0	(22%)	4,885 17.0	(61%)	1,309 7.5	(16%)	8,052 3.5
	pediatric—mother with IV drug use	178 0.1	(15%)	693 2.4	(59%)	268 1.5	(13%)	1,171 0.5
A	female IV drug user	444 5.6	(15%)	1,580 71.8	(53%)	943 55.5	(32%)	2,989 25.3
	pediatric—mother with IV drug use	45 0.6	(9%)	257 11.7	(53%)	178 10.7	(37%)	485 4.1
B	female IV drug user	431 3.1	(24%)	1,199 63.1	(67%)	159 15.9	(9%)	1,796 10.6
	pediatric—mother with IV drug use	50 0.4	(21%)	143 7.5	(60%)	42 4.2	(18%)	240 1.4
C	female IV drug user	150 0.8	(37%)	176 12.6	(44%)	68 22.7	(17%)	401 2.0
	pediatric—mother with IV drug use	8 0.1	(14%)	25 1.8	(44%)	21 7.0	(37%)	57 0.3

9.5 Discussion

Compared to the racial/ethnic distribution of the population in the United States, AIDS cases occur relatively more frequently in blacks and Hispanics than in whites. The relative frequencies of AIDS cases in r/e groups in the U.S. are analyzed in Section 9.1 for adult/adolescent males and females and for children. These values are not given here since the relative frequencies of AIDS in r/e groups for risk categories are more interesting.

The cumulative AIDS cases in homosexual/bisexual males per 100,000 r/e population size are consistently 1.5 to 3 times higher for blacks and Hispanics than for whites in the NE subregions and in the U.S. Moreover, these AIDS case rates are 2 to 3 times higher in New York City than in the rest of the NE region and in the entire U.S. Possible explanations are that males are slightly more likely to be homosexual/bisexual if they are black or Hispanic or if they live in New York City.

Table 9.13. Total consistent pediatric AIDS cases by exposure category and race/ethnicity, through December 1990, with percentages and case rates per 100,000 population in the U.S. and the three NE subregions.

region	exposure category	White, not Hispanic		Black, not Hispanic		Hispanic		Total
		No. rate	(%)	No. rate	(%)	No. rate	(%)	No. rate
US	female–sex with IV drug user	735 0.4	(20%)	1,981 6.9	(54%)	868 4.7	(24%)	3,640 1.6
	pediatric–mother with sex with IV drug user	72 0.0	(16%)	224 0.8	(49%)	142 0.8	(31%)	459 0.2
A	female-sex with IV drug user	146 1.8	(11%)	565 25.7	(44%)	546 32.1	(43%)	1,277 0.8
	pediatric–mother with sex with IV drug user	12 0.2	(7%)	65 3.0	(39%)	83 4.9	(49%)	168 1.4
B	female-sex with IV drug user	166 1.2	(23%)	408 21.5	(58%)	133 13.3	(19%)	709 4.2
	pediatric–mother with sex with IV drug user	13 0.1	(17%)	42 2.2	(54%)	17 1.7	(22%)	78 0.5
C	female-sex with IV drug user	59 0.3	(32%)	80 5.7	(43%)	47 15.7	(25%)	186 0.9
	pediatric–mother with sex with IV drug user	7 0.0	(18%)	14 1.0	(37%)	15 5.0	(39%)	38 0.2

The cumulative AIDS cases in male (heterosexual) and female IVDUs per 100,000 r/e population size are at least 10 times higher for blacks and Hispanics than for whites in the three NE subregions and in the U.S. These AIDS case rates in male (heterosexual) IVDUs are between 3 and 10 times higher than in female IVDUs. The AIDS case rates for black (heterosexual) male IVDUs is highest in regions A and B, and lowest in region C. For Hispanic male (heterosexual) IVDUs, the AIDS case rates are highest in region A and are also quite high in the regions B and C. The data suggest that people are much more likely to be IVDUs or IVDUs who develop AIDS if they are black or Hispanic or if they are males or if they live in the NE region of the U.S.

In the U.S. the cumulative AIDS cases in male homosexual IVDUs per 100,000 r/e population size are 2 to 3 times larger for blacks and Hispanics than for whites. In the three NE subregions, the AIDS case rates for blacks and Hispanics are 4 to 10 times higher than for whites. Since these men have both homosexual behavior and IVDU behavior, it is not surprising that the

Table 9.14. Estimates of the average number E of offspring infected per HIV case in females by race/ethnicity and region in the U.S. and the three NE subregions.

region	estimates of E for female IVDUs			estimates of E for females who had sex with male IVDUs		
	white	black	Hispanic	white	black	Hispanic
U.S.	0.11	0.14	0.20	0.10	0.11	0.16
A	0.10	0.16	0.19	0.08	0.12	0.15
B	0.12	0.12	0.26	0.08	0.10	0.13
C	0.05	0.14	0.31	0.12	0.18	0.32

ratios above comparing r/e groups are between those of homosexual/bisexual men and those of male (heterosexual) IVDUs.

Comparisons of the r/e distributions of AIDS cases in females who have had sex with a bisexual male with AIDS cases in homosexual/bisexual males suggest that black homosexual/bisexual males may be slightly more likely to be bisexual than white or Hispanic homosexual/bisexual males.

With one minor exception described in Section 9.4.2, there is good matching in the three NE subregions and in the U.S. of the r/e percentage distributions of cumulative AIDS cases in male (heterosexual) IVDUs and females who have had sex with male IVDUs. The r/e distributions of cumulative AIDS cases do not match well in any NE subregion or in the U.S. for female IVDUs and (non IVDU) male sexual partners of females IVDUs. A possible explanation is that it is difficult to decide if a male belongs in this exposure category of having a female IVDU sexual partner, but not being an IVDU, so that many misclassifications occur.

In Section 9.2 the average number D of sexual partners infected per HIV case has been defined and an expression for a lower bound on D has been obtained. Estimates in Table 9.4 of these lower bounds range from 0.19 for male (heterosexual) IVDUs and females born in Pattern II countries to 0.06 – 0.09 for hemophiliacs, blood transfusion recipients and males born in Pattern II countries. The data seem to imply that for every 6 new HIV cases in male (heterosexual) IVDUs with female sexual partners, at least one HIV case occurs in their female sexual partners.

The r/e distributions of cumulative AIDS cases in the U.S. match reasonably well in Table 9.3 for the following exposure categories and their sexual partners: 1) males with hemophilia or coagulation disorder, 2) males born in Pattern II countries, 3) males who received blood transfusions, 4) females who received blood transfusions, 5) males in the other/undetermined category and 6) females in the other/undetermined category. The data suggest that black and Hispanic females may receive blood transfusions slightly more frequently than white females.

The r/e distribution of cumulative AIDS cases do not match at all for females born in Pattern II countries and males who have had sex with a female born in a Pattern II country. Nearly all AIDS cases in these females are black, but about half of the AIDS cases in their male sexual partners category are black and half are white. Although some of the white males could be misclassifications, it is more likely that many white males did have sex with blacks females from Pattern II countries.

For many exposure categories of children and females related through perinatal transmission, the racial/ethnic distributions of AIDS cases do not match very well since the percentage of pediatric AIDS cases is consistently low for whites and high for Hispanics. However, as noted in Sections 9.3 and 9.4.3, this pattern can usually be explained since the birth rate for Hispanic females is 1.6 times that for white females. For many exposure categories, the estimates in Table 9.6 suggest that for each 6 or 7 new HIV cases in females, there is approximately 1 new HIV case in a child. Deviations from this pattern noted in Section 9.4.3 suggests that there may be some under or overreporting in pediatric or female cases in some r/e groups in some NE subregions.

CHAPTER 10

REGIONAL COMPARISONS OF HIV AND AIDS IN RISK GROUPS

The goal of this chapter is to use the computer simulation model developed in Chapter 7 to analyze HIV transmission and AIDS in risk groups in the four major regions of the United States shown in Figure 10.1. Each region is divided into three to five subregions based on similarities and differences in AIDS incidences in parts of the region. Whenever there are no significant differences in the time trends in AIDS incidences between racial/ethnic (r/e) groups or subregions, AIDS cases in the groups or subregions are aggregated. Thus the first step in each region is to aggregate into as few subpopulations as possible. Aggregation simplifies the simulation process since it leads to fewer populations to fit. Of course, the HIV and AIDS incidences in the groups or subregions which were aggregated could be recovered at any time by using the fraction of cases which occurred in these groups or subregions.

Each aggregated population is fit using the computer simulation model described in Chapter 7. When male and female IVDUs are aggregated, the fit to AIDS incidences in these IVDUs is found and then the model is fit to AIDS incidences in their heterosexual partners; finally, the model is fit to pediatric AIDS incidences in the children of the female IVDUs and the female heterosexual partners. For each of the four regions, the section in this Chapter devoted to the aggregation process is followed by a section on computer simulations of the aggregated groups. Parameter values in the best fitting simulations are compared among subpopulations, subregions and regions at the end of the Chapter. The different parameter values provide a quantitative measure of the differences in time trends in AIDS incidences.

Data have been furnished by Debra Hanson in the Statistics and Data Management Branch, Division of HIV/AIDS, Center for Infectious Diseases, National Centers for Disease Control. She has sent yearly AIDS incidence estimates for all cases and consistent cases through 1990; these are based on reported AIDS incidences through September 1, 1991 which have been adjusted for reporting delays with redistribution of unclassified cases. Recall from Section 5.4 that the consistent cases are those with a diagnosis (definitive or presumptive) of a disease in the pre–1987 case definition. The expansion of AIDS surveillance definition in 1987 increased the number of patients reported with AIDS. The method used in Section 5.4 is also used here to estimate the total consistent cases by adding the modified nonconsistent cases to the consistent cases. All fitting in this chapter uses these total adjusted consistent case estimates. Data were sent for the major risk groups in subregions in the four regions of the United States. The subregions were chosen to reflect similarities and differences in AIDS incidences in the various parts of each region.

The Northeast (NE) region consists of the New England and Mid–Atlantic states. The North Central (NC) region contains the East and West North Central states. The South (S) region has the South Atlantic and the East and West South Central states. The West (W) region contains the Mountain and Pacific states (including Alaska and Hawaii). The data for the regions, risk groups, subregions and r/e groups are often identified by code words according to

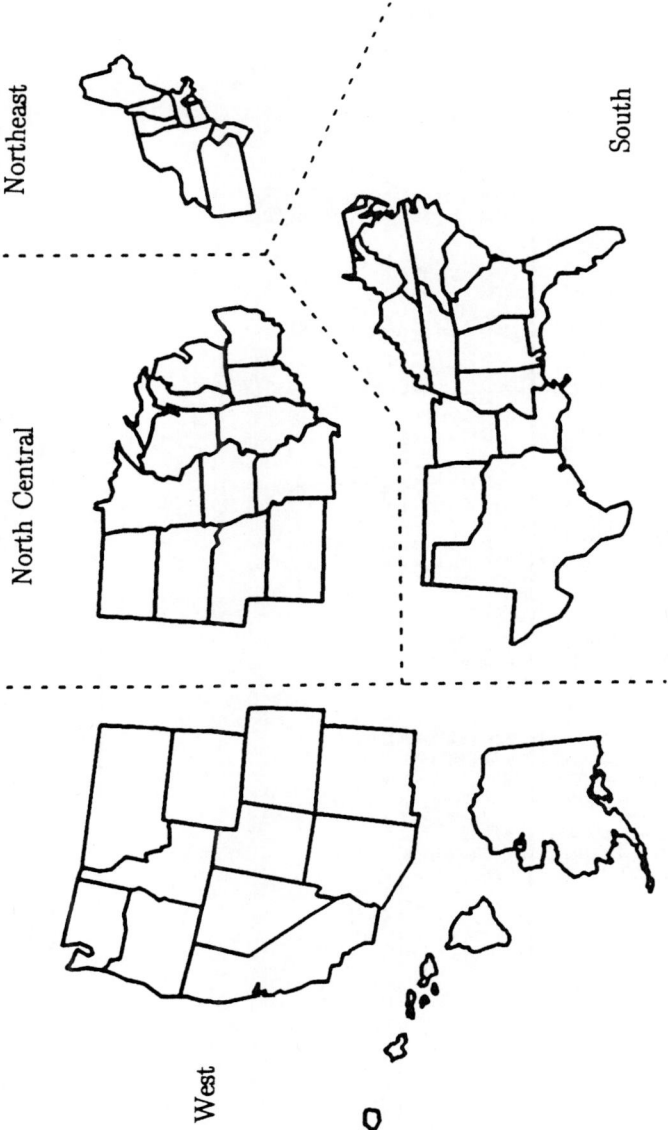

Figure 10.1 The four major regions of the United States.

Table 10.1. Coding scheme for identifying risk groups

First Character(s) (region):
  NE — Northeast
  NC — North Central
  S — South
  W — West

Next Two Characters (risk group):
  01 or 1M — Homosexual and bisexual men, not using IV drugs
  03 or 3M — Homosexual and bisexual male IV drug users (IVDU)
  2M   — Male heterosexual IVDU
  2F   — Female IVDU
  2T   — Male heterosexual and female IVDUs
  5M   — Male sex partners of IVDUs
  5F   — Female sex partners of IVDUs
  5T   — Male and female heterosexual partners of IVDUs
  16   — Perinatal; mother is IVDU
  17   — Perinatal; mother is sex partner of IVDU
  12 or CT — Perinatal; mother is IVDU or sex partner of IVDU

Next Character (subregion):
  T — all subregions (total)
  Northeast:
  A — New York City (NYC) MSA (Metropolitan Statistical Area)
  B — New York (minus NYC), New Jersey (minus Philadelphia MSA),
        Connecticut, Rhode Island
  C — Maine, New Hampshire, Vermont, Massachusetts,
        Pennsylvania, portion of Philadelphia MSA in New Jersey
  North Central:
  A — Chicago MSA
  B — Detroit MSA
  C — Other MSAs with populations over one million
  D — Other MSAs with populations under one million
  South:
  A — Florida
  B — Texas
  C — Washington,D.C. and Baltimore MSA
  D — Other MSAs with populations over one million including Atlanta,
        New Orleans, Norfolk, Charlotte and the part of Cincinnati in Kentucky
  E — All other areas in the South region
  West:
  A — San Francisco and Seattle MSAs
  B — Los Angeles, Oakland, Anaheim, Riverside, and San Jose MSAs
  C — All other areas in the West region

Last Character (racial/ethnic group):
  W — White
  B — Black
  H — Hispanic
  T — All racial/ethnic groups (total)

the scheme given in a Table 10.1. For example, NE01AW refers to the Northeast region, homosexual/bisexual men, subregion A (New York City) and the white racial/ethnic category.

10.1. Simplifications Based on Modeling New York City

Chapter 8 on modeling HIV and AIDS in New York City (NYC) has yielded some useful results. The NYC populations of homosexual men and the heterosexual IVDUs were first fit separately. Then the populations of homosexual men, homosexual IVDUs, and heterosexual IVDUs were fit with both linkages through homosexual and needle–sharing partnerships. The interesting result is that the parameter values for the homosexual men and the heterosexual IVDUs are nearly the same as when these populations are fit separately. Thus the homosexual IVDUs do not serve as an important link in which the HIV epidemic in one population feeds or sustains the epidemic in the other population. Hence the homosexual IVDU linkage is not necessary, and can be eliminated. The time trends in AIDS incidence in homosexual IVDUs are similar to that for homosexual men in NYC so that the simulations for homosexual IVDUs would be similar to those for the homosexual men. Based on the NYC modeling experience, the homosexual men are always fit as a separate population in this regional modeling. Since the AIDS incidence in homosexual IVDUs is much smaller and they have incidence patterns similar to homosexual men, they are not fit explicitly. The heterosexual IVDUs are modeled and fit as a separate population. After parameter values are found for simulation of AIDS incidences in IVDUs, the average number PAP of heterosexual partnerships per month is adjusted to fit the AIDS incidence in heterosexual partners and then the fecundity FC is adjusted to fit the perinatal AIDS incidence. Note that only one parameter is varied in order to fit the AIDS data for heterosexual partners and only one parameter is varied to fit the perinatal AIDS data.

In the NYC modeling the value of PAP which gives the best fit is 0.0318 new partners per month, which corresponds to about one new heterosexual partner per IVDU every 2.6 years. Thus the AIDS incidence in heterosexual partners is consistent with very slow partner turnover. In the NYC modeling the value of the fecundity FC which fit the perinatal data is 0.005 births per female per month. This is close to the reported national birth rate since there are about 70 births per 1000 women per year (World Almanac, 1988) which corresponds to about 0.006 births per female per month. The average probability of transmission during birth by women in the infectious stages is 0.22 in the model.

10.2. The Northeast Region: Aggregation of Racial/Ethnic and Risk Groups

It is important to know in each risk group if the trends over time of the AIDS cases in the r/e groups in the three Northeast (NE) subregions are the same or different. Recall that the three r/e groups and three NE subregions are defined in Table 10.1. If the time trends are the same in the r/e groups or in the subregions, then these groups or subregions can be aggregated together and the larger category can be fit in simulation models. If the time trends in AIDS cases are different in r/e groups or subregions, then they cannot be aggregated and must be modeled separately. Aggregation of groups is a distinct advantage in simulation modeling, since fewer

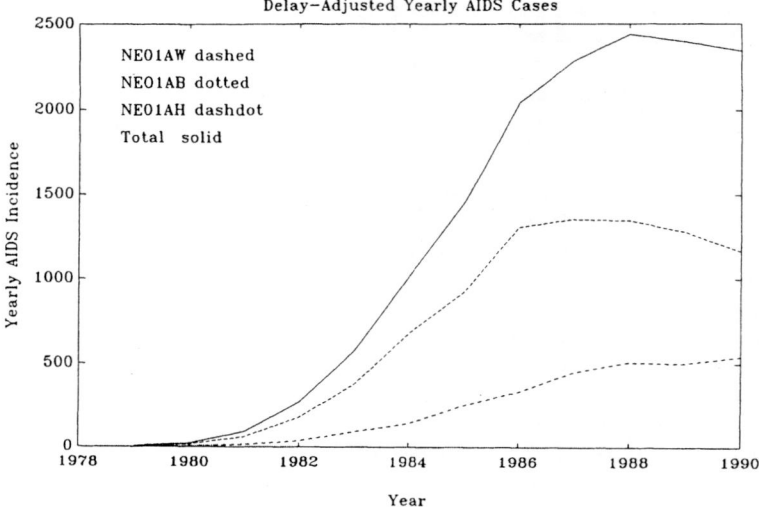

Figure 10.2. AIDS incidence in white, black, and Hispanic homosexual men in NE subregion A (New York City).

groups must be simulated. Of course, the AIDS case incidences in the subgroups which have been aggregated could be recovered at a given time by using the percentages of cases occurring in these subgroups.

First, consider the risk group of homosexual/bisexual males with AIDS case rates in the three r/e groups and the three subregions shown in Figures 10.2 to 10.4. In region A the AIDS cases in all three r/e groups increase steadily until about 1986, after which the AIDS cases continue to increase in blacks and Hispanics, but seem to level off and decrease in whites. Thus in region A (New York City) the time trend in white homosexual males seems to be different from that in black and Hispanic homosexual males. Thus white homosexual/bisexual males should be analyzed separately and should not be aggregated; however, blacks and Hispanics can be aggregated.

For homosexual/bisexual males in regions B and C, the time trends in r/e groups in Figures 10.3 and 10.4 are less clear. Tables giving the r/e percentage distributions each year in each subregion have been printed out, but are not included here. Although there are some differences in 1990, the r/e distributions over time in regions B and C seem to remain reasonably constant. Thus lumping the r/e groups together in each region B and C seems reasonable. Moreover, from the graphs of the total AIDS cases in the regions, it is reasonable to lump regions B and C together. Thus for homosexual/bisexual males the three aggregated groups shown in Figure 10.5 seem to be needed: 1) whites in region A, 2) blacks and Hispanics in region A and 3) all r/e groups in regions B and C.

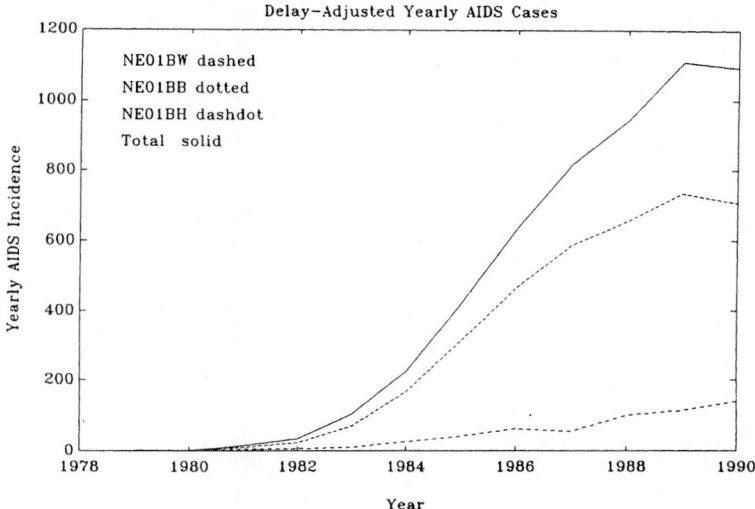

Figure 10.3. AIDS incidence in white, black, and Hispanic homosexual men in NE subregion B.

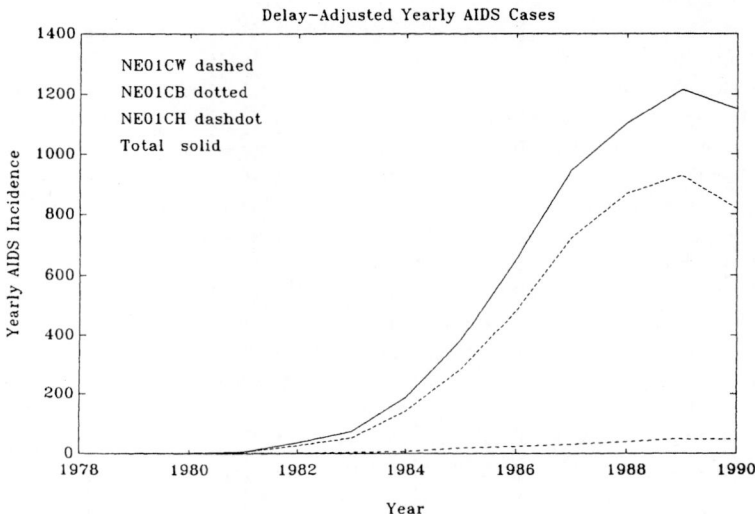

Figure 10.4. AIDS incidence in white, black, and Hispanic homosexual men in NE subregion C.

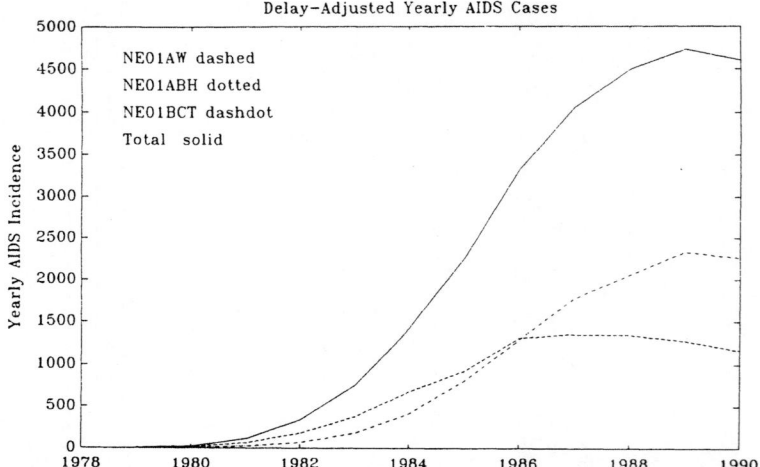

Figure 10.5. AIDS incidence in homosexual men who are whites in NE subregion A (New York City), blacks and Hispanics (other r/e groups) in subregion A, and all r/e groups in subregions B and C (other subregions.)

For homosexual IVDU males, the AIDS incidence in the r/e groups in the NE regions often jumps up and down from year to year in an erratic fashion. These jumps may be due to random fluctuations or may be due to changes in classification or reporting. Conclusions about aggregation or disaggregation in homosexual IVDUs are difficult since clear trends are not evident. Figure 10.6 shows the AIDS incidence for homosexual IVDUs aggregated in the same way as homosexual men in Figure 10.5. The patterns in Figure 10.6 are generally the same as in Figure 10.5 since white males in region A seem to level off in about 1986, but homosexual IVDUs in other r/e groups in region A increase more rapidly up to 1987 and then decrease. In both Figures 10.5 and 10.6, AIDS incidence outside region A increases through 1989. Thus the aggregation of homosexual IVDUs in Figure 10.6 may be reasonable.

For male (heterosexual) IVDUs in Figures 10.7 to 10.9, there do not seem to be any major differences between the r/e groups in the trends in the regions. In region A the r/e distribution is consistently about 15% whites, 43% blacks and 42% Hispanics. In region B the r/e distribution is also uniform over time with 23% whites, 56% blacks and 20% Hispanics. The pattern in region C is slightly erratic, but the r/e distribution does not differ greatly over time from 27% whites, 40% blacks and 31% Hispanics. The graphs of the totals in Figure 10.10 reveal that the AIDS cases are growing together in regions A and B, but are growing faster in region C after 1986. Thus for male (heterosexual) IVDUs, two aggregated groups seem appropriate: 1) all r/e groups in regions A and B, and 2) all r/e groups in region C.

The AIDS incidences in female IVDUs in the r/e groups in the NE regions are smaller, but are similar to those for male (heterosexual) IVDUs so aggregation of r/e groups within the NE

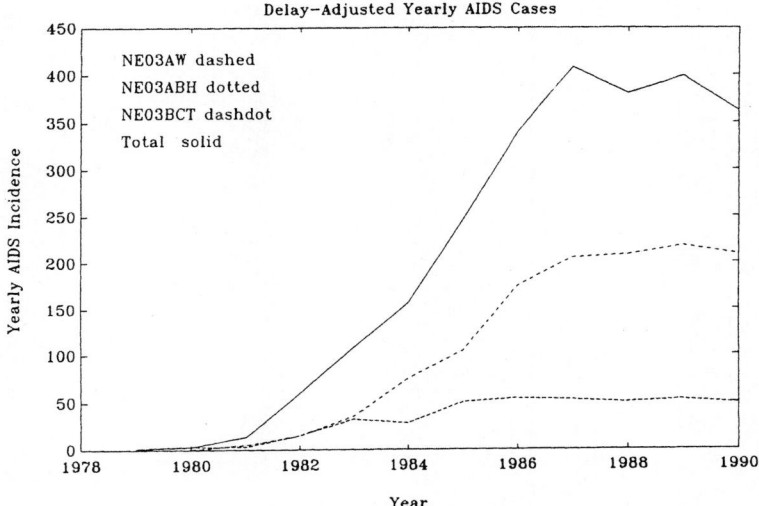

Figure 10.6. AIDS incidence in homosexual IVDUs who are white in NE subregion A (New York City), blacks and Hispanic in subregion A, and all r/e groups in subregions B and C (other subregions).

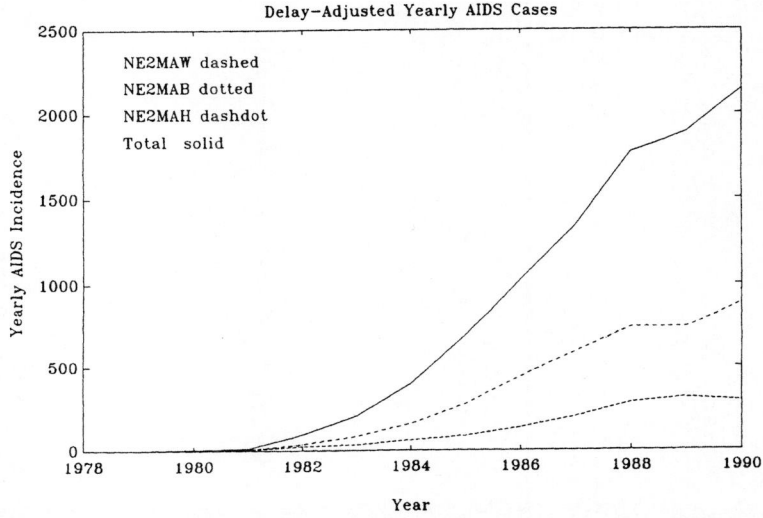

Figure 10.7. AIDS incidence in male (heterosexual) IVDUs who are white, black, and Hispanic in NE subregion A (New York City).

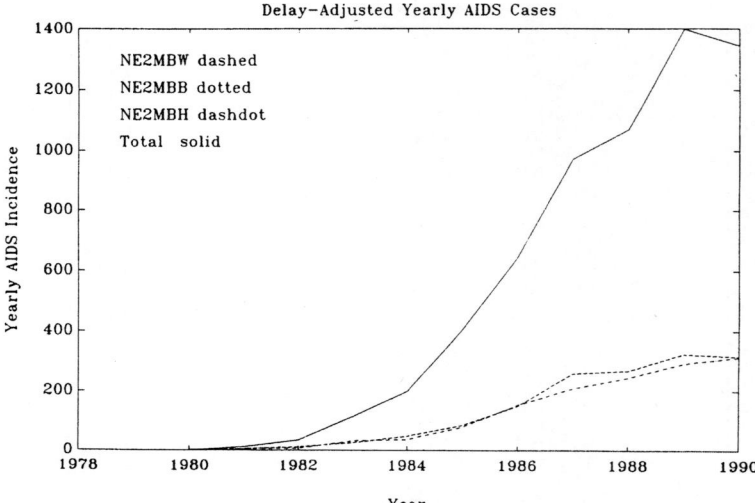

Figure 10.8. AIDS incidence in male (heterosexual) IVDUs who are white, black, and Hispanic in NE subregion B.

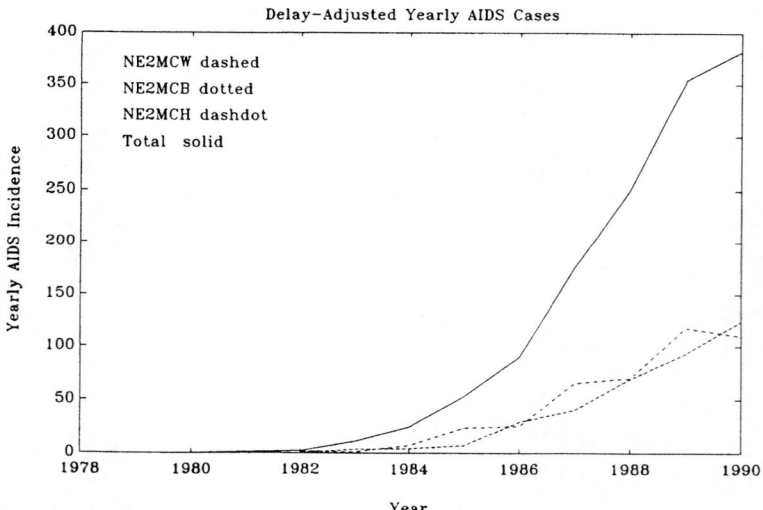

Figure 10.9. AIDS incidence in male (heterosexual) IVDUs who are white, black, and Hispanic in NE subregion C.

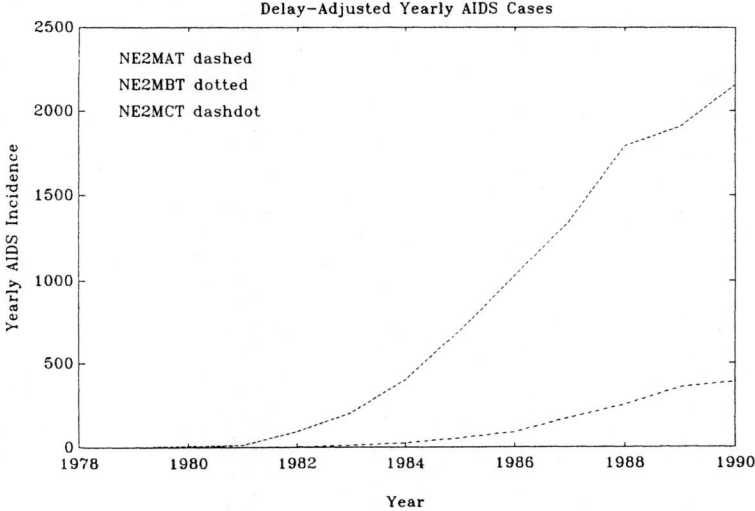

Figure 10.10. AIDS incidence in male (heterosexual) IVDUs in NE subregions A, B, and C.

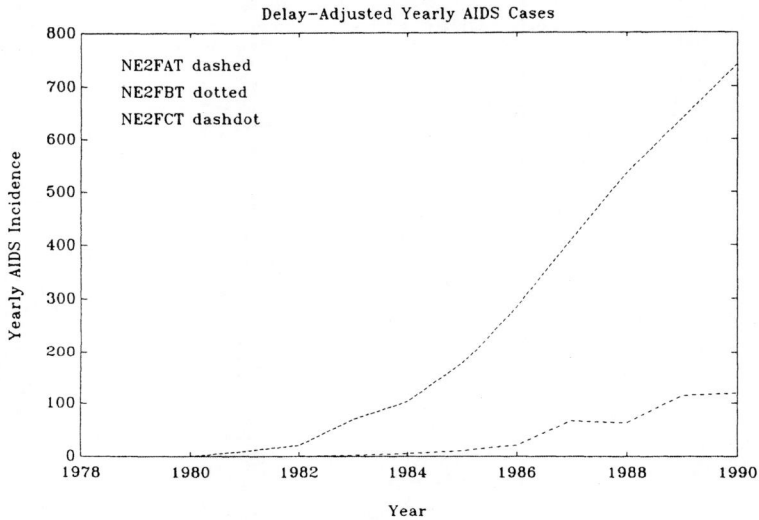

Figure 10.11. AIDS incidence in female IVDUs in NE subregions A, B, and C.

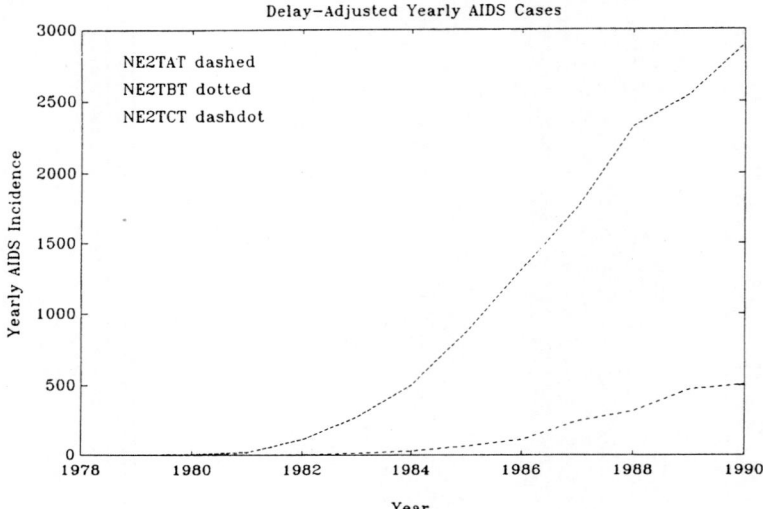

Figure 10.12. AIDS incidence in combined male (heterosexual) and female IVDUs in NE subregions A, B, and C.

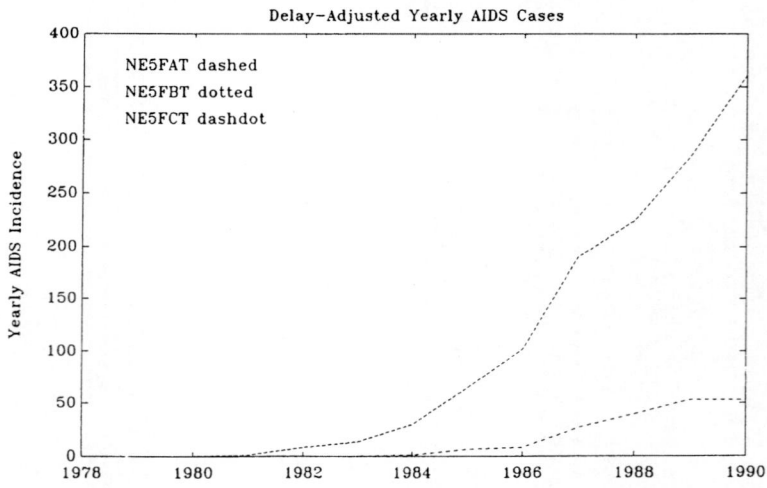

Figure 10.13. AIDS incidence in heterosexual partners of male IVDUs in NE subregions A, B, and C.

regions is reasonable. Figure 10.11 shows the AIDS incidences in female IVDUs in the three NE regions. The time trends are similar to those in Figure 10.10 so the male and female IVDUs can also be aggregated. Figure 10.12 shows the combined male and female IVDUs in the three regions. The AIDS incidence in region C starts lower and then grows faster than in regions A and B. Thus it is reasonable to combine regions A and B, but region C must be treated separately.

Yearly AIDS incidences for female heterosexual partners of IVDUs for the three regions are shown in Figure 10.13. Since the numbers of cases in the r/e groups is small in each region, these r/e groups have been combined. The time trends in Figure 10.13 are similar to those for male (heterosexual) IVDUs in Figure 10.10. Note that in region C the initial growth rate is low, but the growth rate after 1986 is higher in region C than in regions A and B. Figure 10.13 shows that combining regions A and B, but treating C separately, is also reasonable for female heterosexual partners of IVDUs. Yearly AIDS incidences for male sexual partners of female IVDUs are very erratic, especially in regions A and C where there are very few cases. The detailed analysis in Chapter 9 of r/e patterns suggests that many males may be misclassified as heterosexual partners of female IVDUs. Because the number of cases is small and there are no distinct patterns, both female and male heterosexual partners are combined.

Since the AIDS incidences in children in the r/e groups in the three regions are small and subject to random fluctuations and changes in reporting practices, the graphs are rather erratic. Combining r/e groups usually leads to smoother graphs for the larger populations. Figure 10.14 shows the yearly pediatric AIDS cases in children whose mothers are either IVDUs or heterosexual partners of IVDUs. The time trends in Figure 10.14 are roughly similar to those for female IVDUs in Figure 10.11 and for female heterosexual partners of IVDUs in Figure 10.13. The AIDS incidence in children in region B drops down in 1988 primarily due to unexplainable decreases in AIDS cases in black children. Since there is no similar decrease in AIDS cases in black female IVDUs or partners of IVDUs, the lower incidences in 1988 are probably due to a reporting problem in some part of region B. Generally, the combination of cases in regions A and B, but not with region C, also seems reasonable for pediatric cases.

The two primary reasons why the three subregions of the NE region of the U.S. were originally chosen are: 1) the HIV epidemic in homosexual men is different inside and outside New York City and 2) the HIV epidemic in IVDUs is different in regions A and B (New York, New Jersey, Connecticut and Rhode Island) than in region C (the other NE states). The aggregations suggested in this Section by comparing time trends justify these choices of subregions. For homosexual/bisexual males, all r/e groups in regions B and C can be lumped, but region A (New York City) is different. Only for homosexual/bisexual males in New York City is it necessary to analyze time trends for r/e groups separately; namely, the AIDS incidence curve for white males has a different character from the AIDS incidence curve for black and Hispanic males. For male and female IVDUs, all r/e groups can be aggregated in each region and regions A and B can be aggregated, but region C is different. The aggregation into these two groups also seems to work for exposure categories connected to IVDUs; namely, for female sexual partners of male IVDUs, for children with IVDU mothers and for children of female sexual partners of male IVDUs.

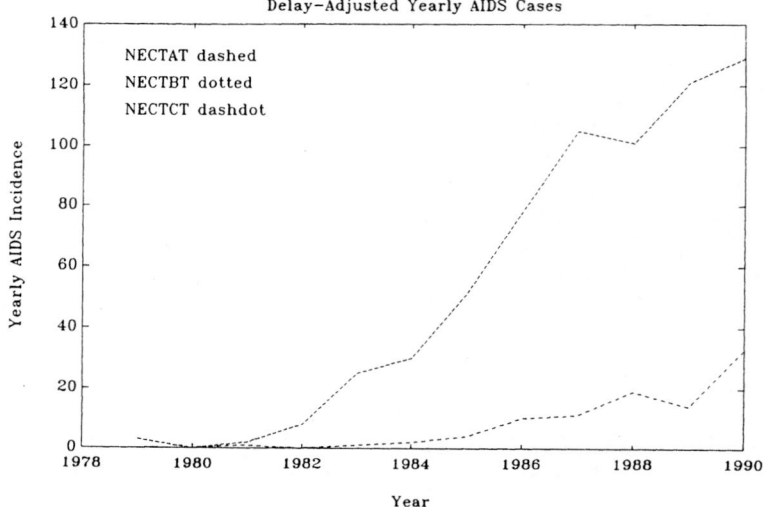

Figure 10.14. AIDS incidence in children of female IVDUs and heterosexual partners of male IVDUs in NE subregions A, B, and C.

10.3. The Northeast Region: Computer Simulations of the Aggregated Groups

The simulation model described in Chapter 7 has been fit to the AIDS incidences of the aggregated groups found in Section 10.2. The parameter values and simulation values for the white homosexual men in New York City (labeled NE01AW) are given in Table 10.2 and the HIV and AIDS incidences are given in Figure 10.15. Table 10.3 and Figure 10.16 correspond to the black and Hispanic homosexual men in NYC (labeled NE01ABH). Table 10.4 and Figure 10.17 correspond to AIDS in all r/e groups in regions B and C (labeled NE01BCT). The NE subregions A, B and C are defined in Table 10.1. Many of the parameter values in the simulation are fixed at the values found from the detailed analysis in Chapter 6 of HIV incidences and AIDS incidences in homosexual men in San Francisco. The parameters which have been varied to fit the AIDS incidences in the NE region are the population size, the epidemic starting year, the external mixing fraction, the average number of partners per month before reduction, the reduction starting and stopping dates, and the yearly reduction factor.

Based on data in Chapter 6 for homosexual men in San Francisco, rules of thumb are used for obtaining crude guesses for two of the parameter values. The homosexual population size is crudely estimated to be 7.67 times the total AIDS cases through 1989. The epidemic starting year is approximately 7 years before the date when the cumulative AIDS cases reach 40. This crude starting date estimate and the population estimate often work reasonably well. For example, the populations of homosexual men at risk for HIV in New York City are estimated to be 60,000 for

145

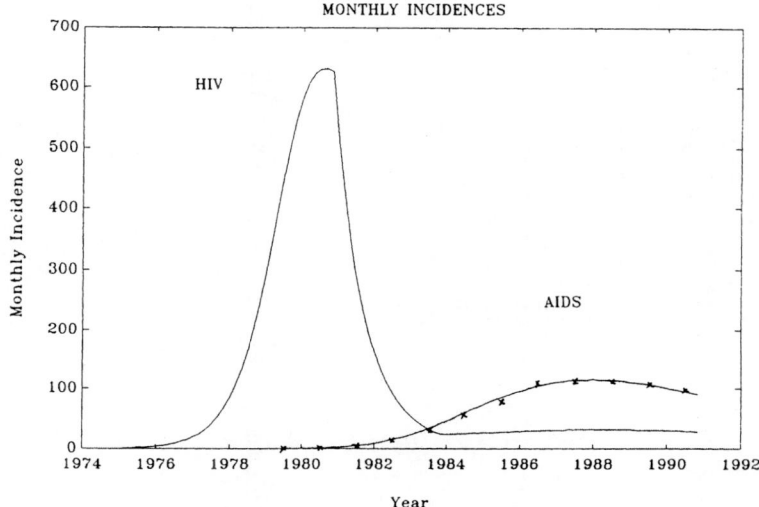

Figure 10.15. Estimated AIDS incidences (*) and simulated HIV and AIDS incidences for white homosexual men in NE subregion A (New York City) corresponding to parameter values in Table 10.2.

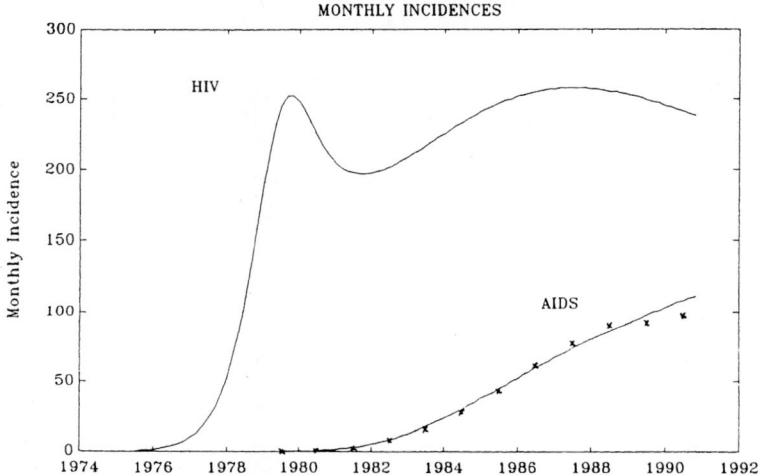

Figure 10.16. Estimated AIDS incidences for black and Hispanic homosexual men in NE subregion A (New York City) corresponding to parameter values in Table 10.3.

Table 10.2 Parameter values and corresponding simulation values for white homosexual men in NYC.

```
THE POPULATION SIZE IS        60000, THE VERY ACTIVE FRACTION IS
   1.000000E-01 AND THE ACTIVITY RATIO IS        10.000000
THE NATURAL MORTALITY RATE XMU IS   5.320000E-04
THE INTERCHANGE RATE  FROM THE VERY ACTIVE CLASS TO THE ACTIVE CLASS IS
   4.166667E-03  AND THE TURNOVER RATE IS DLT =    4.166667E-03
THE NUMBER OF INFECTIOUS STAGES IS  M =        7
THE G PARAMETERS FOR THE TRANSFER BETWEEN STAGES ARE    7.355444E-02
   6.433708E-02     4.867545E-02     4.199281E-02    3.997889E-02
   5.152515E-02     5.398798E-02
THE WEIGHTS OF TRANSMISSION PER INFECTIOUS PARTNER TIMES THE FRACTION STILL
SEXUALLY ACTIVE FOR THE STAGES ARE WRH(I) =        2.000000        1.000000
   1.000000         1.500000         1.500000        1.500000
   7.500000
THE PROBABILITY OF TRANSMISSION IS QH =     5.000000E-02
THE EXTERNAL MIXING FRACTION IS ETA =        1.000000
THE AVERAGE NUMBER OF PARTNERS PER MONTH IS    5.633000E-01 BEFORE        1981
   1, THEN IT IS REDUCED EACH YEAR BY A FACTOR OF    3.401000E-01UNTIL
DEC,    1983
THE STARTING YEAR AND MONTH ARE        1974        4
THE STARTING NUMBER OF VERY ACTIVE INFECTIVES IS   1.000000

          ***********************************************
```

YEAR	HIV INC SIM	HIV PREV	FRACTNAL PREV ALL	V_A ACT	ACT	YR AIDS DATA	INC SIM	AIDS(SIMULATION) PREV	DTHS	OUTSF
1974	5.	5.	.00	.00	.00	*****	0.	0.	0.	0.
1975	23.	28.	.00	.00	.00	*****	0.	0.	0.	0.
1976	103.	128.	.00	.01	.00	*****	0.	0.	0.	0.
1977	455.	567.	.01	.05	.01	*****	0.	0.	0.	0.
1978	1789.	2289.	.04	.19	.02	*****	1.	1.	0.	0.
1979	4947.	7001.	.12	.51	.07	3.	4.	3.	1.	1.
1980	7370.	13798.	.23	.80	.17	16.	16.	15.	5.	2.
1981	4209.	17102.	.29	.85	.22	62.	58.	54.	19.	9.
1982	1350.	17412.	.29	.81	.23	178.	170.	161.	62.	31.
1983	475.	16762.	.28	.75	.23	377.	383.	380.	164.	82.
1984	304.	15816.	.26	.68	.22	677.	677.	714.	343.	174.
1985	337.	14731.	.25	.61	.21	918.	984.	1112.	585.	302.
1986	366.	13498.	.22	.54	.19	1305.	1225.	1492.	845.	445.
1987	384.	12150.	.20	.48	.17	1354.	1355.	1779.	1069.	575.
1988	390.	10753.	.18	.42	.15	1347.	1369.	1931.	1217.	670.
1989	380.	9378.	.16	.36	.13	1278.	1291.	1947.	1275.	718.
1990	359.	8089.	.13	.31	.12	1166.	1155.	1851.	1250.	722.

CHISQ =   11.852450

Table 10.3 Parameter values and corresponding simulation values for black and Hispanic homosexual men in NYC.

```
THE POPULATION SIZE IS        40000, THE VERY ACTIVE FRACTION IS
  1.000000E-01 AND THE ACTIVITY RATIO IS        10.000000
THE NATURAL MORTALITY RATE XMU IS    5.320000E-04
THE INTERCHANGE RATE   FROM THE VERY ACTIVE CLASS TO THE ACTIVE CLASS IS
  4.166667E-03   AND THE TURNOVER RATE IS DLT =    4.166667E-03
THE NUMBER OF INFECTIOUS STAGES IS  M =        7
THE G PARAMETERS FOR THE TRANSFER BETWEEN STAGES ARE     7.355444E-02
  6.433708E-02     4.867545E-02     4.199281E-02     3.997889E-02
  5.152515E-02     5.398798E-02
THE WEIGHTS OF TRANSMISSION PER INFECTIOUS PARTNER TIMES THE FRACTION STILL
SEXUALLY ACTIVE FOR THE STAGES ARE WRH(I) =        2.000000      1.000000
  1.000000        1.500000        1.500000        1.500000
  7.500000
THE PROBABILITY OF TRANSMISSION IS QH =    5.000000E-02
THE EXTERNAL MIXING FRACTION IS ETA =    4.168000E-01
THE AVERAGE NUMBER OF PARTNERS PER MONTH IS    4.581000E-01 BEFORE        2222
  1, THEN IT IS REDUCED EACH YEAR BY A FACTOR OF        1.000000UNTIL
DEC,     2222
THE STARTING YEAR AND MONTH ARE        1974        12
THE STARTING NUMBER OF VERY ACTIVE INFECTIVES IS      1.000000

           ***************************************************
```

YEAR	HIV INC SIM	HIV PREV	FRACTNAL PREV ALL	V_A	ACT	YR AIDS DATA	INC SIM	AIDS(SIMULATION) PREV	DTHS	OUTSF
1974	0.	1.	.00	.00	.00	*****	0.	0.	0.	0.
1975	8.	9.	.00	.00	.00	*****	0.	0.	0.	0.
1976	47.	55.	.00	.01	.00	*****	0.	0.	0.	0.
1977	261.	308.	.01	.06	.00	*****	0.	0.	0.	0.
1978	1169.	1438.	.04	.27	.01	*****	0.	0.	0.	0.
1979	2722.	4016.	.10	.66	.04	2.	2.	2.	0.	0.
1980	2770.	6490.	.16	.88	.08	7.	9.	8.	2.	1.
1981	2406.	8467.	.21	.92	.13	32.	34.	31.	11.	5.
1982	2420.	10327.	.26	.93	.18	93.	95.	91.	36.	18.
1983	2587.	12198.	.30	.93	.24	195.	203.	204.	90.	45.
1984	2782.	14070.	.35	.92	.29	335.	351.	374.	181.	92.
1985	2948.	15885.	.40	.89	.34	529.	523.	589.	307.	159.
1986	3056.	17567.	.44	.87	.39	738.	699.	831.	457.	240.
1987	3097.	19051.	.48	.83	.44	932.	868.	1080.	619.	330.
1988	3076.	20286.	.51	.80	.48	1089.	1023.	1323.	780.	422.
1989	3008.	21248.	.53	.76	.51	1115.	1164.	1552.	935.	513.
1990	2908.	21932.	.55	.73	.53	1174.	1289.	1761.	1079.	599.

CHISQ =   25.353680

Table 10.4 Parameter values and corresponding simulation values for homosexual men in NE subregions B and C.

```
THE POPULATION SIZE IS        250000, THE VERY ACTIVE FRACTION IS
   1.000000E-01 AND THE ACTIVITY RATIO IS        10.000000
THE NATURAL MORTALITY RATE XMU IS    5.320000E-04
THE INTERCHANGE RATE  FROM THE VERY ACTIVE CLASS TO THE ACTIVE CLASS IS
   4.166667E-03  AND THE TURNOVER RATE IS DLT =     4.166667E-03
THE NUMBER OF INFECTIOUS STAGES IS  M =        7
THE G PARAMETERS FOR THE TRANSFER BETWEEN STAGES ARE    7.355444E-02
   6.433708E-02    4.867545E-02    4.199281E-02    3.997889E-02
   5.152515E-02    5.398798E-02
THE WEIGHTS OF TRANSMISSION PER INFECTIOUS PARTNER TIMES THE FRACTION STILL
SEXUALLY ACTIVE FOR THE STAGES ARE WRH(I) =           2.000000        1.000000
       1.000000        1.500000        1.500000        1.500000
       7.500000
THE PROBABILITY OF TRANSMISSION IS QH =     5.000000E-02
THE EXTERNAL MIXING FRACTION IS ETA =     2.960000E-02
THE AVERAGE NUMBER OF PARTNERS PER MONTH IS     3.287000E-01 BEFORE          1984
       7, THEN IT IS REDUCED EACH YEAR BY A FACTOR OF     3.809000E-01UNTIL
DEC,       1987
THE STARTING YEAR AND MONTH ARE         1975          1
THE STARTING NUMBER OF VERY ACTIVE INFECTIVES IS        1.000000

        ************************************************
```

YEAR	HIV INC SIM	HIV PREV	FRACTNAL PREV ALL	V_A ACT	PREV	YR AIDS DATA	INC SIM	AIDS(SIMULATION) PREV	DTHS	OUTSF
1975	4.	5.	.00	.00	.00	*****	0.	0.	0.	0.
1976	20.	24.	.00	.00	.00	*****	0.	0.	0.	0.
1977	88.	109.	.00	.00	.00	*****	0.	0.	0.	0.
1978	391.	486.	.00	.02	.00	*****	0.	0.	0.	0.
1979	1638.	2066.	.01	.08	.00	2.	1.	1.	0.	0.
1980	5480.	7317.	.03	.28	.00	2.	3.	3.	1.	0.
1981	9964.	16630.	.07	.61	.01	21.	14.	13.	4.	2.
1982	8019.	23495.	.09	.83	.01	69.	55.	51.	17.	8.
1983	4953.	26965.	.11	.90	.02	176.	176.	165.	61.	30.
1984	3641.	28858.	.12	.90	.03	412.	431.	421.	175.	87.
1985	1865.	28713.	.11	.85	.03	806.	827.	853.	395.	200.
1986	986.	27418.	.11	.77	.04	1288.	1300.	1428.	725.	372.
1987	507.	25364.	.10	.68	.04	1772.	1752.	2058.	1123.	586.
1988	403.	22961.	.09	.59	.04	2060.	2095.	2629.	1523.	810.
1989	470.	20459.	.08	.51	.03	2337.	2277.	3050.	1856.	1008.
1990	513.	17950.	.07	.43	.03	2264.	2290.	3268.	2072.	1149.

CHISQ =   14.260470

149

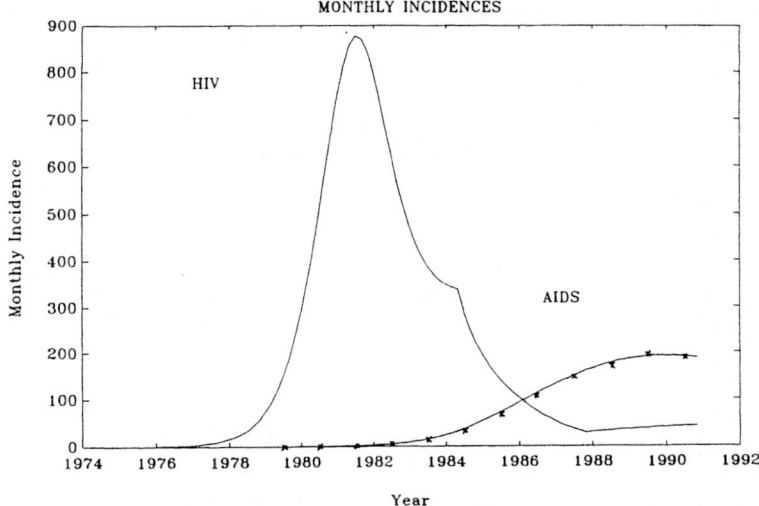

Figure 10.17. Estimated AIDS incidences (*) and simulated HIV and AIDS incidences for homosexual men in all r/e groups in NE subregions B and C corresponding to parameter values in Table 10.4.

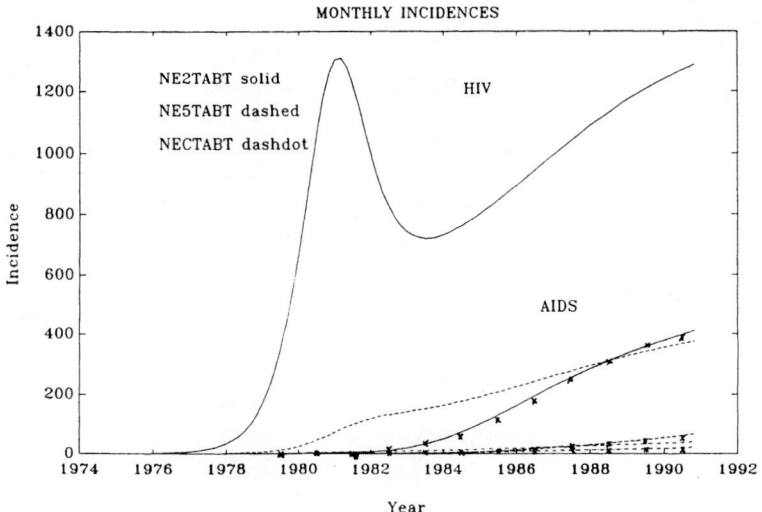

Figure 10.18. Estimated AIDS incidences (*) and simulated HIV and AIDS incidences for IVDUs, their heterosexual partners, and related pediatric cases in NE subregions A and B corresponding to parameter values in Table 10.5.

whites and 40,000 for blacks and Hispanics. The total of 100,000 homosexual men at risk in New York City is the same as the estimate in Chapter 8 on New York City.

A computer program (see Appendix), which varies the values of the external mixing fraction ETA, the average number of partners PAS and the yearly reduction factor RDN, has been used to find these values for various reduction starting and stopping dates. Comparisons of outputs of these computer runs leads to the best fitting simulations in the sense that the chi–square value for fitting the AIDS incidence curve is minimized. The simulations shown in Figures 10.15–10.17 are not meant to be predictive since other simulations also yield adequate fits. More specifically, the HIV incidences in recent years may not be as high as shown in Figure 10.16; the HIV incidences shown occur because the AIDS incidences have not yet shown a clear decrease. A detailed sensitivity analysis has not been carried out for each data set. However, the other adequate simulations usually have similar parameter values so comparisons of the parameter values can be enlightening.

Rather than go through Tables 10.2 to 10.4 individually, it is more interesting to compare parameter values in these Tables. The epidemic starting dates are April 1974 for whites in NYC, December 1974 for blacks and Hispanics in NYC and January 1975 for homosexual men in regions B and C. The slightly later start in blacks and Hispanics in NYC and in homosexual men outside NYC is not surprising. The population estimates of 100,000 homosexual men at risk inside NYC and 250,000 in the NE outside NYC seem plausible.

The average number of partners per month before reduction is 0.56 for white homosexual men in NYC, 0.46 for black and Hispanic men in NYC, and 0.33 for homosexual men in NE outside NYC. This suggests that the initial growth rate was fastest in white homosexual men in NYC, slower for NYC blacks and Hispanics and slowest outside NYC.

A striking difference is that the AIDS incidence for the blacks and Hispanics in NYC have been fit without any reductions in sexual behavior, but reductions have been necessary to fit the white homosexual men in NYC. This difference is consistent with the AIDS incidence graphs in Figure 10.5. For homosexual men in regions B and C, the best fit involves a reduction in high risk behavior, but the fit without any change in behavior is almost as good. For NYC white homosexual men, the reduction factor of 0.34 per year from January 1981 through 1983 yields an overall reduction factor of 0.039 over the 3 year period. Thus the decrease in AIDS incidence in white homosexual men in NYC in recent years can be explained by a precipitous decrease in high risk sexual behavior, starting in 1981. The other two populations of homosexual men have been fit adequately without such precipitous decreases, but recent decreases in AIDS incidence suggest that change in behavior may have occurred later in these populations.

The external mixing fraction, ETA, is different in Tables 10.2 to 10.4. For white homosexual men in NYC, ETA is 1, which corresponds to proportional mixing (random mixing) between the very active and active risk groups. For black and Hispanic homosexual men in NYC, ETA is 0.42 which means the very active and active risk groups are less strongly connected. For homosexual men outside NYC, the connection between the very active and active groups is very weak since ETA = 0.03. One reason why ETA is small is that the population size is large (250,000) and most of the AIDS cases so far have occurred in the one—tenth (25,000) that are in the very active group. Indeed, in some reasonably good fits, ETA was zero so there was no connection between the very active and active groups. The weak connection implies that there could be a biphasic epidemic with the first epidemic in the very active group and the second, later epidemic in the active risk group. It is interesting that fits to the homosexual men outside NYC with smaller population sizes had larger values of ETA so the active and very active groups were more closely linked.

For IVDUs in the NE the two aggregated groups from Section 10.2 are all IVDUs in regions A and B (labeled NE2TOT) and all IVDUs in region C (labeled NE2TCT). Many of the parameter values in the simulations of AIDS incidence in IVDUs are the same as those used for homosexual men. For example, HIV—infected IVDUs are assumed to progress towards AIDS and death in the same way as homosexual men. Simulations which fit the AIDS incidence data for the two IVDU groups are shown in Tables 10.5 and 10.6 and in Figures 10.18 and 10.19. Only the parameter values which are varied to fit the data are compared and discussed.

The population size estimates are 300,000 IVDUs at risk in regions A and B and 100,000 IVDUs in region C. These estimates are educated guesses. They use information such as the estimate in Chapter 8 on NYC that there are 150,000 IVDUs in NYC (region A). In Chapter 9 on r/e patterns it was estimated that 3/4 of IVDU are men, 2/3 of IVDU men have a female sexual partner who is not an IVDU and almost no female IVDUs have a non—IVDU male sexual partner. Since $(3/4)(2/3) = 1/2$, the population sizes of heterosexual partners are set at half of the IVDU population sizes. In the NE subregions A and B, 23% of AIDS cases in IVDUs are women and 86% of AIDS cases in heterosexual partners are women; these percentages are 23% and 70% in subregion C.

In Table 10.5 corresponding to subregions A and B, the IVDUs are fit without any reduction in needle—sharing partnership rates. The connection between the very active and active groups is somewhat weak since ETA = 0.15, but this seems to be due to the large population size. In Table 10.6 corresponding to subregion C, the initial number of needle—sharing partners per month is higher than in Table 10.5, but there is a yearly reduction of 0.72 starting in July 1981. In Table 10.6, ETA = 1 so the high and low activity groups are very closely connected. The epidemic starting date in regions A and B is January 1975, but it is January 1977 in region C. Visually the differences in the behaviors and fits don't seem that much different in Figures 10.18 and 10.19 except that the peak HIV incidence is about 3 years later in subregion C than in subregions A and B. As in Figure 10.16 the high HIV incidences in recent years are not predictions; they occur because the observed AIDS incidences have not yet indicated that there has been a decrease in needle—sharing partnerships.

152

Table 10.5 Parameter values and corresponding simulation values for IVDUs, heterosexual partners and related pediatric cases in NE subregions A and B.

```
THE IVDU & HTRO POPULATION SIZES ARE      300000      150000
THE VERY ACTIVE FRACTION IS    1.000000E-01
THE ACTIVITY RATIO IS     10.000000
THE NATURAL MORTALITY RATE XMU IS   5.320000E-04
THE INTERCHANGE RATE  FROM THE VERY ACTIVE CLASS TO THE ACTIVE CLASS IS
  4.166667E-03  AND THE TURNQVER RATE IS DLT =   4.166667E-03
THE NUMBER OF INFECTIOUS STAGES IS  M =      7
THE G PARAMETERS FOR THE TRANSFER BETWEEN ADULT STAGES ARE    7.355444E-02
  6.433708E-02    4.867545E-02    4.199281E-02   3.997889E-02
  5.152515E-02    5.398798E-02
THE WEIGHTS OF TRANSMISSION PER INFECTIOUS PARTNER TIMES THE FRACTION STILL
SEXUALLY ACTIVE FOR THE STAGES ARE WRH(I) =         2.000000        1.000000
  1.000000            1.500000        1.500000        1.500000
  7.500000
THE PROBABILITIES OF TRANSMISSION ARE QH, QHP & QC =    5.000000E-02
  1.000000E-01    1.000000E-01
THE EXTERNAL MIXING FRACTION IS ETA =    1.518000E-01
THE AVERAGE NUMBER OF NEEDLE-SHARING PARTNERS PER MONTH IS    3.766000E-01
BEFORE       2222        2, THEN IT IS REDUCED EACH YEAR BY A FACTOR OF
  1.000000 UNTIL DEC,    2222
THE FRACTION OF IVDU WHO ARE WOMEN IS   2.300000E-01
THE FRACTION OF HETEROSEXUALS WHO ARE WOMEN IS    8.600000E-01
THE AVERAGE NUMBER OF IVDU PARTNERS OF HETEROSEXUALS PER MONTH IS
  2.700000E-02
THE FRACTION    3.400000E-01 OF CHILDREN PROGRESS RAPIDLY TO AIDS WITH RATE
CONSTANT   8.000000E-02. OTHERS MOVE THROUGH M STAGES WITH SPEED FACTOR
  1.550000
THE FECUNDITY FC (CHILDREN/MONTH) IS    5.900000E-03
THE STARTING YEAR AND MONTH ARE     1975          0
THE STARTING NUMBER OF VERY ACTIVE INFECTIVES IS     1.000000
****************************************************

THE SIMULATED INCIDENCES ARE GIVEN ON THE NEXT PAGE
```

153

YEAR	CLASS	HIV INC	HIV PREV	FRACTNAL_PREV ALL	V_A	PREV ACT	YR AIDS DATA	INC SIM	AIDS(SIMULATION) PREV	DTHS	OUTSF
1975	IVDU	6.	7.	.00	.00	.00	0.	0.	0.	0.	0.
	HTRO	0.	0.	.00	-	-	****	0.	0.	0.	0.
	PED	0.	0.	-	-	-	0.	0.	0.	0.	
1976	IVDU	32.	39.	.00	.00	.00	0.	0.	0.	0.	0.
	HTRO	1.	1.	.00	-	-	0.	0.	0.	0.	0.
	PED	0.	0.	-	-	-	0.	0.	0.	0.	
1977	IVDU	166.	199.	.00	.01	.00	0.	0.	0.	0.	0.
	HTRO	5.	6.	.00	-	-	0.	0.	0.	0.	0.
	PED	0.	0.	-	-	-	0.	0.	0.	0.	
1978	IVDU	837.	1009.	.00	.03	.00	0.	0.	0.	0.	0.
	HTRO	26.	31.	.00	-	-	0.	0.	0.	0.	0.
	PED	1.	2.	-	-	-	0.	0.	0.	0.	
1979	IVDU	3796.	4676.	.02	.14	.00	0.	1.	1.	0.	0.
	HTRO	123.	150.	.00	-	-	0.	0.	1.	0.	0.
	PED	7.	8.	-	-	-	3.	1.	1.	0.	
1980	IVDU	11473.	15639.	.05	.45	.01	5.	6.	3.	2.	1.
	HTRO	479.	611.	.00	-	-	0.	0.	3.	0.	0.
	PED	27.	34.	-	-	-	1.	3.	4.	2.	
1981	IVDU	14793.	29175.	.10	.78	.02	34.	29.	9.	8.	4.
	HTRO	1108.	1659.	.01	-	-	1.	1.	9.	0.	0.
	PED	66.	95.	-	-	-	5.	9.	12.	6.	
1982	IVDU	10497.	37750.	.13	.89	.04	162.	118.	19.	37.	18.
	HTRO	1540.	3069.	.02	-	-	9.	4.	19.	1.	1.
	PED	100.	181.	-	-	-	11.	19.	24.	14.	
1983	IVDU	8748.	44078.	.15	.92	.06	414.	360.	31.	129.	64.
	HTRO	1796.	4647.	.03	-	-	17.	15.	31.	5.	2.
	PED	127.	283.	-	-	-	36.	31.	37.	25.	
1984	IVDU	9063.	50162.	.17	.92	.08	744.	824.	45.	349.	174.
	HTRO	2086.	6412.	.04	-	-	47.	41.	45.	16.	8.
	PED	157.	402.	-	-	-	45.	45.	52.	38.	
1985	IVDU	10032.	56494.	.19	.91	.11	1386.	1484.	63.	741.	376.
	HTRO	2448.	8409.	.06	-	-	99.	92.	63.	40.	20.
	PED	194.	543.	-	-	-	82.	63.	72.	54.	
1986	IVDU	11188.	63094.	.21	.90	.13	2158.	2243.	86.	1294.	667.
	HTRO	2858.	10656.	.07	-	-	203.	171.	86.	84.	43.
	PED	239.	708.	-	-	-	121.	86.	96.	74.	
1987	IVDU	12353.	69868.	.23	.87	.16	3026.	2990.	113.	1949.	1021.
	HTRO	3280.	13127.	.09	-	-	319.	278.	113.	153.	78.
	PED	288.	897.	-	-	-	162.	113.	126.	98.	
1988	IVDU	13437.	76707.	.26	.84	.19	3712.	3658.	144.	2631.	1402.
	HTRO	3683.	15768.	.11	-	-	423.	409.	144.	246.	128.
	PED	341.	1110.	-	-	-	144.	144.	159.	128.	
1989	IVDU	14382.	83507.	.28	.81	.22	4344.	4229.	179.	3281.	1778.
	HTRO	4049.	18513.	.12	-	-	541.	560.	179.	363.	191.
	PED	395.	1344.	-	-	-	171.	179.	196.	161.	
1990	IVDU	15162.	90165.	.30	.78	.25	4655.	4724.	218.	3872.	2129.
	HTRO	4370.	21295.	.14	-	-	635.	728.	218.	501.	267.
	PED	449.	1595.	-	-	-	190.	218.	236.	198.	

CHISQD =   49.249570
CHISQP =   32.489760
CHISQC =   51.331530
SUM OF CHISQ-D,P,C =   133.070800

Table 10.6 Parameter values and corresponding simulation values for IVDUs, heterosexual partners and related pediatric cases in NE subregion C.

```
THE IVDU & HTRO POPULATION SIZES ARE        100000        50000
THE VERY ACTIVE FRACTION IS     1.000000E-01
THE ACTIVITY RATIO IS        10.000000
THE NATURAL MORTALITY RATE XMU IS    5.320000E-04
THE INTERCHANGE RATE   FROM THE VERY ACTIVE CLASS TO THE ACTIVE CLASS IS
    4.166667E-03   AND THE TURNOVER RATE IS DLT =     4.166667E-03
THE NUMBER OF INFECTIOUS STAGES IS  M =      7
THE G PARAMETERS FOR THE TRANSFER BETWEEN ADULT STAGES ARE    7.355444E-02
    6.433708E-02     4.867545E-02     4.199281E-02    3.997889E-02
    5.152515E-02     5.398798E-02
THE WEIGHTS OF TRANSMISSION PER INFECTIOUS PARTNER TIMES THE FRACTION STILL
SEXUALLY ACTIVE FOR THE STAGES ARE WRH(I) =        2.000000      1.000000
    1.000000         1.500000         1.500000         1.500000
    7.500000
THE PROBABILITIES OF TRANSMISSION ARE QH, QHP & QC =     5.000000E-02
    1.000000E-01     1.000000E-01
THE EXTERNAL MIXING FRACTION IS ETA =        1.000000
THE AVERAGE NUMBER OF NEEDLE-SHARING PARTNERS PER MONTH IS    4.852000E-01
BEFORE     1981          7, THEN IT IS REDUCED EACH YEAR BY A FACTOR OF
    7.150000E-01 UNTIL DEC,      1987
THE FRACTION OF IVDU WHO ARE WOMEN IS     2.300000E-01
THE FRACTION OF HETEROSEXUALS WHO ARE WOMEN IS     7.000000E-01
THE AVERAGE NUMBER OF IVDU PARTNERS OF HETEROSEXUALS PER MONTH IS
    4.600000E-02
THE FRACTION    3.400000E-01 OF CHILDREN PROGRESS RAPIDLY TO AIDS WITH RATE
CONSTANT     8.000000E-02. OTHERS MOVE THROUGH M STAGES WITH SPEED FACTOR
    1.550000
THE FECUNDITY FC (CHILDREN/MONTH) IS     6.200000E-03
THE STARTING YEAR AND MONTH ARE        1977          1
THE STARTING NUMBER OF VERY ACTIVE INFECTIVES IS       1.000000
*******************************************************

THE SIMULATED INCIDENCES ARE GIVEN ON THE NEXT PAGE
```

ne2tct.m ne2tct.m ne2tct.m ne2tct.m ne2tct.m
****

YEAR	CLASS	HIV INC	HIV PREV	FRACTNAL PREV ALL	V_A	ACT	YR AIDS DATA	INC SIM	AIDS(SIMULATION) PREV	DTHS	OUTSF
1977	IVDU	6.	6.	.00	.00	.00	0.	0.	0.	0.	0.
	HTRO	0.	0.	.00	-	-	****	0.	0.	0.	0.
	PED	0.	0.	-	-	-	0.	0.	0.	0.	
1978	IVDU	20.	25.	.00	.00	.00	0.	0.	0.	0.	0.
	HTRO	1.	1.	.00	-	-	0.	0.	0.	0.	0.
	PED	0.	0.	-	-	-	0.	0.	0.	0.	
1979	IVDU	70.	93.	.00	.00	.00	0.	0.	0.	0.	0.
	HTRO	4.	6.	.00	-	-	0.	0.	0.	0.	0.
	PED	0.	0.	-	-	-	0.	0.	0.	0.	
1980	IVDU	248.	331.	.00	.02	.00	0.	0.	0.	0.	0.
	HTRO	16.	21.	.00	-	-	0.	0.	0.	0.	0.
	PED	1.	1.	-	-	-	0.	0.	0.	0.	
1981	IVDU	791.	1087.	.01	.05	.01	1.	1.	0.	0.	0.
	HTRO	56.	75.	.00	-	-	0.	0.	0.	0.	0.
	PED	2.	3.	-	-	-	1.	0.	0.	0.	
1982	IVDU	1465.	2456.	.02	.12	.01	2.	3.	1.	1.	0.
	HTRO	146.	213.	.00	-	-	0.	0.	1.	0.	0.
	PED	6.	8.	-	-	-	0.	1.	1.	0.	
1983	IVDU	1798.	4071.	.04	.19	.02	13.	.9.	2.	3.	1.
	HTRO	264.	459.	.01	-	-	0.	1.	2.	0.	0.
	PED	11.	18.	-	-	-	1.	2.	2.	1.	
1984	IVDU	1719.	5512.	.06	.25	.03	30.	27.	3.	10.	5.
	HTRO	377.	801.	.02	-	-	1.	2.	3.	1.	0.
	PED	17.	32.	-	-	-	2.	3.	4.	2.	
1985	IVDU	1439.	6584.	.07	.29	.04	64.	67.	6.	27.	14.
	HTRO	466.	1210.	.02	-	-	6.	6.	6.	2.	1.
	PED	22.	50.	-	-	-	4.	6.	6.	4.	
1986	IVDU	1134.	7268.	.07	.31	.05	112.	134.	8.	62.	31.
	HTRO	536.	1660.	.03	-	-	10.	13.	8.	5.	3.
	PED	28.	71.	-	-	-	10.	8.	9.	7.	
1987	IVDU	872.	7606.	.08	.31	.05	244.	226.	11.	120.	61.
	HTRO	593.	2136.	.04	-	-	35.	26.	11.	12.	6.
	PED	33.	95.	-	-	-	11.	11.	13.	10.	
1988	IVDU	794.	7778.	.08	.31	.05	316.	333.	15.	199.	103.
	HTRO	643.	2623.	.05	-	-	55.	47.	15.	24.	12.
	PED	39.	121.	-	-	-	19.	15.	17.	13.	
1989	IVDU	848.	7908.	.08	.31	.05	469.	437.	19.	291.	153.
	HTRO	697.	3120.	.06	-	-	76.	73.	19.	42.	21.
	PED	46.	150.	-	-	-	14.	19.	21.	17.	
1990	IVDU	897.	7994.	.08	.30	.06	504.	523.	24.	385.	206.
	HTRO	746.	3615.	.07	-	-	82.	106.	24.	65.	34.
	PED	52.	181.	-	-	-	33.	24.	26.	21.	

CHISQD =   11.419700
CHISQP =   11.762620
CHISQC =   10.166080
SUM OF CHISQ-D,P,C =   33.348400

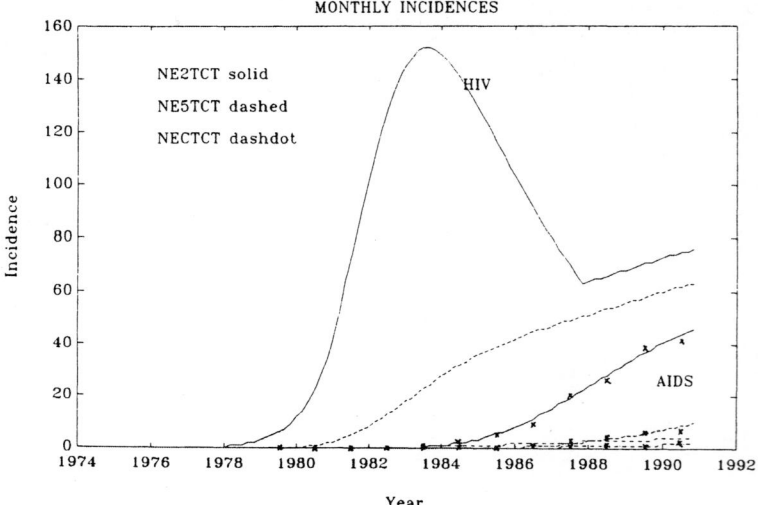

Figure 10.19. Estimated AIDS incidences (*) and simulated HIV and AIDS incidences for IVDUs, their heterosexual partners, and related pediatric cases in NE subregion C corresponding to parameter values in Table 10.6.

In Chapter 9 on r/e patterns, it was found that the AIDS incidence in heterosexual partners relative to that in IVDUs is higher in region C than in regions A and B. Thus it is not surprising that the average number of heterosexual partners per month of IVDUs in region C is 70% higher than that in regions A and B. The values of the fecundity which give the best fit to the pediatric AIDS incidence are almost the same in Tables 10.5 and 10.6. The near equality of these fecundity values suggests that the differences in the heterosexual partnership parameter values may be realistic and not just due to reporting differences. That is, the modeling suggests that IVDUs in region C are about twice as likely to have non–IVDU heterosexual partners or are twice as likely to transmit HIV infection to their heterosexual partners as IVDUs in regions A and B. It may be that IVDUs in regions A and B tend to have sex partners who are also IVDUs. The fecundities of about 0.006 births per female per month are consistent with birth rate data of 70 births per 1000 women per year (World Almanac, 1988).

10.4. The North Central Region: Aggregation of Racial/Ethnic and Risk Groups

The four subregions of the North Central region defined in Table 10.1 are Chicago (A), Detroit (B), large cities (C) and small cities (D). In regions A, C and D the time trends for AIDS incidences for homosexual/bisexual men in the r/e groups are the same in the sense that the percentages in each r/e group remain roughly the same over time. For example, the time trends in whites, blacks and Hispanics in Chicago are shown in Figure 10.20. The time trends for AIDS

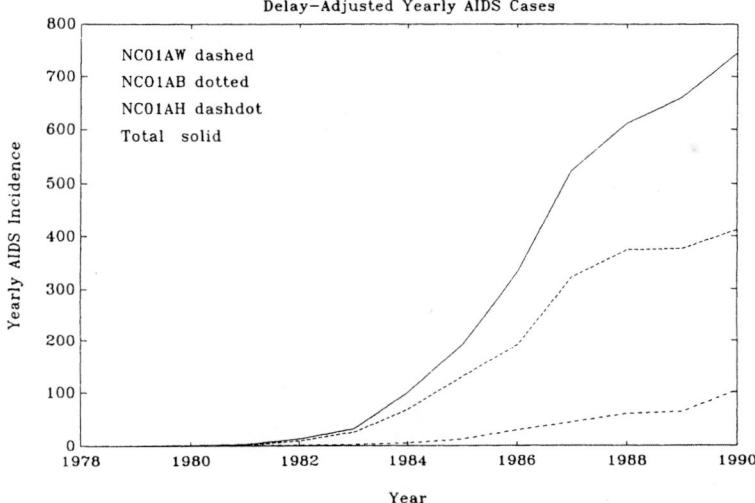

Figure 10.20. AIDS incidences in white, black, and Hispanic homosexual men in NC subregion A (Chicago).

in homosexual men in Detroit shown in Figure 10.21 are somewhat different for whites and blacks, however, since both are increasing and the numbers are small, it seems reasonable to combine them. Thus the r/e groups of homosexual men can be lumped together in all four subregions. The r/e percentages are 61% white (W), 30% black (B) and 7% Hispanic (H) in Chicago, 56% W and 44% B in Detroit, 83% W and 17% B in large cities, and 94% W and 9% B in small cities.

The time trends for AIDS are shown in Figure 10.22 for homosexual men in the four NC subregions. Some erratic changes have occurred in the last few years. The Chicago (A) time trend is somewhat different and it suggests that AIDS has not grown quite as fast in this group in recent years. However, the trend is increasing in all subregions so the Chicago homosexual men are not analyzed separately. Examination of the percentages of AIDS cases in each subregion over time shows that AIDS cases are growing at similar rates in all four subregions so that they can be combined. For AIDS cases in homosexual men in the NC region, 30% are from Chicago, 6% from Detroit, 37% from large cities and 27% from small cities.

In the four NC subregions the AIDS incidences in r/e subgroups of homosexual IVDUs are small and erratic so that there is no indication of differences between the subgroups; thus the r/e subgroups can be combined. Cumulative AIDS incidences in homosexual IVDUs are 6% of that in homosexual men in Chicago, 11% in Detroit, 7% in large cities and 14% in small cities. The time trends for NC homosexual IVDUs are similar to those for NC homosexual men and AIDS incidence in homosexual IVDUs is about 7% of AIDS incidence in homosexual men.

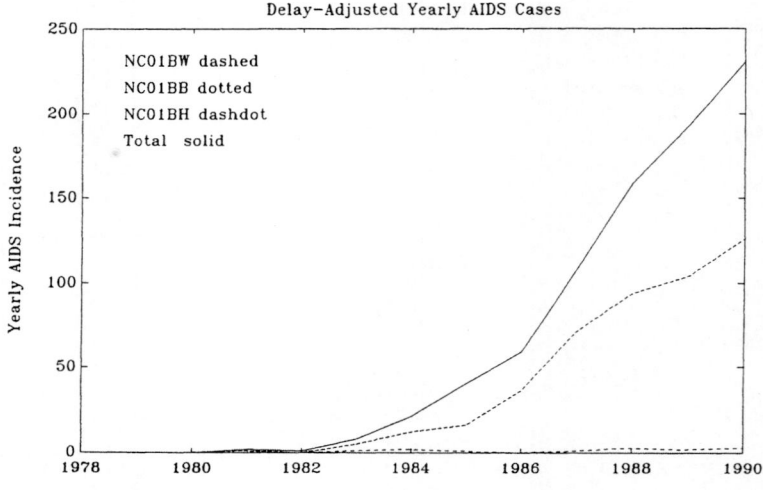

Figure 10.21. AIDS incidence in white, black, and Hispanic homosexual men in NC subregion B (Detroit).

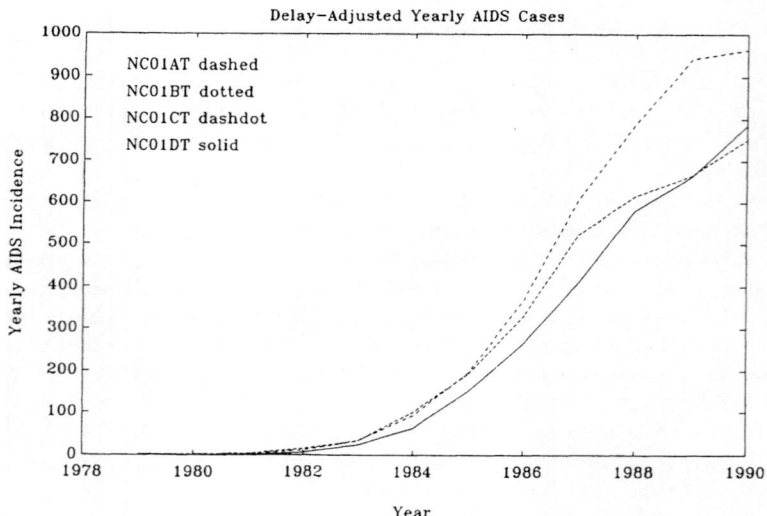

Figure 10.22. AIDS incidence in homosexual men in the four NC subregions: Chicago (A), Detroit (B), other large cities (C), and small cities (D).

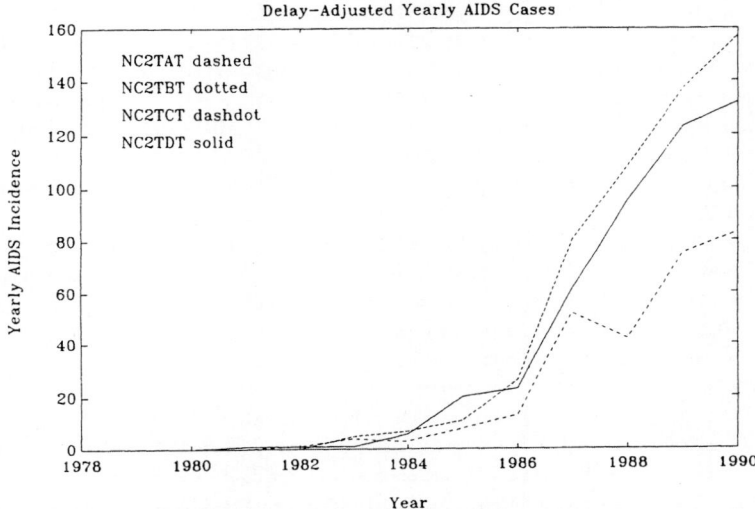

Figure 10.23. AIDS incidence in combined male (heterosexual) and female IVDUs in the four NC regions: Chicago (A), Detroit (B), large cities (C), and small cities (D).

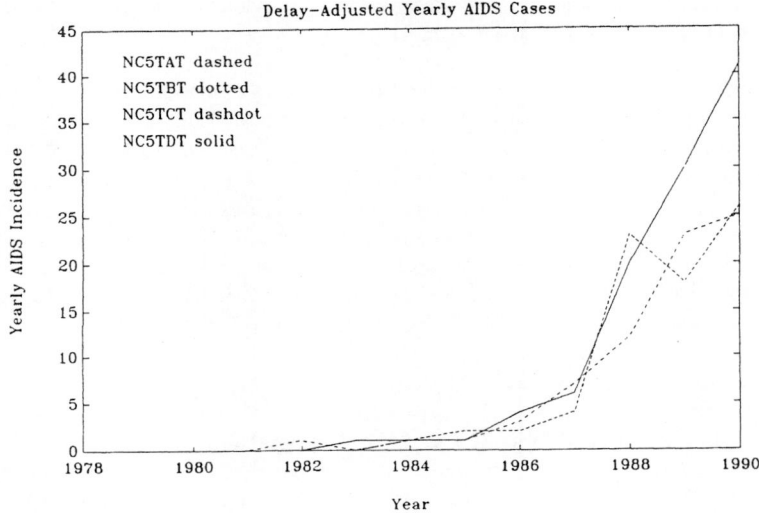

Figure 10.24. AIDS incidence in heterosexual partners of IVDUs in the four NC subregions: Chicago (A), Detroit (B), other large cities (C), and small cities (D).

The AIDS incidences for IVDUs in NC subregions are small and erratic, particularly for females. The variability of the incidence data is probably due to random effects in incidence and reporting. Since trends cannot be detected in erratic data, aggregation is necessary so that the yearly incidences are large enough to give smooth time trends. Thus the r/e groups are lumped together for male IVDUs and female IVDUs in each subregion. For AIDS cases in male IVDUs the r/e percentages are 28% W, 43% B and 30% H in Chicago, 4% W and 96%B in Detroit, 43% W and 56% B in large cities, and 38% W and 62% B in small cities. Since the time trends in female IVDUs are similar to those in male IVDUs, these risk groups are combined. The percentages of AIDS cases who are women are 20% in Chicago, 29% in Detroit, 20% in large cities (with very few white females) and 16% in small cities. Figure 10.23 shows the male and female heterosexual IVDUs by subregion. The AIDS incidences seem to be increasing slower in large cities and Detroit so these regions (B and C) are combined. Chicago and small cities (A and D) are lumped since the AIDS growth is faster in these cities.

For heterosexual partners (male and female) of IVDUs the AIDS incidences shown in Figure 10.24 in the subregions are somewhat erratic, but the growth rate is slowest in Detroit, somewhat faster in larger cities, faster in small cities and fastest in Chicago. This ordering is the same as for the IVDUs in the regions, as would be expected. The downward trend after 1988 in Chicago and the low incidences in 1988 and 1989 in Detroit are hard to explain, but they are probably due to reporting problems.

The number of perinatal AIDS cases is small enough so that it is impossible to determine time trends in r/e subgroups or in the subregions. Thus it is assumed that the aggregations used for IVDUs and heterosexual partners also apply.

10.5. The North Central Region: Computer Simulations of the Aggregated Groups

The simulation model in Chapter 7 has been fit to the combined groups given in Section 10.4. Recall that all homosexual men in the NC region have been combined into one group. The AIDS incidences for this group have been fit as shown in Table 10.7 and Figure 10.25. The estimate of 500,000 has been used for the population size of homosexual men at risk in the North Central region. The sexual behavior parameters are similar to those for homosexual men in NYC; namely, the average number of partners before reduction is 0.55, the yearly reduction starts in January 1981, and the activity level groups are mixing randomly. The epidemic starting date of January 1976 is later than any of the NE starting dates for homosexual men.

Table 10.8 and Figure 10.26 show the simulations for IVDUs, their heterosexual partners and related pediatric cases in the combined regions A and D. Table 10.9 and Figure 10.27 correspond to combined regions B and C. The populations sizes are different, but many of the parameter values are similar in Tables 10.8 and 10.9. Although the epidemic starting date is 6 months earlier in regions A and D, both dates are near the beginning of 1978, the average numbers of new needle–sharing partners per month are about 0.5 and the changes in behavior start in July 1981. In the North Central subregions AD and BC, respectively 19% and 26% of AIDS cases in IVDUs are women and 59% and 68% of AIDS cases in heterosexual partners are women. The average numbers of new heterosexual partners per month are both close to the value for IVDUs in

Table 10.7 Parameter values and corresponding simulation values for all homosexual men in NC region.

```
THE POPULATION SIZE IS        500000, THE VERY ACTIVE FRACTION IS
  1.000000E-01 AND THE ACTIVITY RATIO IS      10.000000
THE NATURAL MORTALITY RATE XMU IS    5.320000E-04
THE INTERCHANGE RATE  FROM THE VERY ACTIVE CLASS TO THE ACTIVE CLASS IS
  4.166667E-03  AND THE TURNOVER RATE IS DLT =     4.166667E-03
THE NUMBER OF INFECTIOUS STAGES IS  M =         7
THE G PARAMETERS FOR THE TRANSFER BETWEEN STAGES ARE     7.355444E-02
  6.433708E-02   4.867545E-02   4.199281E-02   3.997889E-02
  5.152515E-02   5.398798E-02
THE WEIGHTS OF TRANSMISSION PER INFECTIOUS PARTNER TIMES THE FRACTION STILL
SEXUALLY ACTIVE FOR THE STAGES ARE WRH(I) =          2.000000        1.000000
  1.000000          1.500000          1.500000          1.500000
  7.500000
THE PROBABILITY OF TRANSMISSION IS QH =    5.000000E-02
THE EXTERNAL MIXING FRACTION IS ETA =     1.000000
THE AVERAGE NUMBER OF PARTNERS PER MONTH IS    5.539000E-01 BEFORE      1981
        1, THEN IT IS REDUCED EACH YEAR BY A FACTOR OF    6.346000E-01UNTIL
DEC,      1990
THE STARTING YEAR AND MONTH ARE         1975          12
THE STARTING NUMBER OF VERY ACTIVE INFECTIVES IS        1.000000

      *************************************************
```

YEAR	HIV INC SIM	HIV PREV	FRACTN ALL	AL_PREV V_A	ACT	YR AIDS DATA	INC SIM	AIDS(SIMULATION) PREV	DTHS	OUTSF
1975	0.	1.	.00	.00	.00	*****	0.	0.	0.	0.
1976	8.	9.	.00	.00	.00	*****	0.	0.	0.	0.
1977	36.	44.	.00	.00	.00	*****	0.	0.	0.	0.
1978	157.	196.	.00	.00	.00	*****	0.	0.	0.	0.
1979	691.	863.	.00	.01	.00	1.	0.	0.	0.	0.
1980	2975.	3734.	.01	.04	.00	1.	1.	1.	0.	0.
1981	7819.	11167.	.02	.11	.01	6.	6.	5.	2.	1.
1982	9992.	20283.	.04	.19	.02	32.	25.	23.	7.	4.
1983	8655.	27565.	.06	.25	.03	99.	93.	86.	30.	15.
1984	6263.	32049.	.06	.28	.04	275.	267.	254.	99.	49.
1985	4254.	34184.	.07	.29	.04	575.	595.	592.	257.	129.
1986	2841.	34568.	.07	.28	.05	1022.	1066.	1122.	536.	272.
1987	1885.	33636.	.07	.27	.05	1650.	1607.	1798.	931.	480.
1988	1236.	31700.	.06	.24	.04	2145.	2116.	2520.	1394.	731.
1989	794.	29028.	.06	.21	.04	2463.	2503.	3172.	1851.	989.
1990	497.	25875.	.05	.19	.04	2733.	2718.	3658.	2232.	1216.

CHISQ =   9.766908

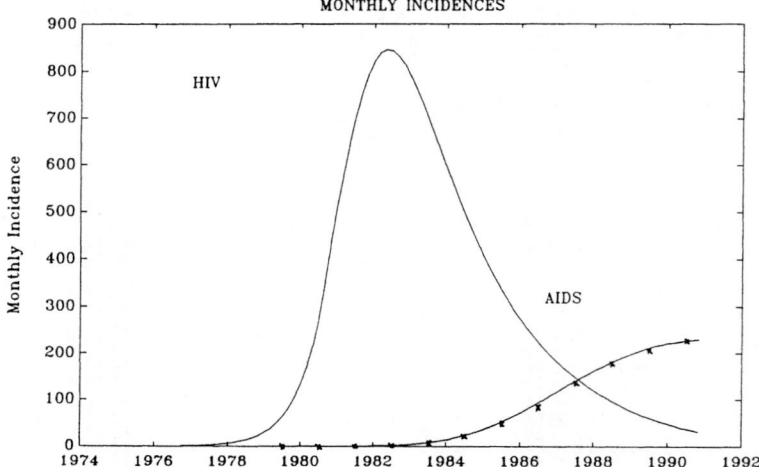

Figure 10.25. Estimated AIDS incidences (*) and simulated HIV and AIDS incidences for homosexual men in the NC region corresponding to parameter values in Table 10.7.

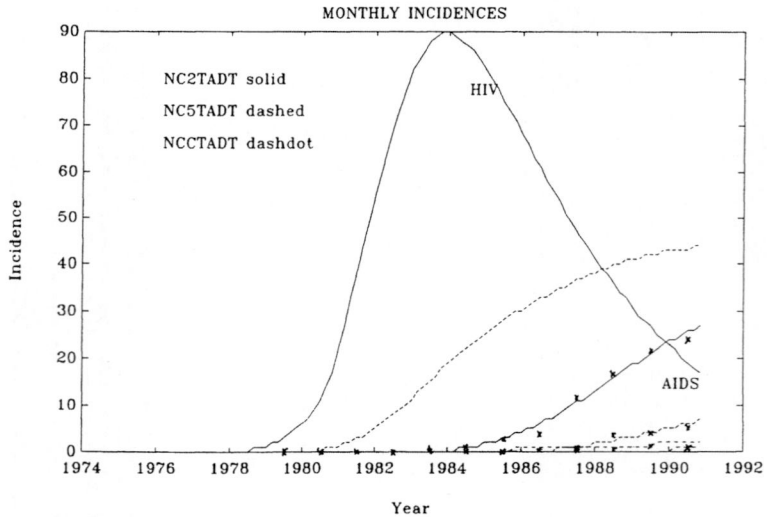

Figure 10.26. Estimated AIDS incidences (*) and simulates HIV and AIDS incidences for IVDUs, their heterosexual partners, and related pediatric cases in combined NC subregions A and D corresponding to parameter values in Table 10.8.

Table 10.8 Parameter values and corresponding simulation values for IVDUs, heterosexual partners and related pediatric cases in NC subregions A and D.

```
THE IVDU & HTRO POPULATION SIZES ARE          100000          50000
THE VERY ACTIVE FRACTION IS      1.000000E-01
THE ACTIVITY RATIO IS        10.000000
THE NATURAL MORTALITY RATE XMU IS     5.320000E-04
THE INTERCHANGE RATE  FROM THE VERY ACTIVE CLASS TO THE ACTIVE CLASS IS
   4.166667E-03  AND THE TURNOVER RATE IS DLT =    4.166667E-03
THE NUMBER OF INFECTIOUS STAGES IS  M =         7
THE G PARAMETERS FOR THE TRANSFER BETWEEN ADULT STAGES ARE    7.355444E-02
   6.433708E-02    4.867545E-02    4.199281E-02    3.997889E-02
   5.152515E-02    5.398798E-02
THE WEIGHTS OF TRANSMISSION PER INFECTIOUS PARTNER TIMES THE FRACTION STILL
SEXUALLY ACTIVE FOR THE STAGES ARE WRH(I) =          2.000000          1.000000
   1.000000        1.500000        1.500000        1.500000
   7.500000
THE PROBABILITIES OF TRANSMISSION ARE QH, QHP & QC =    5.000000E-02
   1.000000E-01    1.000000E-01
THE EXTERNAL MIXING FRACTION IS ETA =          1.000000
THE AVERAGE NUMBER OF NEEDLE-SHARING PARTNERS PER MONTH IS    4.827000E-01
BEFORE      1981            7, THEN IT IS REDUCED EACH YEAR BY A FACTOR OF
   7.160000E-01 UNTIL DEC,      1990
THE FRACTION OF IVDU WHO ARE WOMEN IS    1.900000E-01
THE FRACTION OF HETEROSEXUALS WHO ARE WOMEN IS    5.900000E-01
THE AVERAGE NUMBER OF IVDU PARTNERS OF HETEROSEXUALS PER MONTH IS
   5.600000E-02
THE FRACTION    3.400000E-01 OF CHILDREN PROGRESS RAPIDLY TO AIDS WITH RATE
CONSTANT    8.000000E-02. OTHERS MOVE THROUGH M STAGES WITH SPEED FACTOR
   1.550000
THE FECUNDITY FC (CHILDREN/MONTH) IS     5.800000E-03
THE STARTING YEAR AND MONTH ARE      1977            7
THE STARTING NUMBER OF VERY ACTIVE INFECTIVES IS        1.000000
***************************************************

THE SIMULATED INCIDENCES ARE GIVEN ON THE NEXT PAGE
```

nc2tadt.m nc2tadt.m nc2tadt.m nc2tadt.m nc2tadt.m
****

YEAR	CLASS	HIV INC	HIV PREV	FRACTNAL_PREV ALL	V_A	ACT	YR AIDS DATA	INC SIM	AIDS(SIMULATION) PREV	DTHS	OUTSF
1977	IVDU	2.	3.	.00	.00	.00	****	0.	0.	0.	0.
	HTRO	0.	0.	.00	-	-	****	0.	0.	0.	0.
	PED	0.	0.	-	-	-	0.	0.	0.	0.	
1978	IVDU	10.	13.	.00	.00	.00	0.	0.	0.	0.	0.
	HTRO	1.	1.	.00	-	-	****	0.	0.	0.	0.
	PED	0.	0.	-	-	-	0.	0.	0.	0.	
1979	IVDU	36.	48.	.00	.00	.00	0.	0.	0.	0.	0.
	HTRO	3.	4.	.00	-	-	0.	0.	0.	0.	0.
	PED	0.	0.	-	-	-	0.	0.	0.	0.	
1980	IVDU	128.	171.	.00	.01	.00	0.	0.	0.	0.	0.
	HTRO	10.	13.	.00	-	-	0.	0.	0.	0.	0.
	PED	0.	0.	-	-	-	0.	0.	0.	0.	
1981	IVDU	413.	566.	.01	.03	.00	1.	0.	0.	0.	0.
	HTRO	35.	47.	.00	-	-	0.	0.	0.	0.	0.
	PED	1.	1.	-	-	-	0.	0.	0.	0.	
1982	IVDU	796.	1312.	.01	.07	.01	1.	1.	0.	0.	0.
	HTRO	94.	136.	.00	-	-	0.	0.	0.	0.	0.
	PED	2.	3.	-	-	-	0.	0.	0.	0.	
1983	IVDU	1039.	2251.	.02	.11	.01	6.	5.	1.	2.	1.
	HTRO	176.	301.	.01	-	-	1.	0.	1.	0.	0.
	PED	5.	8.	-	-	-	0.	1.	1.	1.	
1984	IVDU	1058.	3153.	.03	.15	.02	13.	14.	2.	5.	3.
	HTRO	261.	538.	.01	-	-	2.	1.	2.	0.	0.
	PED	8.	14.	-	-	-	0.	2.	2.	1.	
1985	IVDU	930.	3872.	.04	.18	.02	31.	35.	3.	14.	7.
	HTRO	333.	832.	.02	-	-	3.	4.	3.	1.	1.
	PED	11.	23.	-	-	-	0.	3.	3.	2.	
1986	IVDU	757.	4365.	.04	.19	.03	49.	72.	4.	33.	17.
	HTRO	391.	1164.	.02	-	-	6.	8.	4.	4.	2.
	PED	14.	34.	-	-	-	7.	4.	4.	3.	
1987	IVDU	592.	4641.	.05	.20	.03	141.	125.	5.	65.	33.
	HTRO	438.	1520.	.03	-	-	10.	17.	5.	8.	4.
	PED	17.	46.	-	-	-	5.	5.	6.	5.	
1988	IVDU	452.	4724.	.05	.20	.03	203.	188.	7.	110.	57.
	HTRO	478.	1887.	.04	-	-	43.	31.	7.	16.	8.
	PED	20.	60.	-	-	-	6.	7.	8.	6.	
1989	IVDU	339.	4642.	.05	.19	.03	260.	252.	9.	165.	87.
	HTRO	508.	2252.	.05	-	-	48.	50.	9.	28.	14.
	PED	23.	75.	-	-	-	15.	9.	10.	8.	
1990	IVDU	249.	4424.	.04	.17	.03	289.	308.	12.	222.	119.
	HTRO	526.	2600.	.05	-	-	67.	73.	12.	45.	23.
	PED	26.	90.	-	-	-	11.	12.	13.	11.	

CHISQD = 14.597640
CHISQP = 10.765990
CHISQC = 10.959110
SUM OF CHISQ-D,P,C = 36.322740

165

Table 10.9 Parameter values and corresponding simulation values for IVDUs, heterosexual partners and related pediatric cases in NC subregions B and C.

```
THE IVDU & HTRO POPULATION SIZES ARE        50000        25000
THE VERY ACTIVE FRACTION IS     1.000000E-01
THE ACTIVITY RATIO IS        10.000000
THE NATURAL MORTALITY RATE XMU IS    5.320000E-04
THE INTERCHANGE RATE   FROM THE VERY ACTIVE CLASS TO THE ACTIVE CLASS IS
   4.166667E-03  AND THE TURNOVER RATE IS DLT =    4.166667E-03
THE NUMBER OF INFECTIOUS STAGES IS  M =          7
THE G PARAMETERS FOR THE TRANSFER BETWEEN ADULT STAGES ARE    7.355444E-02
   6.433708E-02    4.867545E-02    4.199281E-02    3.997889E-02
   5.152515E-02    5.398798E-02
THE WEIGHTS OF TRANSMISSION PER INFECTIOUS PARTNER TIMES THE FRACTION STILL
SEXUALLY ACTIVE FOR THE STAGES ARE WRH(I) =        2.000000        1.000000
   1.000000        1.500000        1.500000        1.500000
   7.500000
THE PROBABILITIES OF TRANSMISSION ARE QH, QHP & QC =    5.000000E-02
   1.000000E-01    1.000000E-01
THE EXTERNAL MIXING FRACTION IS ETA =         1.000000
THE AVERAGE NUMBER OF NEEDLE-SHARING PARTNERS PER MONTH IS    5.027000E-01
BEFORE        1981         7, THEN IT IS REDUCED EACH YEAR BY A FACTOR OF
   6.958000E-01 UNTIL DEC,        1990
THE FRACTION OF IVDU WHO ARE WOMEN IS    2.600000E-01
THE FRACTION OF HETEROSEXUALS WHO ARE WOMEN IS    6.800000E-01
THE AVERAGE NUMBER OF IVDU PARTNERS OF HETEROSEXUALS PER MONTH IS
   5.900000E-02
THE FRACTION    3.400000E-01 OF CHILDREN PROGRESS RAPIDLY TO AIDS WITH RATE
CONSTANT    8.000000E-02. OTHERS MOVE THROUGH M STAGES WITH SPEED FACTOR
   1.550000
THE FECUNDITY FC (CHILDREN/MONTH) IS    5.400000E-03
THE STARTING YEAR AND MONTH ARE        1978        1
THE STARTING NUMBER OF VERY ACTIVE INFECTIVES IS        1.000000
*******************************************************

THE SIMULATED INCIDENCES ARE GIVEN ON THE NEXT PAGE
```

nc2tbct.m nc2tbct.m nc2tbct.m nc2tbct.m nc2tbct.m
****

YEAR	CLASS	HIV INC	HIV PREV	FRACTNAL_PREV ALL	V_A	ACT	YR AIDS DATA	INC SIM	AIDS(SIMULATION) PREV	DTHS	OUTSF
1978	IVDU	6.	7.	.00	.00	.00	0.	0.	0.	0.	0.
	HTRO	0.	0.	.00	–	–	****	0.	0.	0.	0.
	PED	0.	0.	–	–	–	0.	0.	0.	0.	
1979	IVDU	22.	28.	.00	.00	.00	0.	0.	0.	0.	0.
	HTRO	2.	2.	.00	–	–	0.	0.	0.	0.	0.
	PED	0.	0.	–	–	–	0.	0.	0.	0.	
1980	IVDU	83.	108.	.00	.01	.00	0.	0.	0.	0.	0.
	HTRO	7.	8.	.00	–	–	0.	0.	0.	0.	0.
	PED	0.	0.	–	–	–	0.	0.	0.	0.	
1981	IVDU	279.	375.	.01	.04	.00	0.	0.	0.	0.	0.
	HTRO	24.	32.	.00	–	–	0.	0.	0.	0.	0.
	PED	1.	1.	–	–	–	0.	0.	0.	0.	
1982	IVDU	531.	873.	.02	.09	.01	1.	1.	0.	0.	0.
	HTRO	66.	94.	.00	–	–	1.	0.	0.	.0.	0.
	PED	2.	3.	–	–	·–	0.	0.	0.	0.	
1983	IVDU	656.	1463.	.03	.14	.02	6.	3.	1.	1.	0.
	HTRO	122.	208.	.01	–	–	0.	0.	1.	0.	0.
	PED	4.	6.	–	–	–	0.	1.	1.	0.	
1984	IVDU	624.	1987.	.04	.18	.02	8.	9.	1.	3.	2.
	HTRO	174.	366.	.01	–	–	1.	1.	1.	0.	0.
	PED	6.	11.	–	–	–	1.	1.	1.	1.	
1985	IVDU	515.	2371.	.05	.21	.03	14.	23.	2.	9.	5.
	HTRO	215.	555.	.02	–	–	1.	2.	2.	1.	0.
	PED	8.	18.	–	–	–	0.	2.	2.	2.	
1986	IVDU	397.	2607.	.05	.23	.03	39.	47.	3.	22.	11.
	HTRO	247.	763.	.03	–	–	4.	6.	3.	2.	1.
	PED	10.	26.	–	–	–	4.	3.	3.	2.	
1987	IVDU	297.	2713.	.05	.23	.03	98.	81.	4.	42.	22.
	HTRO	272.	982.	.04	–	–	14.	12.	4.	5.	3.
	PED	12.	35.	–	–	–	5.	4.	5.	3.	
1988	IVDU	219.	2711.	.05	.22	.04	110.	119.	5.	71.	37.
	HTRO	293.	1203.	.05	–	–	17.	21.	5.	11.	6.
	PED	14.	44.	–	–	–	4.	5.	6.	5.	
1989	IVDU	158.	2619.	.05	.21	.04	165.	157.	7.	104.	55.
	HTRO	307.	1419.	.06	–	–	33.	34.	7.	19.	10.
	PED	16.	55.	–	–	–	11.	7.	8.	6.	
1990	IVDU	112.	2457.	.05	.19	.03	181.	188.	9.	138.	74.
	HTRO	315.	1620.	.06	–	–	44.	48.	9.	30.	16.
	PED	18.	65.	–	–	–	8.	9.	9.	8.	

```
CHISQD =        13.813320
CHISQP =        19.807490
CHISQC =         6.232977
SUM OF CHISQ-D,P,C =      39.853790
```

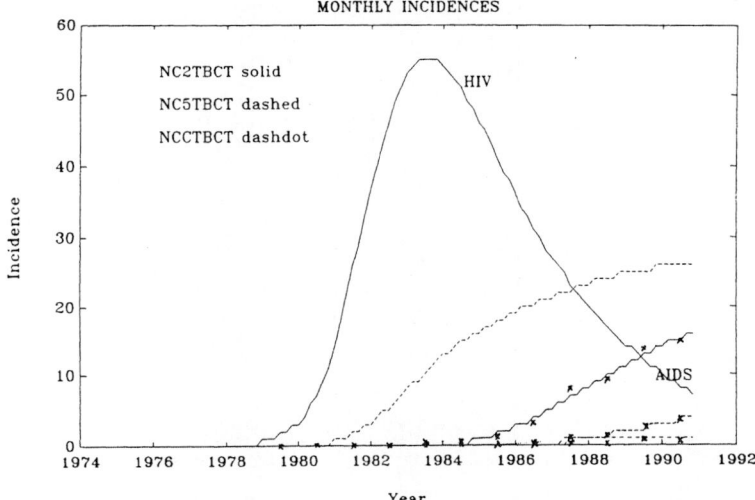

Figure 10.27. Estimated AIDS incidences (*) and simulated HIV and AIDS incidences for IVDUs, their heterosexual partners, and related pediatric cases in combined NC subregions B and C corresponding to parameter values in Table 10.9.

the NE region C. The fecundity of 0.0058 births per woman per month in regions A and D is close to the value of 0.0054 in regions B and C; these values are very close to the values in the NE region. The similar parameter values indicate that AIDS incidence in IVDUs in the combined regions A and D are really similar to those in the combined regions B and C so that it would be reasonable to combine all IVDUs in the NC region.

10.6. The South Region: Aggregation of Racial/Ethnic and Risk Groups

The five subregions of the South (S) region are Florida (A), Texas (B), Washington, D.C. and Baltimore (C), other cities over one million (D) and all other areas (E). Figure 10.28 shows the time trends in white, black and Hispanic homosexual men in Florida (A). These r/e groups in region A can be combined since the time trends are similar with 70% white, 13% black and 17% Hispanic. In Figure 10.29 for Texas (B) there are kinks in the AIDS incidence in white homosexual men; but these kinks may be due to reporting problems or to the 1987 AIDS definition change. Although the AIDS incidence in white homosexual men in subregion B (also in subregions C and D) seems to be increasing less rapidly than in blacks and Hispanics, the implications of these differences are not pursued here. Thus all r/e groups in Texas (B) can also be combined with about 76% white, 11% black and 13% Hispanic homosexual men. Figures 10.30 to 10.32 corresponding to subregions C, D, and E suggest that the r/e groups of homosexual men in each

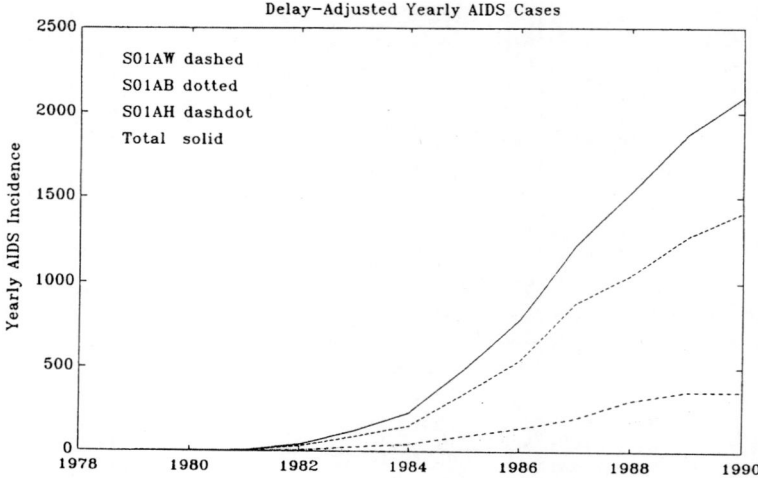

Figure 10.28. AIDS incidence in racial/ethnic groups of homosexual men in South subregion A (Florida).

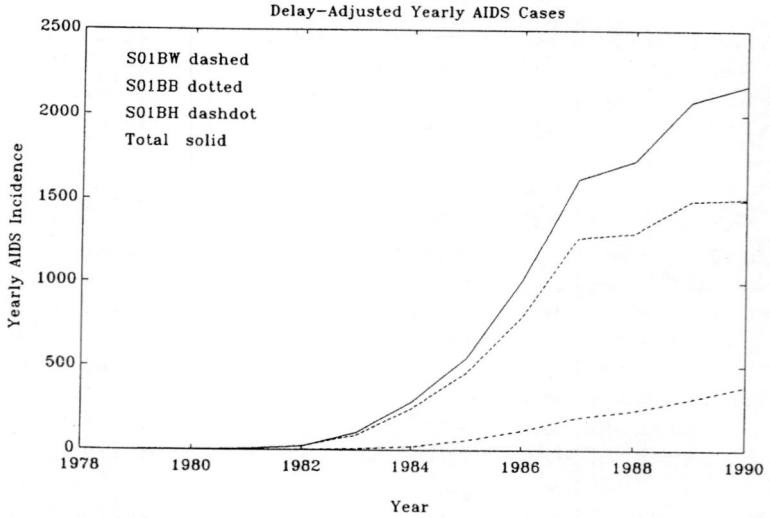

Figure 10.29. AIDS incidence in racial/ethnic groups of homosexual men in South subregion B (Texas).

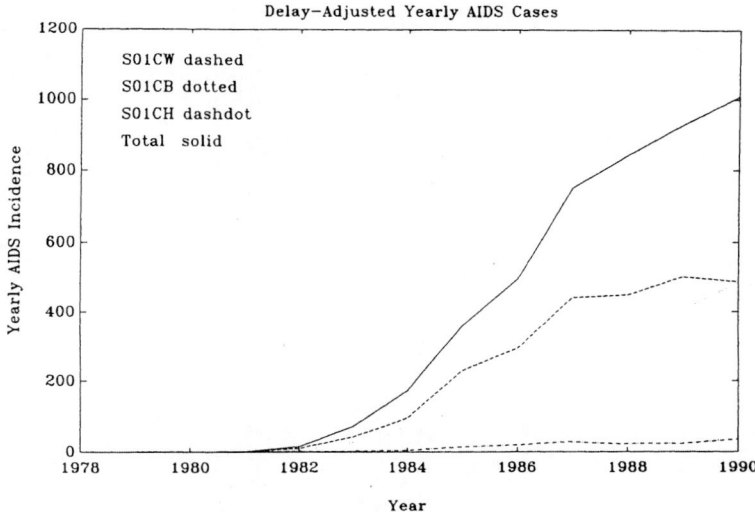

Figure 10.30. AIDS incidence in racial/ethnic groups of homosexual men in South subregion C (Washington, D.C. and Baltimore).

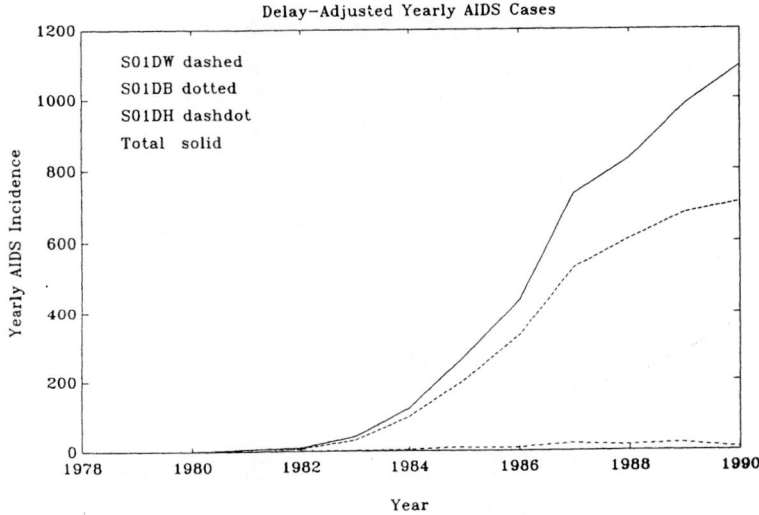

Figure 10.31. AIDS incidence in racial/ethnic groups of homosexual men in South subregion D (other cities over 1 million).

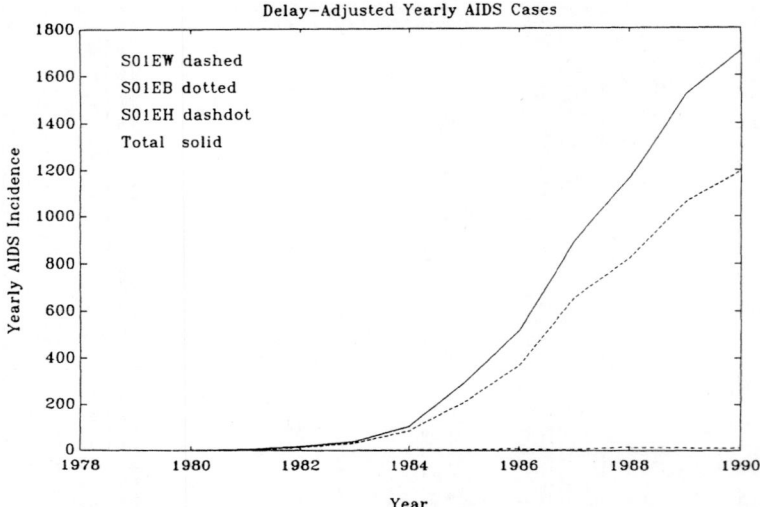

Figure 10.32. AIDS incidence in racial/ethnic groups of homosexual men in South subregion E (all other areas).

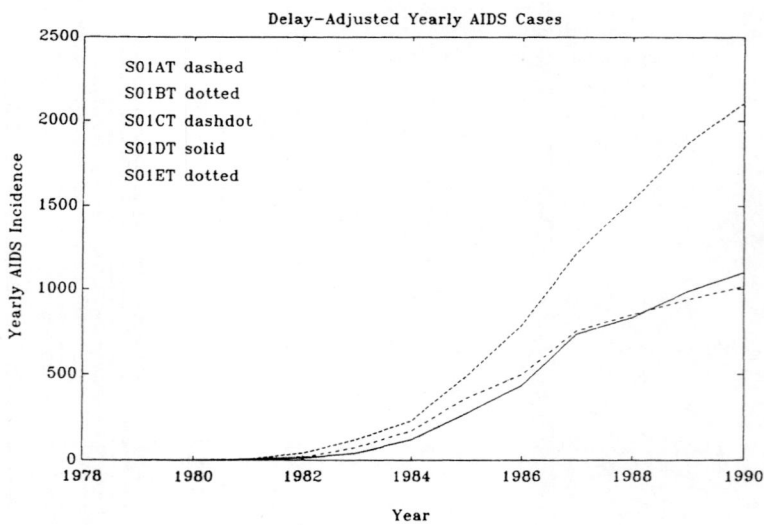

Figure 10.33. AIDS incidence in homosexual men in the five South subregions.

subregion can be lumped together. The r/e distributions are 55% W and 41% B in subregion C, 72% W and 25% B in subregion D, and 70% W and 28% B in subregion E.

Figure 10.33 shows the time trends of AIDS incidence in homosexual men in the five subregions of the South region. The time trends are generally similar for all regions except region C (Washington DC and Baltimore) where the growth rate is slower. Thus subregions A, B, D and E can be combined, but subregion C is considered separately.

The time trends in r/e groups of male (heterosexual) IVDUs in the five subregions are shown in Figures 10.34 to 10.38. Although there are some irregularities, the AIDS incidences in the r/e subgroups in each subregion are generally similar so that they can be combined. The r/e distributions are about 21%W, 67% B and 12% H in Florida (A), 37% W, 44% B and 19% H in Texas (B), 10% W and 90% B in Washington DC and Baltimore (C), 21% W and 79%B in other cities over one million (D), and 25% W and 75% B in all other areas (E). The AIDS incidences in female IVDUs are smaller and hence somewhat more erratic than in male IVDUs, but the time trends in r/e subgroups are generally similar in each subregion so that the r/e subgroups can be combined. Moreover, the male (heterosexual) and female IVDUs can be combined since they have similar AIDS incidence patterns. Figure 10.39 shows AIDS incidences for the combined male and female IVDUs in the five South subregions. The AIDS incidences in these subregions are all increasing together in a parallel pattern so that these five subregions can be combined. Figure 10.40 shows the AIDS incidences for heterosexual partners of IVDUs in the five South subregions. Although the time trends are not as smooth as for IVDUs, they are generally parallel so that all heterosexual partners of IVDUs in the South are combined together. Perinatal cases are also combined in the South region.

10.7. The South Region: Computer Simulations of the Aggregated Groups

The combined groups in Section 10.6 have been fit by the simulation model presented in Chapter 7. Recall that four subregions of homosexual men have been combined, but subregion C (Washington, D.C. and Baltimore) has not been combined because the growth rate there seemed to be slower. The simulated HIV and AIDS incidences for the four combined subregions and for subregion C are shown in Figures 10.41 and 10.42 and Tables 10.10 and 10.11. Note that there is no reduction in sexual behavior over time in the four combined subregions, but there is some reduction starting in January 1982 in subregion C. The population size of 500,000 in combined regions A, B, D and E is about 10 times the size of 50,000 for region C. The epidemic starting date of February 1975 for the combined subregions is 14 months earlier than the epidemic starting date of April 1976 in subregion C. The average number of new sexual partners and the external mixing fraction are smaller for the combined subregions than in subregion C. In summary, the AIDS incidences in subregion C (Washington D.C., and Baltimore) suggest that changes in behavior may have occurred there, but there is no evidence for changes in behavior in homosexual men in the four combined regions. Note that the high HIV incidences in recent years in Figure 10.41 are not predictions, but they do represent the situation if there have been no changes in sexual behavior in recent years.

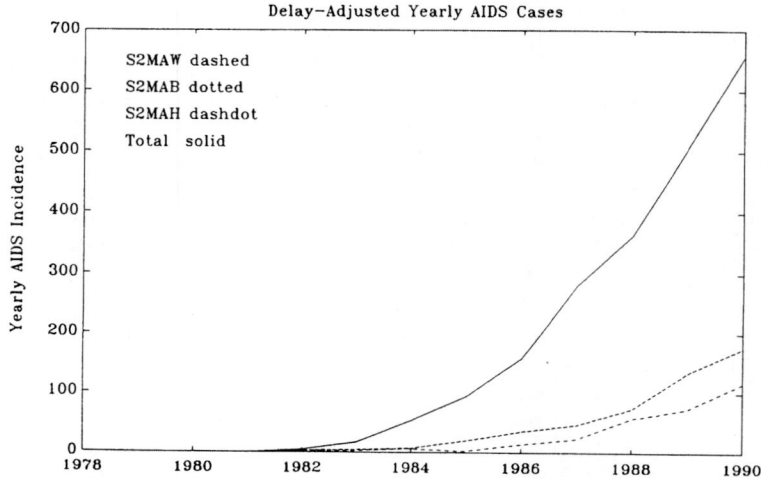

Figure 10.34. AIDS incidence in racial/ethnic groups of male (heterosexual) IVDUs in South subregion A (Florida).

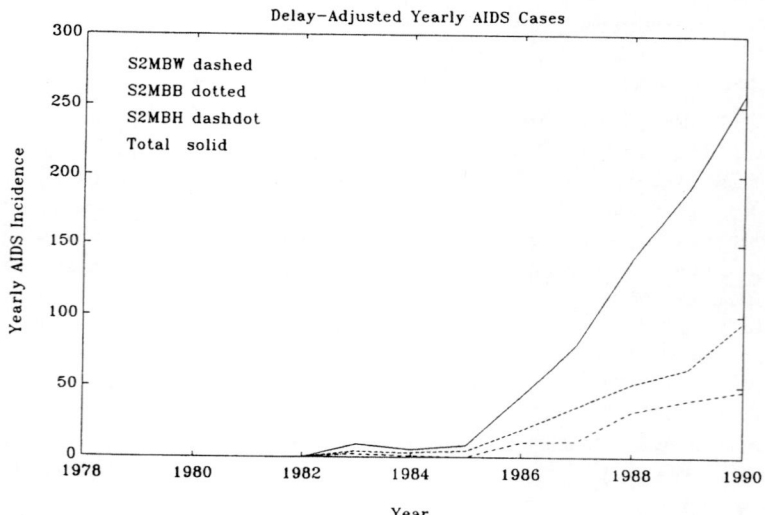

Figure 10.35. AIDS incidence in racial/ethnic groups of male (heterosexual) IVDUs in South subregion B (Texas).

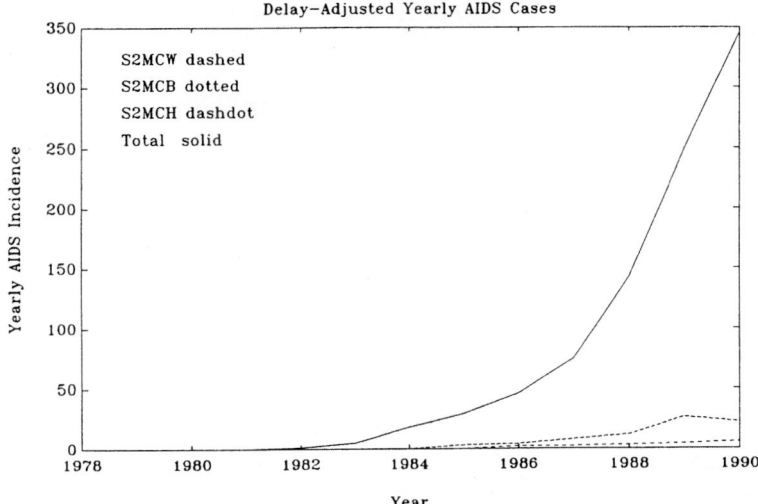

Figure 10.36. AIDS incidence in racial/ethnic groups of male (heterosexual) IVDUs in South subregion C (Washington, D.C. and Baltimore).

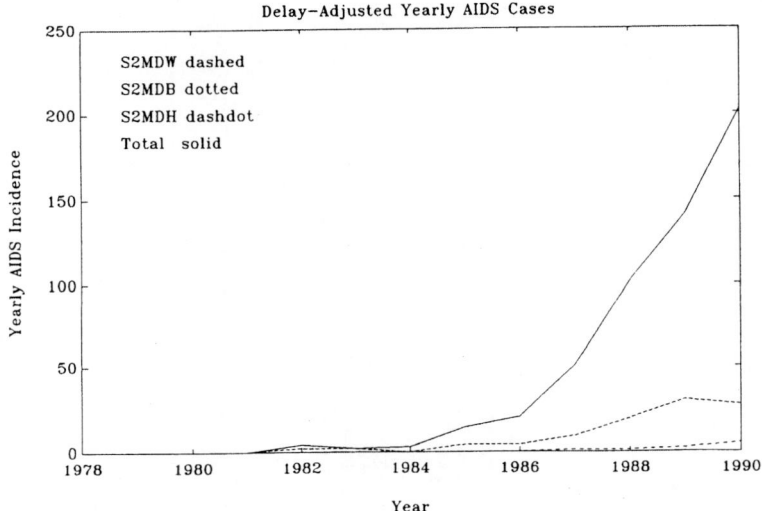

Figure 10.37. AIDS incidences in racial/ethnic groups of male (heterosexual) IVDUs in South subregion D (other cities over 1 million).

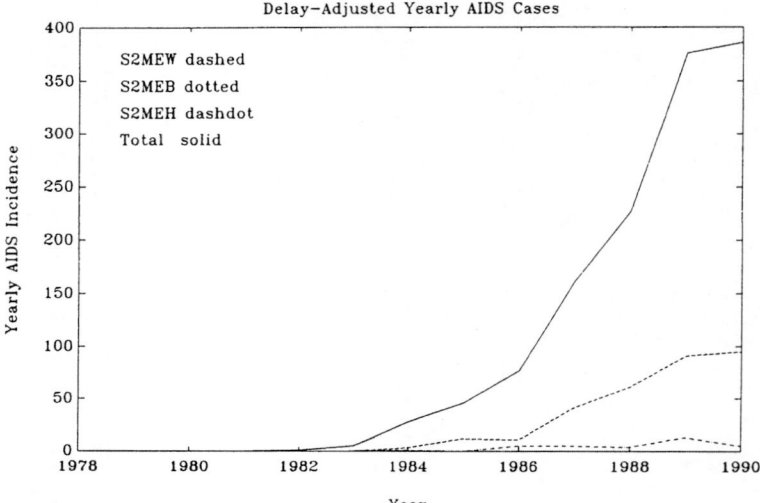

Figure 10.38. AIDS incidences in racial/ethnic groups of male (heterosexual) IVDUs in South subregion E (all other areas).

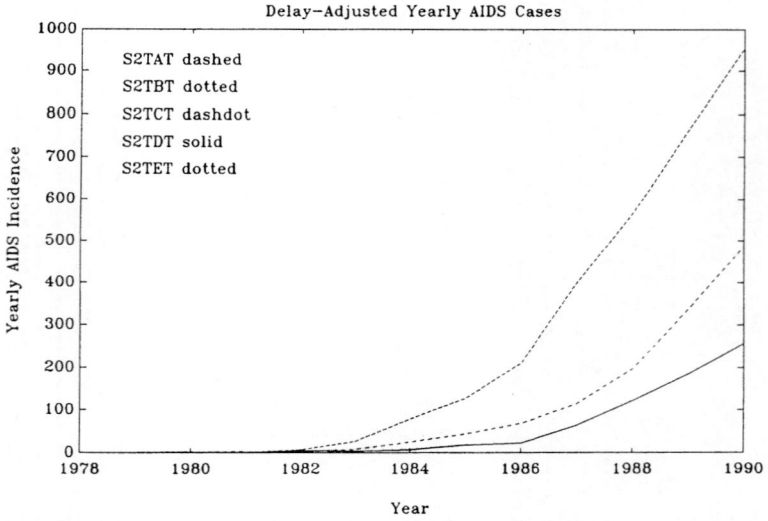

Figure 10.39. AIDS incidence in IVDUs in the five South subregions.

175

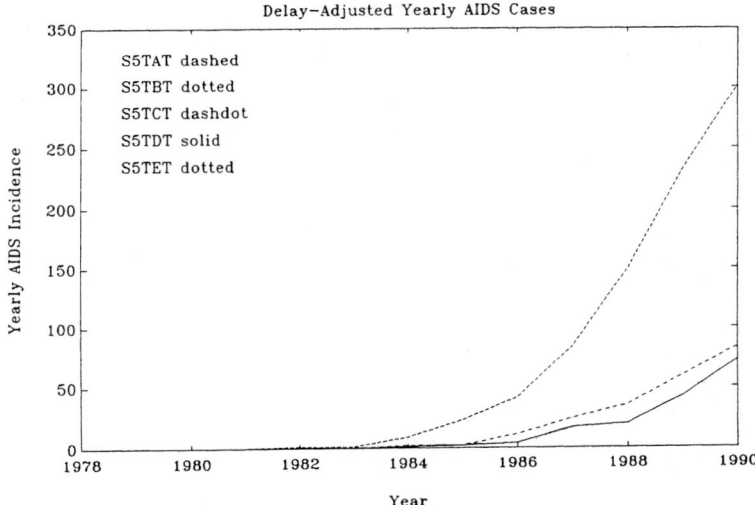

Figure 10.40. AIDS incidence in heterosexual partners of IVDUs in the five South subgroups.

Recall that the male and female IVDUs in the five South subregions have been combined into one group. Table 10.12 and Figure 10.43 show the simulated HIV and AIDS incidences for this aggregated group. The epidemic starting date of January 1975 is similar to that for IVDUs in the NE regions A and B, but earlier than in the NC regions. As in the NE regions the fits are obtained without any reduction in needle–sharing behavior over time. The average number of new needle–sharing partners per month of 0.26 is lower than the values in the other regions. The average number of new heterosexual partners of IVDUs per month of 0.76 is somewhat larger than in the NE and NC regions. The fecundity of 0.0045 births per woman per month is lower than in the other regions. In the South 26% of AIDS cases in IVDUs are women and 57% of AIDS cases in heterosexual partners of IVDUs are women.

10.8. The West Region: Aggregation of Racial/Ethnic and Risk Groups

The three subregions of the West region described in Table 10.1 are A (San Francisco and Seattle), B (Los Angeles, Oakland, Anaheim, Riverside and San Jose) and C (all other areas). AIDS incidences in homosexual men in subregion A are given for r/e groups in Figure 10.44. Figures 10.45 and 10.46 contain AIDS incidences for subregions B and C. All three show some kinks for white homosexual males, but the kink around 1987 is primarily due to reporting practices before and after the 1987 AIDS definition change. If the kinks are smoothed out, then the time trends in r/e groups are similar so that they can be combined in each subregion. The AIDS incidences are about 91% W, 4% B, and 5% H in region A, 72% W, 13% B and 15% H in region B, and 92% W, 5% B, and 3% H in region C.

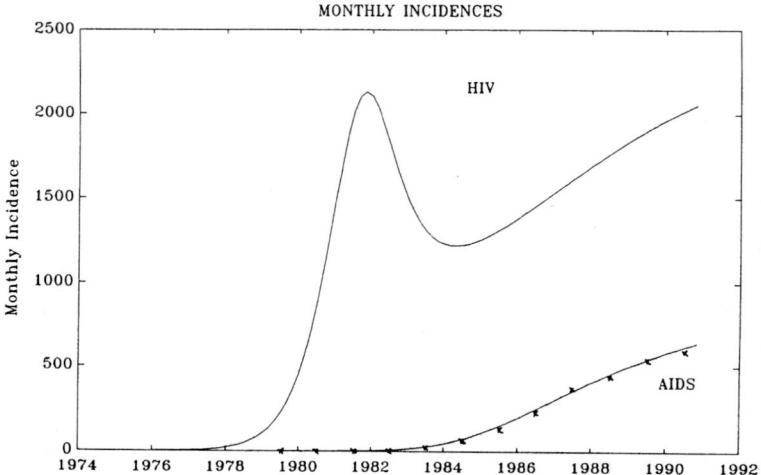

Figure 10.41. Estimated AIDS incidences (*) and simulated HIV and AIDS incidences for homosexual men in combined South subregions A, B, D, and E corresponding to parameters in Table 10.10.

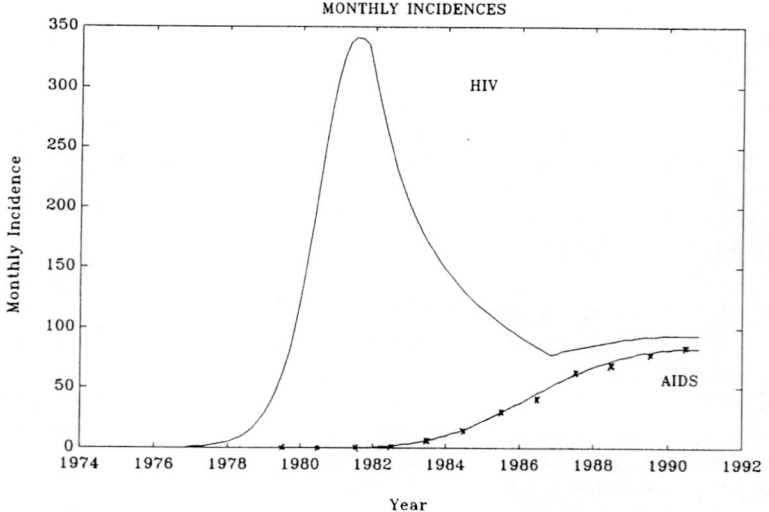

Figure 10.42. Estimated AIDS incidences (*) and simulated HIV and AIDS incidences for homosexual men in South subregion C (Washington, D.C. and Baltimore) corresponding to parameters in Table 10.11.

Table 10.10 Parameter values and corresponding simulation values for homosexual men in South subregions A, B, D, and E.

```
THE POPULATION SIZE IS      500000, THE VERY ACTIVE FRACTION IS
  1.000000E-01 AND THE ACTIVITY RATIO IS        10.000000
THE NATURAL MORTALITY RATE XMU IS    5.320000E-04
THE INTERCHANGE RATE  FROM THE VERY ACTIVE CLASS TO THE ACTIVE CLASS IS
  4.166667E-03  AND THE TURNOVER RATE IS DLT =    4.166667E-03
THE NUMBER OF INFECTIOUS STAGES IS  M =       7
THE G PARAMETERS FOR THE TRANSFER BETWEEN STAGES ARE     7.355444E-02
  6.433708E-02    4.867545E-02    4.199281E-02   3.997889E-02
  5.152515E-02    5.398798E-02
THE WEIGHTS OF TRANSMISSION PER INFECTIOUS PARTNER TIMES THE FRACTION STILL
SEXUALLY ACTIVE FOR THE STAGES ARE WRH(I) =      2.000000       1.000000
  1.000000        1.500000        1.500000        1.500000
  7.500000
THE PROBABILITY OF TRANSMISSION IS QH =     5.000000E-02
THE EXTERNAL MIXING FRACTION IS ETA =    1.612000E-01
THE AVERAGE NUMBER OF PARTNERS PER MONTH IS   3.665000E-01 BEFORE        2222
  2, THEN IT IS REDUCED EACH YEAR BY A FACTOR OF       1.000000UNTIL
DEC,    2222
THE STARTING YEAR AND MONTH ARE       1975      2
THE STARTING NUMBER OF VERY ACTIVE INFECTIVES IS       1.000000

     *************************************************
```

YEAR	HIV INC SIM	HIV PREV	FRACTN ALL	AL_PREV V_A	ACT	YR AIDS DATA	INC SIM	AIDS(SIMULATION) PREV	DTHS	OUTSF
1975	4.	5.	.00	.00	.00	*****	0.	0.	0.	0.
1976	22.	26.	.00	.00	.00	*****	0.	0.	0.	0.
1977	106.	129.	.00	.00	.00	*****	0.	0.	0.	0.
1978	515.	628.	.00	.01	.00	*****	0.	0.	0.	0.
1979	2402.	2950.	.01	.05	.00	0.	1.	1.	0.	0.
1980	9499.	12097.	.02	.21	.00	3.	4.	4.	1.	1.
1981	22205.	33113.	.07	.56	.01	24.	19.	17.	5.	3.
1982	22639.	53299.	.11	.82	.03	90.	82.	75.	24.	12.
1983	16326.	66173.	.13	.90	.05	304.	293.	272.	96.	47.
1984	14705.	76579.	.15	.92	.07	744.	801.	767.	306.	151.
1985	15586.	86859.	.17	.92	.09	1600.	1677.	1690.	754.	378.
1986	17267.	97531.	.20	.91	.12	2753.	2840.	3040.	1490.	759.
1987	19155.	108554.	.22	.89	.14	4476.	4112.	4681.	2470.	1279.
1988	21003.	119755.	.24	.86	.17	5282.	5327.	6424.	3585.	1889.
1989	22679.	130951.	.26	.83	.20	6485.	6396.	8106.	4713.	2526.
1990	24107.	141973.	.28	.80	.23	7106.	7309.	9642.	5773.	3142.

CHISQ =   53.533080

Table 10.11 Parameter values and corresponding simulation values for homosexual men in South subregions C (Washington D.C. and Baltimore).

```
THE POPULATION SIZE IS         50000, THE VERY ACTIVE FRACTION IS
  1.000000E-01 AND THE ACTIVITY RATIO IS      10.000000
THE NATURAL MORTALITY RATE XMU IS    5.320000E-04
THE INTERCHANGE RATE  FROM THE VERY ACTIVE CLASS TO THE ACTIVE CLASS IS
  4.166667E-03  AND THE TURNOVER RATE IS DLT =    4.166667E-03
THE NUMBER OF INFECTIOUS STAGES IS  M =          7
THE G PARAMETERS FOR THE TRANSFER BETWEEN STAGES ARE    7.355444E-02
  6.433708E-02   4.867545E-02    4.199281E-02   3.997889E-02
  5.152515E-02   5.398798E-02
THE WEIGHTS OF TRANSMISSION PER INFECTIOUS PARTNER TIMES THE FRACTION STILL
SEXUALLY ACTIVE FOR THE STAGES ARE WRH(I) =        2.000000      1.000000
  1.000000          1.500000          1.500000          1.500000
  7.500000
THE PROBABILITY OF TRANSMISSION IS QH =     5.000000E-02
THE EXTERNAL MIXING FRACTION IS ETA =    5.312000E-01
THE AVERAGE NUMBER OF PARTNERS PER MONTH IS    4.640000E-01 BEFORE        1982
          1, THEN IT IS REDUCED EACH YEAR BY A FACTOR OF    7.283000E-01UNTIL
DEC,      1986
THE STARTING YEAR AND MONTH ARE        1976        3
THE STARTING NUMBER OF VERY ACTIVE INFECTIVES IS       1.000000
```

****

YEAR	HIV INC SIM	HIV PREV	FRACTNAL_PREV ALL	V_A	ACT	YR AIDS DATA	INC SIM	AIDS(SIMULATION) PREV	DTHS	OUTSF
1976	5.	6.	.00	.00	.00	*****	0.	0.	0.	0.
1977	27.	32.	.00	.00	.00	*****	0.	0.	0.	0.
1978	140.	168.	.00	.02	.00	*****	0.	0.	0.	0.
1979	668.	813.	.02	.11	.01	0.	0.	0.	0.	0.
1980	2327.	3047.	.06	.40	.02	1.	1.	1.	0.	0.
1981	3953.	6733.	.13	.75	.07	2.	5.	4.	1.	1.
1982	3177.	9447.	.19	.87	.11	16.	21.	19.	6.	3.
1983	2160.	11007.	.22	.88	.15	74.	71.	66.	24.	12.
1984	1625.	11917.	.24	.87	.17	171.	175.	170.	71.	35.
1985	1288.	12367.	.25	.83	.18	359.	335.	345.	160.	81.
1986	1040.	12426.	.25	.79	.19	496.	528.	579.	294.	151.
1987	991.	12287.	.25	.74	.19	753.	715.	838.	456.	238.
1988	1068.	12079.	.24	.70	.19	847.	865.	1081.	623.	331.
1989	1117.	11801.	.24	.67	.19	938.	961.	1274.	768.	416.
1990	1137.	11464.	.23	.63	.18	1015.	1001.	1400.	875.	483.

CHISQ =   10.268390

Table 10.12 Parameter values and corresponding simulation values for IVDUs, heterosexual partners and related pediatric cases in the South region.

```
THE IVDU & HTRO POPULATION SIZES ARE        300000       150000
THE VERY ACTIVE FRACTION IS    1.000000E-01
THE ACTIVITY RATIO IS        10.000000
THE NATURAL MORTALITY RATE XMU IS   5.320000E-04
THE INTERCHANGE RATE  FROM THE VERY ACTIVE CLASS TO THE ACTIVE CLASS IS
   4.166667E-03  AND THE TURNOVER RATE IS DLT =    4.166667E-03
THE NUMBER OF INFECTIOUS STAGES IS  M =       7
THE G PARAMETERS FOR THE TRANSFER BETWEEN ADULT STAGES ARE    7.355444E-02
   6.433708E-02    4.867545E-02    4.199281E-02    3.997889E-02
   5.152515E-02    5.398798E-02
THE WEIGHTS OF TRANSMISSION PER INFECTIOUS PARTNER TIMES THE FRACTION STILL
SEXUALLY ACTIVE FOR THE STAGES ARE WRH(I) =      2.000000       1.000000
   1.000000        1.500000        1.500000        1.500000
   7.500000
THE PROBABILITIES OF TRANSMISSION ARE QH, QHP & QC =    5.000000E-02
   1.000000E-01    1.000000E-01
THE EXTERNAL MIXING FRACTION IS ETA =     6.290000E-02
THE AVERAGE NUMBER OF NEEDLE-SHARING PARTNERS PER MONTH IS   2.641000E-01
BEFORE       2222        2, THEN IT IS REDUCED EACH YEAR BY A FACTOR OF
   1.000000 UNTIL DEC,       2222
THE FRACTION OF IVDU WHO ARE WOMEN IS   2.600000E-01
THE FRACTION OF HETEROSEXUALS WHO ARE WOMEN IS   5.700000E-01
THE AVERAGE NUMBER OF IVDU PARTNERS OF HETEROSEXUALS PER MONTH IS
   7.600000E-02
THE FRACTION   3.400000E-01 OF CHILDREN PROGRESS RAPIDLY TO AIDS WITH RATE
CONSTANT    8.000000E-02. OTHERS MOVE THROUGH M STAGES WITH SPEED FACTOR
   1.550000
THE FECUNDITY FC (CHILDREN/MONTH) IS    4.500000E-03
THE STARTING YEAR AND MONTH ARE       1975        1
THE STARTING NUMBER OF VERY ACTIVE INFECTIVES IS        1.000000
*****************************************************

THE SIMULATED INCIDENCES ARE GIVEN ON THE NEXT PAGE
```

s2ttt.m   s2ttt.m   s2ttt.m   s2ttt.m   s2ttt.m
****

YEAR	CLASS	HIV INC	HIV PREV	FRACTNAL_PREV ALL	V_A	ACT	YR AIDS DATA	INC SIM	AIDS(SIMULATION) PREV	DTHS	OUTSF
1975	IVDU	3.	4.	.00	.00	.00	0.	0.	0.	0.	0.
	HTRO	0.	0.	.00	–	–	****	0.	0.	0.	0.
	PED	0.	0.	–	–	–	0.	0.	0.	0.	
1976	IVDU	9.	12.	.00	.00	.00	0.	0.	0.	0.	0.
	HTRO	1.	1.	.00	–	–	0.	0.	0.	0.	0.
	PED	0.	0.	–	–	–	0.	0.	0.	0.	
1977	IVDU	28.	38.	.00	.00	.00	0.	0.	0.	0.	0.
	HTRO	3.	4.	.00	–	–	0.	0.	0.	0.	0.
	PED	0.	0.	–	–	–	0.	0.	0.	0.	
1978	IVDU	87.	121.	.00	.00	.00	0.	0.	0.	0.	0.
	HTRO	10.	14.	.00	–	–	0.	0.	0.	0.	0.
	PED	0.	0.	–	–	–	0.	0.	0.	0.	
1979	IVDU	272.	381.	.00	.01	.00	0.	0.	0.	0.	0.
	HTRO	32.	45.	.00	–	–	0.	0.	0.	0.	0.
	PED	1.	1.	–	–	–	0.	0.	0.	0.	
1980	IVDU	832.	1175.	.00	.04	.00	1.	1.	0.	0.	0.
	HTRO	99.	139.	.00	–	–	0.	0.	0.	0.	0.
	PED	2.	3.	–	–	–	0.	0.	0.	0.	
1981	IVDU	2380.	3439.	.01	.11	.00	2.	3.	1.	1.	1.
	HTRO	297.	423.	.00	–	–	0.	0.	1.	0.	0.
	PED	6.	8.	–	–	–	0.	1.	1.	0.	
1982	IVDU	5672.	8793.	.03	.27	.00	13.	11.	2.	4.	2.
	HTRO	805.	1187.	.01	–	–	1.	1.	2.	0.	0.
	PED	16.	23.	–	–	–	2.	2.	3.	1.	
1983	IVDU	9279.	17353.	.06	.52	.01	53.	33.	6.	12.	6.
	HTRO	1752.	2832.	.02	–	–	2.	4.	6.	1.	1.
	PED	36.	56.	–	–	–	6.	6.	7.	4.	
1984	IVDU	9334.	25453.	.08	.73	.01	148.	94.	12.	35.	17.
	HTRO	2801.	5407.	.04	–	–	13.	12.	12.	4.	2.
	PED	63.	110.	–	–	–	6.	12.	14.	8.	
1985	IVDU	7102.	30876.	.10	.84	.02	260.	239.	20.	96.	48.
	HTRO	3500.	8511.	.06	–	–	43.	32.	20.	12.	6.
	PED	88.	183.	–	–	–	14.	20.	24.	15.	
1986	IVDU	5725.	34540.	.12	.88	.03	444.	516.	30.	229.	115.
	HTRO	3953.	11866.	.08	–	–	77.	79.	30.	33.	16.
	PED	110.	268.	–	–	–	27.	30.	35.	25.	
1987	IVDU	5409.	37474.	.12	.88	.04	882.	936.	43.	470.	239.
	HTRO	4391.	15425.	.10	–	–	190.	168.	43.	76.	38.
	PED	135.	367.	–	–	–	53.	43.	48.	36.	
1988	IVDU	5605.	40111.	.13	.88	.05	1348.	1452.	58.	826.	426.
	HTRO	4873.	19185.	.13	–	–	316.	309.	58.	154.	78.
	PED	163.	481.	–	–	–	71.	58.	65.	50.	
1989	IVDU	5991.	42575.	.14	.86	.06	1995.	1983.	76.	1267.	663.
	HTRO	5362.	23101.	.15	–	–	503.	503.	76.	277.	142.
	PED	194.	608.	–	–	–	104.	76.	84.	66.	
1990	IVDU	6424.	44895.	.15	.84	.07	2530.	2454.	97.	1740.	926.
	HTRO	5801.	27072.	.18	–	–	709.	744.	97.	447.	233.
	PED	227.	749.	–	–	–	95.	97.	107.	86.	

```
CHISQD =      69.209290
CHISQP =       9.932351
CHISQC =      19.184600
SUM OF CHISQ-D,P,C =      98.326240
```

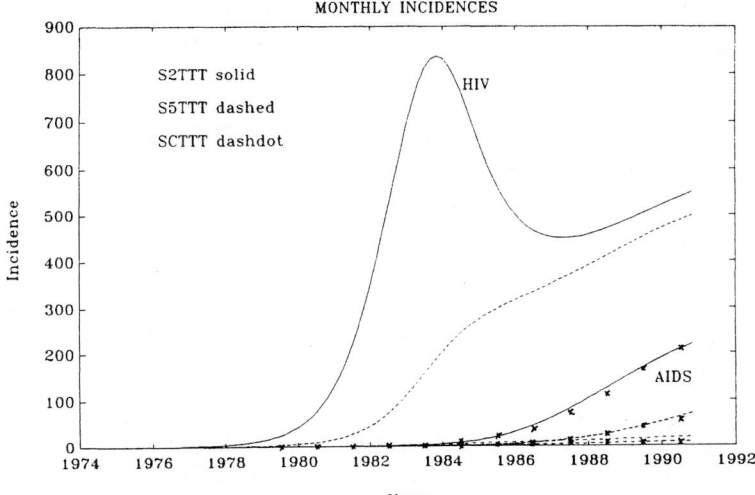

Figure 10.43. Estimated AIDS incidences (*) and simulated HIV and AIDS incidences for IVDUs, their heterosexual partners, and related pediatric cases in the entire South region corresponding to parameter values in Table 10.12.

The AIDS incidences in homosexual men in the three subregions are shown in Figure 10.47. The subregions B and C are similar so they can be combined, but subregion A (San Francisco and Seattle) has a different AIDS incidence pattern so it must be considered separately. In the combined B and C group, 61% are from subregion B and 39% are from subregion C. Figure 10.48 shows the AIDS incidences in homosexual IVDUs in the three subregions; the patterns are similar to those in Figure 10.47 so the subregions B and C can be combined, but subregion A has slower growth after 1986. Figure 10.49 shows AIDS incidences in homosexual men in the four aggregated groups in the South and West regions. It looks like the all other South group has the fastest growing incidence with slower growth in the all other West group and the San Francisco and Seattle group. The epidemic seems to start later and grow slower in the Washington DC and Baltimore group.

The general time trends for r/e groups of male IVDUs in each subregion are similar so they can be combined in each region. Moreover, the general patterns are similar for male IVDUs and female IVDUs in each subregion so they are combined. Figure 10.50 shows the AIDS incidences for the combined male and female IVDUs in the three West subregions. The growth rates in the three subregions are roughly the same since the AIDS incidence curves are approximately parallel. Thus the three subregions can be combined. Figure 10.51 for heterosexual partners of IVDUs also shows that the patterns are similar so the three subregions can be aggregated.

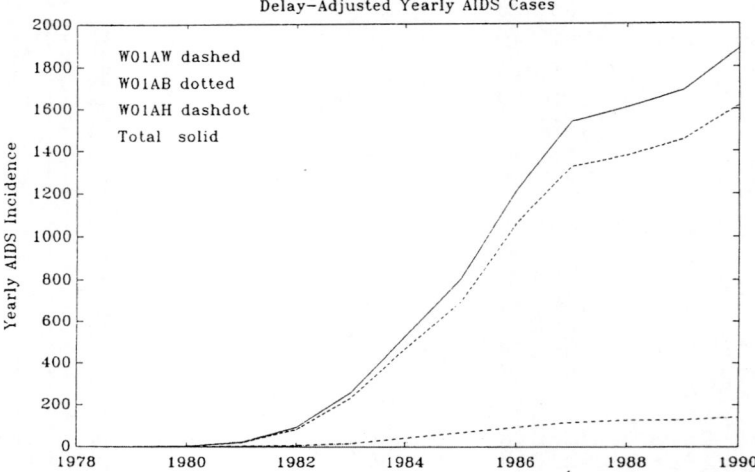

Figure 10.44. AIDS incidence in racial/ethnic groups of homosexual men in West subregion A (San Francisco and Seattle).

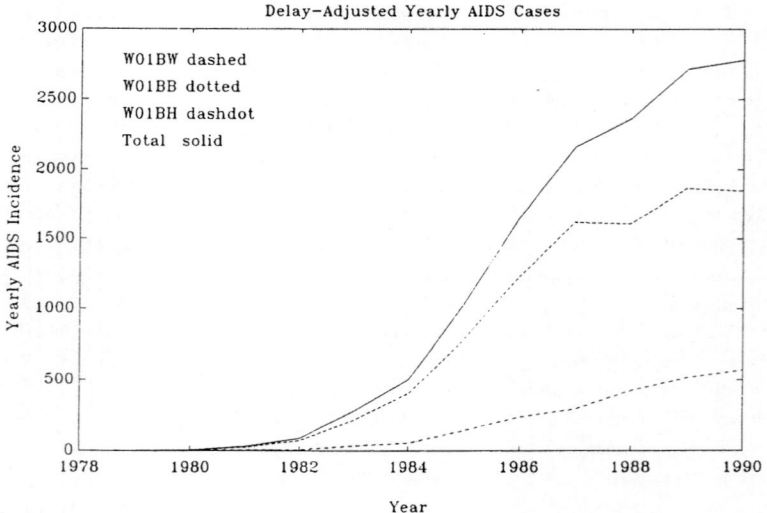

Figure 10.45. AIDS incidence in racial/ethnic groups of homosexual men in West subregion B (Los Angeles, Oakland, Anaheim, Riverside, and San Jose).

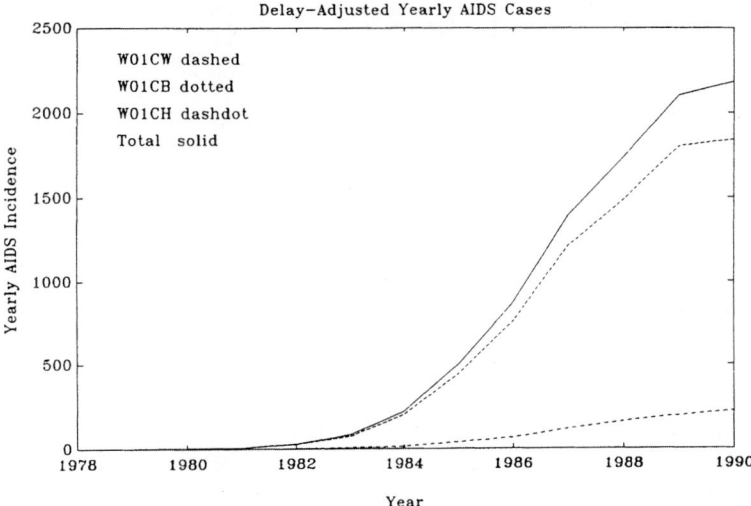

Figure 10.46. AIDS incidence in racial/ethnic groups of homosexual men in West subregion C (all other areas).

10.9. The West Region: Computer Simulations of the Aggregated Groups

Recall that the aggregated groups are homosexual men in subregion A (SF and Seattle), homosexual men in other West subregions and all IVDUs in the West. The simulated HIV and AIDS incidences in homosexual men in subregion A are given in Table 10.13 and Figure 10.52; the simulation for homosexual men in combined subregions B and C are given in Table 10.14 and Figure 10.53. The estimated population size for regions B and C is five times that of region A. The epidemic starting dates are both near the beginning of 1975. The average numbers of new sexual partners per month are similar and the external mixing fractions are both 1. Moreover, the yearly reduction factors and reduction starting dates are very similar. Although the best fit in region A has behavior change stopping in 1983 and the best fit in regions B and C has this change continuing through 1990, this difference is not significant since the actual behavior change in recent years cannot be determined reliably from current AIDS incidence data. Thus there seem to have been similar changes in sexual behavior in SF and Seattle and elsewhere in the West.

The simulations for the IVDUs in the West region are given in Table 10.15 and Figure 10.54. The best fit occurs when there is a yearly decrease in needle–sharing with a factor of 0.8 starting in July 1978. Although changes starting in 1978 would not have been motivated by AIDS, the decrease in needle–sharing is different than several other regions. It is not possible to fit the AIDS incidence data without changes in needle–sharing behavior. The population size estimate of 200,000 is an educated guess, but is adequate for the data so far since the epidemic starting date of August 1977 is late. The average number 0.72 of new needle–sharing partners

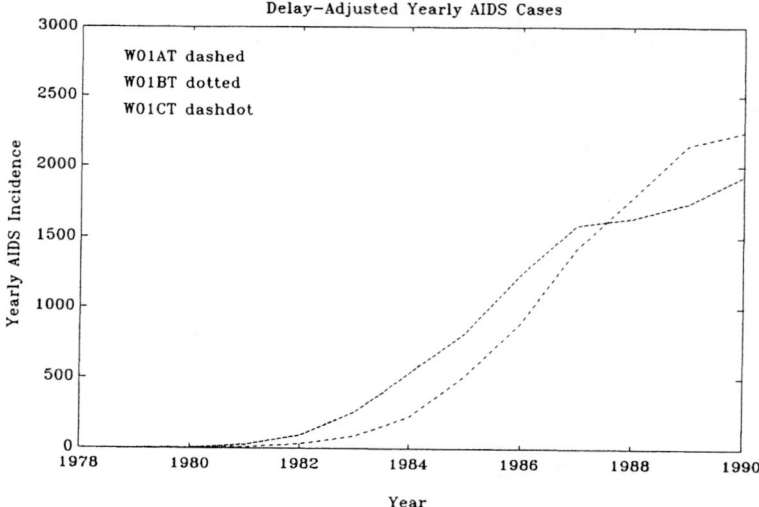

Figure 10.47. AIDS incidence in homosexual men in the three West subregions.

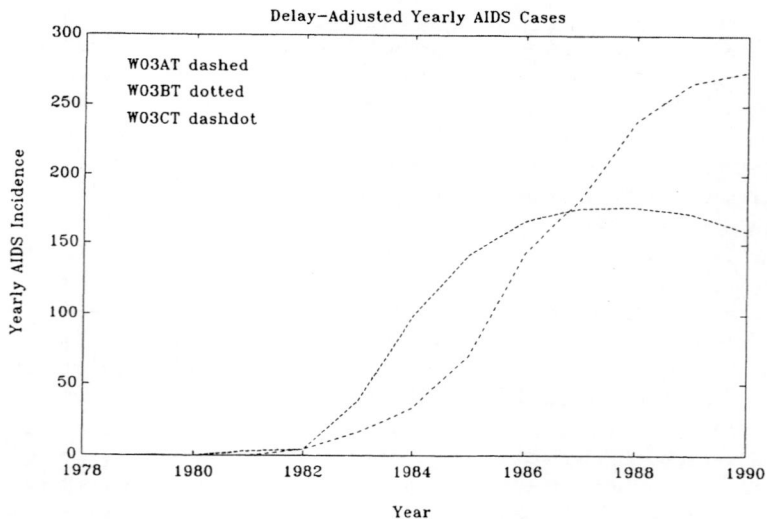

Figure 10.48. AIDS incidence in homosexual IVDUs in the three West subregions.

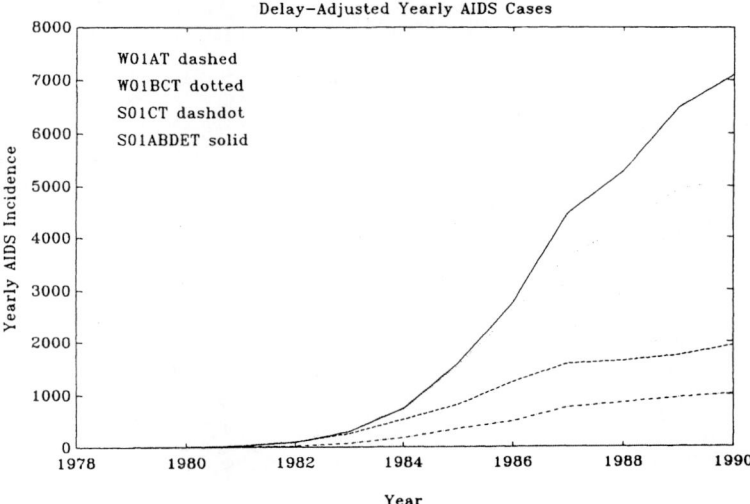

Figure 10.49. AIDS incidence in homosexual men in the four aggregated groups in the South and West regions.

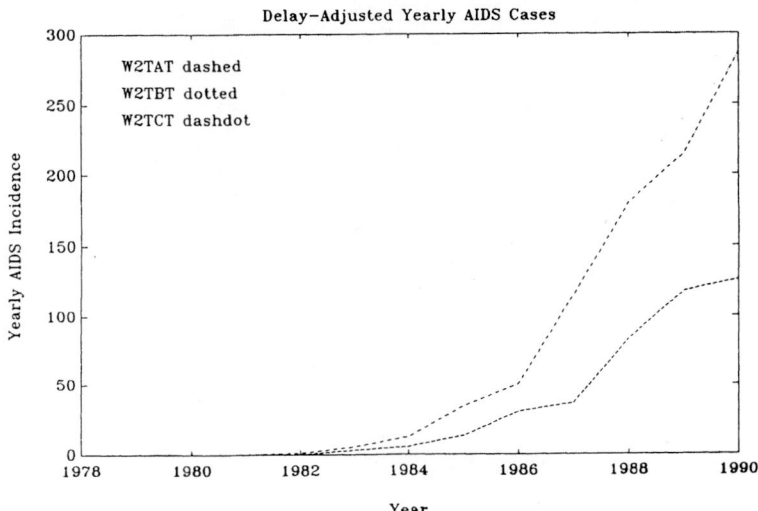

Figure 10.50. AIDS incidence in racial/ethnic groups of the combined male (heterosexual) and female IVDUs in the three West subregions.

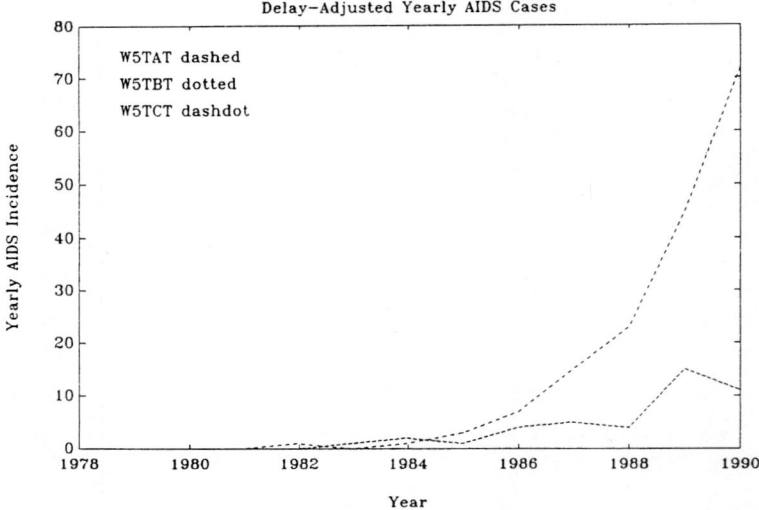

Figure 10.51. AIDS incidence in heterosexual partners of IVDUs in the three West subregions.

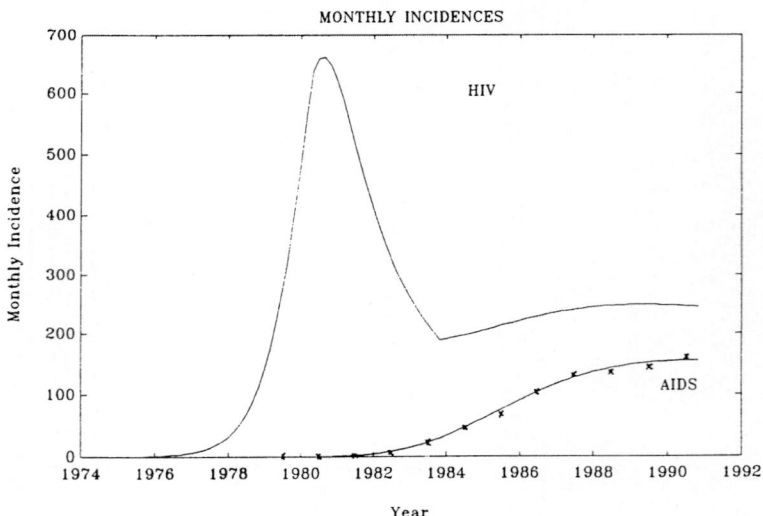

Figure 10.52. Estimated AIDS incidences (*) and simulated HIV and AIDS incidences for homosexual men in West subregion A corresponding to parameter values in Table 10.13.

Table 10.13 Parameter values and corresponding simulation values for homosexual men in West subregion A (San Francisco and Seattle).

```
THE POPULATION SIZE IS        80000, THE VERY ACTIVE FRACTION IS
   1.000000E-01 AND THE ACTIVITY RATIO IS        10.000000
THE NATURAL MORTALITY RATE XMU IS   5.320000E-04
THE INTERCHANGE RATE  FROM THE VERY ACTIVE CLASS TO THE ACTIVE CLASS IS
   4.166667E-03  AND THE TURNOVER RATE IS DLT =    4.166667E-03
THE NUMBER OF INFECTIOUS STAGES IS  M =        7
THE G PARAMETERS FOR THE TRANSFER BETWEEN STAGES ARE     7.355444E-02
   6.433708E-02     4.867545E-02     4.199281E-02    3.997889E-02
   5.152515E-02     5.398798E-02
THE WEIGHTS OF TRANSMISSION PER INFECTIOUS PARTNER TIMES THE FRACTION STILL
SEXUALLY ACTIVE FOR THE STAGES ARE WRH(I) =        2.000000        1.000000
   1.000000         1.500000         1.500000         1.500000
   7.500000
THE PROBABILITY OF TRANSMISSION IS QH =     5.000000E-02
THE EXTERNAL MIXING FRACTION IS ETA =        1.000000
THE AVERAGE NUMBER OF PARTNERS PER MONTH IS    5.829000E-01 BEFORE      1980
        7, THEN IT IS REDUCED EACH YEAR BY A FACTOR OF    6.602000E-01UNTIL
DEC,     1983
THE STARTING YEAR AND MONTH ARE        1975        2
THE STARTING NUMBER OF VERY ACTIVE INFECTIVES IS     1.000000
```

```
        ***********************************************
```

YEAR	HIV INC SIM	HIV PREV	FRACTNAL PREV ALL	V_A	ACT	YR AIDS DATA	INC SIM	AIDS(SIMULATION) PREV	DTHS	OUTSF
1975	7.	8.	.00	.00	.00	*****	0.	0.	0.	0.
1976	34.	40.	.00	.00	.00	*****	0.	0.	0.	0.
1977	160.	195.	.00	.01	.00	*****	0.	0.	0.	0.
1978	741.	912.	.01	.06	.01	*****	0.	0.	0.	0.
1979	2982.	3785.	.05	.23	.03	0.	1.	1.	0.	0.
1980	7199.	10603.	.13	.56	.08	2.	6.	5.	2.	1.
1981	6515.	16351.	.20	.74	.14	24.	25.	23.	8.	4.
1982	4190.	19499.	.24	.79	.18	94.	92.	85.	30.	15.
1983	2737.	20999.	.26	.79	.20	259.	252.	241.	96.	48.
1984	2353.	21918.	.27	.77	.22	533.	522.	527.	236.	118.
1985	2536.	22755.	.28	.76	.23	818.	866.	932.	461.	235.
1986	2724.	23465.	.29	.74	.24	1242.	1215.	1399.	748.	388.
1987	2870.	24001.	.30	.72	.25	1583.	1506.	1851.	1053.	557.
1988	2954.	24342.	.30	.70	.26	1633.	1707.	2228.	1329.	717.
1989	2978.	24497.	.31	.68	.27	1737.	1818.	2501.	1545.	849.
1990	2956.	24495.	.31	.65	.27	1931.	1861.	2670.	1692.	947.

CHISQ =   21.086610

Table 10.14 Parameter values and corresponding simulation values for homosexual men in West subregions B and C.

```
THE POPULATION SIZE IS        400000, THE VERY ACTIVE FRACTION IS
  1.000000E-01 AND THE ACTIVITY RATIO IS        10.000000
THE NATURAL MORTALITY RATE XMU IS   5.320000E-04
THE INTERCHANGE RATE  FROM THE VERY ACTIVE CLASS TO THE ACTIVE CLASS IS
  4.166667E-03  AND THE TURNOVER RATE IS DLT =      4.166667E-03
THE NUMBER OF INFECTIOUS STAGES IS  M =        7
THE G PARAMETERS FOR THE TRANSFER BETWEEN STAGES ARE      7.355444E-02
  6.433708E-02       4.867545E-02     4.199281E-02    3.997889E-02
  5.152515E-02     5.398798E-02
THE WEIGHTS OF TRANSMISSION PER INFECTIOUS PARTNER TIMES THE FRACTION STILL
SEXUALLY ACTIVE FOR THE STAGES ARE WRH(I) =        2.000000          1.000000
  1.000000        1.500000        1.500000        1.500000
  7.500000
THE PROBABILITY OF TRANSMISSION IS QH =     5.000000E-02
THE EXTERNAL MIXING FRACTION IS ETA =        1.000000
THE AVERAGE NUMBER OF PARTNERS PER MONTH IS    5.494000E-01 BEFORE        1980
         7, THEN IT IS REDUCED EACH YEAR BY A FACTOR OF     6.916000E-01UNTIL
DEC,      1990
THE STARTING YEAR AND MONTH ARE        1974        11
THE STARTING NUMBER OF VERY ACTIVE INFECTIVES IS     1.000000
```

`****************************************************`

YEAR	HIV INC SIM	HIV PREV	FRACTNAL_PREV ALL V_A ACT			YR AIDS DATA	INC SIM	AIDS(SIMULATION) PREV DTHS OUTSF		
1974	1.	2.	.00	.00	.00	*****	0.	0.	0.	0.
1975	9.	10.	.00	.00	.00	*****	0.	0.	0.	0.
1976	39.	48.	.00	.00	.00	*****	0.	0.	0.	0.
1977	170.	212.	.00	.00	.00	*****	0.	0.	0.	0.
1978	735.	921.	.00	.01	.00	*****	0.	0.	0.	0.
1979	3094.	3905.	.01	.05	.01	0.	1.	1.	0.	0.
1980	10718.	14180.	.04	.17	.02	8.	6.	6.	2.	1.
1981	17670.	30627.	.08	.35	.05	35.	27.	24.	8.	4.
1982	17052.	45516.	.11	.48	.07	114.	105.	97.	33.	16.
1983	13066.	55618.	.14	.55	.09	363.	334.	313.	117.	58.
1984	9454.	61448.	.15	.57	.11	729.	816.	797.	333.	166.
1985	6859.	64042.	.16	.57	.11	1560.	1581.	1627.	751.	379.
1986	5025.	64114.	.16	.55	.12	2568.	2536.	2770.	1393.	714.
1987	3680.	62131.	.16	.51	.12	3631.	3511.	4080.	2201.	1147.
1988	2663.	58488.	.15	.47	.11	4195.	4334.	5355.	3059.	1622.
1989	1888.	53595.	.13	.41	.10	4939.	4887.	6407.	3835.	2072.
1990	1304.	47886.	.12	.36	.09	5118.	5127.	7111.	4424.	2436.

CHISQ =   27.206620

189

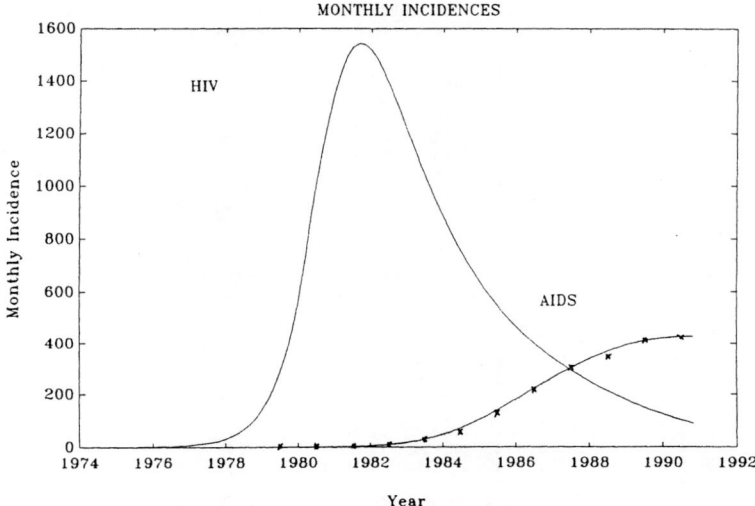

Figure 10.53. Estimated AIDS incidences (*) and simulated HIV and AIDS incidences for homosexual men in combined West subregions B and C corresponding to parameter values in Table 10.14.

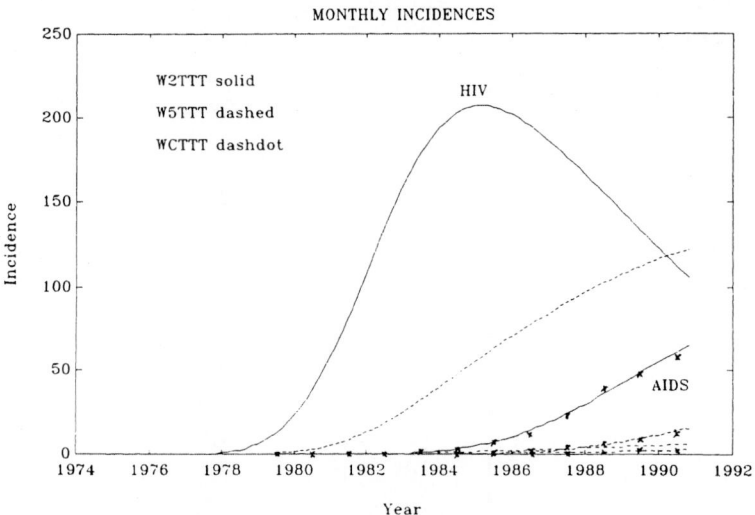

Figure 10.54. Estimated AIDS incidences (*) and simulated HIV and AIDS incidences for IVDUs, their heterosexual partners, and related pediatric cases in the entire West region corresponding to parameter values in Table 10.15.

Table 10.15 Parameter values and corresponding simulation values for IVDUs, heterosexual partners and related pediatric cases in the West region.

```
THE IVDU & HTRO POPULATION SIZES ARE      200000      100000
THE VERY ACTIVE FRACTION IS    1.000000E-01
THE ACTIVITY RATIO IS        10.000000
THE NATURAL MORTALITY RATE XMU IS   5.320000E-04
THE INTERCHANGE RATE  FROM THE VERY ACTIVE CLASS TO THE ACTIVE CLASS IS
   4.166667E-03  AND THE TURNOVER RATE IS DLT =    4.166667E-03
THE NUMBER OF INFECTIOUS STAGES IS  M =        7
THE G PARAMETERS FOR THE TRANSFER BETWEEN ADULT STAGES ARE    7.355444E-02
   6.433708E-02     4.867545E-02     4.199281E-02    3.997889E-02
   5.152515E-02     5.398798E-02
THE WEIGHTS OF TRANSMISSION PER INFECTIOUS PARTNER TIMES THE FRACTION STILL
SEXUALLY ACTIVE FOR THE STAGES ARE WRH(I) =        2.000000       1.000000
   1.000000        1.500000        1.500000        1.500000
   7.500000
THE PROBABILITIES OF TRANSMISSION ARE QH, QHP & QC =    5.000000E-02
   1.000000E-01    1.000000E-01
THE EXTERNAL MIXING FRACTION IS ETA =    1.000000
THE AVERAGE NUMBER OF NEEDLE-SHARING PARTNERS PER MONTH IS    7.177000E-01
BEFORE       1978        7, THEN IT IS REDUCED EACH YEAR BY A FACTOR OF
   8.012000E-01 UNTIL DEC,       1990
THE FRACTION OF IVDU WHO ARE WOMEN IS    2.200000E-01
THE FRACTION OF HETEROSEXUALS WHO ARE WOMEN IS    5.500000E-01
THE AVERAGE NUMBER OF IVDU PARTNERS OF HETEROSEXUALS PER MONTH IS
   5.500000E-02
THE FRACTION    3.400000E-01 OF CHILDREN PROGRESS RAPIDLY TO AIDS WITH RATE
CONSTANT    8.000000E-02. OTHERS MOVE THROUGH M STAGES WITH SPEED FACTOR
   1.550000
THE FECUNDITY FC (CHILDREN/MONTH) IS    6.000000E-03
THE STARTING YEAR AND MONTH ARE       1977        7
THE STARTING NUMBER OF VERY ACTIVE INFECTIVES IS       1.000000
*********************************************************

THE SIMULATED INCIDENCES ARE GIVEN ON THE NEXT PAGE
```

w2ttt.m   w2ttt.m   w2ttt.m   w2ttt.m   w2ttt.m
****

YEAR	CLASS	HIV INC	HIV PREV	FRACTNAL_PREV ALL	V_A	ACT	YR AIDS DATA	AIDS INC SIM	AIDS(SIMULATION) PREV	DTHS	OUTSF
1977	IVDU	4.	4.	.00	.00	.00	****	0.	0.	0.	0.
	HTRO	0.	0.	-	-	-	****	0.	0.	0.	0.
	PED	0.	0.	-	-	-	0.	0.	0.	0.	
1978	IVDU	32.	35.	.00	.00	.00	0.	0.	0.	0.	0.
	HTRO	2.	2.	.00	-	-	****	0.	0.	0.	0.
	PED	0.	0.	-	-	-	0.	0.	0.	0.	
1979	IVDU	140.	171.	.00	.00	.00	0.	0.	0.	0.	0.
	HTRO	9.	11.	.00	-	-	0.	0.	0.	0.	0.
	PED	0.	0.	-	-	-	0.	0.	0.	0.	
1980	IVDU	419.	572.	.00	.01	.00	1.	0.	0.	0.	0.
	HTRO	35.	45.	.00	-	-	0.	0.	0.	0.	0.
	PED	1.	1.	-	-	-	2.	0.	0.	0.	
1981	IVDU	917.	1436.	.01	.04	.00	1.	1.	0.	0.	0.
	HTRO	97.	137.	.00	-	-	0.	0.	0.	0.	0.
	PED	3.	4.	-	-	-	0.	0.	0.	0.	
1982	IVDU	1539.	2859.	.01	.07	.01	5.	4.	1.	1.	1.
	HTRO	208.	332.	.00	-	-	1.	0.	1.	0.	0.
	PED	6.	10.	-	-	-	1.	1.	1.	1.	
1983	IVDU	2087.	4733.	.02	.11	.01	15.	14.	2.	5.	2.
	HTRO	364.	669.	.01	-	-	2.	1.	2.	0.	0.
	PED	12.	20.	-	-	-	2.	2.	3.	1.	
1984	IVDU	2406.	6805.	.03	.16	.02	33.	38.	4.	15.	7.
	HTRO	546.	1164.	.01	-	-	3.	3.	4.	1.	1.
	PED	19.	36.	-	-	-	5.	4.	5.	3.	
1985	IVDU	2475.	8809.	.04	.20	.03	85.	86.	6.	37.	19.
	HTRO	733.	1812.	.02	-	-	7.	9.	6.	4.	2.
	PED	26.	57.	-	-	-	4.	6.	7.	5.	
1986	IVDU	2363.	10553.	.05	.23	.03	143.	164.	10.	79.	40.
	HTRO	911.	2593.	.03	-	-	24.	20.	10.	9.	4.
	PED	35.	84.	-	-	-	5.	10.	11.	8.	
1987	IVDU	2153.	11932.	.06	.26	.04	273.	276.	14.	148.	76.
	HTRO	1074.	3480.	.03	-	-	48.	40.	14.	19.	10.
	PED	44.	117.	-	-	-	14.	14.	16.	11.	
1988	IVDU	1901.	12901.	.06	.27	.04	461.	415.	19.	245.	127.
	HTRO	1219.	4443.	.04	-	-	73.	70.	19.	36.	18.
	PED	54.	155.	-	-	-	16.	19.	21.	16.	
1989	IVDU	1640.	13449.	.07	.27	.04	571.	569.	25.	367.	193.
	HTRO	1341.	5448.	.05	-	-	111.	111.	25.	62.	32.
	PED	63.	196.	-	-	-	32.	25.	27.	21.	
1990	IVDU	1386.	13595.	.07	.27	.05	695.	720.	31.	504.	269.
	HTRO	1435.	6456.	.06	-	-	146.	164.	31.	99.	52.
	PED	73.	242.	-	-	-	28.	31.	34.	28.	

CHISQD =   14.197060
CHISQP =   7.680979
CHISQC =   33.935920
SUM OF CHISQ-D,P,C =   55.813960

before changes start is similar to values in other regions; also similar are the average number 0.055 of new heterosexual partners per month of IVDUs and the fecundity 0.006. In the West 22% of AIDS cases in IVDUs are women and 55% of AIDS cases in heterosexual partners of IVDUs are women.

10.10. Discussion of Regional Comparisons

One major advantage of simulation modeling of AIDS incidence in risk groups in different regions is that the parameter values in the simulations can be compared. The simulation model fits for homosexual men in the subregions are summarized in Table 10.16. The theoretical epidemic starting dates give some insight into the relative possible starting times. Good estimates are usually obtained from the rule of thumb that the epidemic in the simulation model started approximately seven years before the date when the cumulative AIDS cases reached 40. The starting dates range from April 1974 for white homosexual men in New York City to March 1976 for homosexual men in Washington, D.C. and Baltimore. In Table 10.16 note that the HIV incidence increased in all groups until 1980 to 1982 before plateauing or declining. Thus the time trend patterns in the groups of homosexual men are quite similar; the starting dates are in a two year period, all of the HIV incidences increase until about 1980 to 1982 and then they all level off or decrease. Comparing population size estimates is not very enlightening since they are only crude approximations. Recall from Section 6.4.1 that the simulations are not sensitive to the population size estimates.

In the simulations the average numbers of new homosexual partners per month (before reduction if any occurs) range from a high of 0.58 in homosexual men in SF and Seattle to a low of 0.33 in the NE region outside NYC. Although these estimates are somewhat different, the similarity of these parameter values suggests that the growth of HIV infections in homosexual populations throughout the U.S. has been similar. Of course, the HIV epidemic seems to have started earlier in some locations than in others. Recent decreases in the growth rate of AIDS incidences in some locations and r/e groups suggests that there has been a reduction in risky homosexual behavior in these places and groups.

A major difference between simulations of AIDS incidence in homosexual men in regions is that some can be fit without any changes over time in sexual behavior while others require reductions in sexual partnership rates. In Table 10.16 only two groups could be fit without any reduction in sexual partnership rates; namely, black and Hispanic homosexual men in NYC and homosexual men in the South outside Washington, D.C. and Baltimore. It is possible that changes in behavior have occurred in these regions, but that these changes have not yet led to a slowing down of the AIDS incidence.

When the population size is very large and the AIDS incidence has been relatively low, the best fitting simulations can have a low initial monthly partnership rate, reductions in this partnership rate and a weak connection between the high risk group of sexually very active homosexual men and the lower risk group of active homosexual men. This type of fit occurs for the large populations of homosexual men in the NE outside NYC and in the South outside Washington, D.C. and Baltimore. In the two large homosexual populations in the NC region and

Table 10.16 Summary of Simulation Model Fits for Homosexual Men in Subregions of the US

region	size	epidemic starting date	initial partners per month	reduction starting date	reduction factor	external mixing fraction	first HIV incidence peak (year)	HIV prevalence in 1990
NYC (whites)	60,000	4/74	.56	1/81	.34	1	7,400 (1980)	8,100
NYC (nonwhites)	40,000	12/74	.46	none	none	.42	2,800 (1980)	22,000
Other NE	250,000	1/75	.33	7/84	.38	.30	10,000 (1981)	18,000
North Central	500,000	12/75	.55	1/81	.63	1	10,000 (1982)	26,900
Wash DC & Balt.	50,000	3/76	.46	1/82	.73	.53	4,000 (1981)	11,500
Other South	500,000	2/75	.37	none	none	.16	22,600 (1982)	142,000
SF & Seattle	80,000	2/75	.58	7/80	.66	1	7,200 (1980)	24,500
Other West	400,000	11/74	.55	7/80	.69	1	17,700 (1981)	48,000
Total	1,880,000							301,000

in the West outside SF and Seattle, the best fitting simulations have typical initial monthly partnership rates (0.55) and strongly connected very active and active risk groups, but they have reduction in the partnership rates starting very early (1/81 and 7/80).

The external mixing fractions in Table 10.16 are often near 1 corresponding to proportionate mixing, but lower values are obtained in two NE groups and in the South. External mixing fractions near 1 correspond to more mixing between high and low risk groups while lower values correspond to more internal mixing within the low and high risk groups.

It is important to recognize the limitations of the results in Table 10.16, since they reflect the best fits, but do not show nearby parameter sets for which the fit is almost as good. In particular the amount and stopping year for the reduction in sexual behavior are not reliable since changes in recent years have almost no impact on current AIDS incidence. This is consistent with the principle observed in Chapter 6 that HIV incidences in the last approximately six years cannot be estimated from current AIDS incidence data. Thus the HIV prevalences in 1990 in Table 10.16 must be viewed as possibilities instead of predictions. The value 142,000 for 1990 HIV prevalence in the South region outside Washington, D.C. and Baltimore is particularly suspect since it assumes that no changes of behavior occurred, but there may have been undetectable behavior changes in recent years in this region. Indeed, a careful examination of Figures 10.28 to 10.31 suggests that changes in behavior may have started to occur in white homosexual men in several subregions.

A summary of the results for AIDS in homosexual men in the regions follows. The three aggregated groups in the NE region really are different from each other. The epidemic started early in white homosexual men in NYC and the growth rate has slowed recently. The growth rate in black and Hispanic men in NYC was later and slower, but steady. The growth in the rest of the NE region was later and slowest. The growth pattern is the same throughout the NC region and is similar to that in white homosexual men in NYC, but it started later. The growth in AIDS incidence in homosexual men in Washington, D.C. and Baltimore seems to have slowed down, but there is not much evidence so far of behavior changes in other parts of the South. In the West the early rapid growth in homosexual men in San Francisco and Seattle has decreased recently; the pattern in the rest of the West is quite similar.

In Section 8.8 it is described how the simulation modeling in NYC of homosexual men, homosexual–IVDUs and IVDUs led to the conclusion that the homosexual–IVDUs do not constitute a crucial link between the epidemics in homosexual men and IVDUs. Since the epidemic in one population is not feeding or driving the epidemic in the other population, the homosexual men and IVDUs can be simulated separately. The AIDS incidence in homosexual–IVDUs is always less than 10% of that in homosexual men and the time trends are usually similar. Since simulation modeling of homosexual–IVDUs would not lead to new insights, these simulations have not been done.

For IVDUs the theoretical epidemic starting dates range from 1975 in the NE region to 1978 in subregions B and C of the NC region. The estimated population sizes of IVDUs at risk are only educated guesses. These population sizes may differ from actual at–risk population sizes, but it is shown in Section 6.4.1 that the simulation fits are not sensitive to the population size

Table 10.17 Summary of Simulation Model Fits for IVDUs in Subregions of the US

region	size	epidemic starting date	initial partners per month	reduction starting date	reduction factor	external mixing fraction	1990 HIV prevalence	heterosexual partners per month	fecundity per month
NY,NJ,CT,RI	300,000	1/75	.38	none	none	.15	90,200	.027	.0059
Other NE	100,000	1/77	.49	7/81	.72	1	8,000	.046	.0062
Chicago + small cities	100,000	7/77	.48	7/81	.72	1	4,400	.056	.0058
other NC	50,000	1/78	.50	7/81	.70	1	2,500	.059	.0054
South	300,000	1/75	.26	none	none	.63	44,900	.076	.0045
West	200,000	7/77	.72	7/78	.80	1	13,600	.055	.0060
Total	1,050,000						163,600		

estimates.

When the AIDS incidence in a population has slowed down in recent years, the simulation modeling can fit this by either a reduction in the needle–sharing partnership rate or a weak linkage between the risk groups so the HIV epidemic in the very active risk group goes up and down before the HIV epidemic in the active risk group starts to go up. Since it is possible to fit an AIDS incidence curve with either of the two patterns above, the type of pattern which gives the best fit may depend on minor differences and may not reflect major differences in behavior. In Table 10.17 the four groups with smaller population sizes have the former pattern and the two groups with the largest population sizes (300,000) have the latter pattern.

In the best fits for three of the groups with changes in needle–sharing behavior, the initial number of needle–sharing partners per month is 0.48 to 0.50 with a yearly reduction factor of 0.70 to 0.72 which starts in July 1981. In the West the initial partnership rate is 0.72, but the yearly reduction factor starts early (in July 1978) so that the partnership rate in mid–1980 is 0.46 which is similar to the value in the three groups above. In all four groups the very active and active risk groups mix randomly so they are strongly connected.

In the two groups with population sizes of 300,000 located in NE subregions A and B and in the South, the best fitting simulations have low monthly partnership rates of 0.38 and 0.27, respectively, but there are no changes in these partnership rates. The very active and active risk groups are weakly connected since the external mixing fractions are less than one. For these two regions it is clear from Figures 10.18 and 10.43 that the HIV epidemic on the very active risk group goes up and down before the HIV epidemic starts to increase in the active risk group. The downside of the HIV epidemic in the very active risk group leads to a slowdown in the AIDS incidence, but this is temporary since the HIV epidemic is biphasic so the AIDS incidence will also be biphasic with a later higher AIDS incidence peak. If this simulation fitting corresponds to what is actually happening in these regions, then the slowing down or leveling in the AIDS incidence is only temporary since it will soon start increasing again.

The net result of the simulation modeling fits to the AIDS incidence in IVDUs in different regions is that there are many more similarities in the parameter sets and patterns than differences. Although the HIV epidemic starting dates range over three years in the simulations, the growth in the AIDS incidences in IVDUs in these subregions are similar. Although the simulation modeling suggests that reduction in needle–sharing partnerships have occurred, it is not possible to determine the magnitude and extent of these changes from the current AIDS incidence data. It is important to recognize the limitations of the values in Table 10.17. These values correspond to the best fits to the AIDS data, but they do not reflect the nearby parameter values for fits which are almost as good.

Nationally, 23% of the AIDS cases in IVDUs are women. This percentage is between 19% and 26% in the aggregated groups. Nationally, 71% of the AIDS cases in heterosexual partners of IVDUs are women. This percentage is 86% in the NE, 59% in NC subregions A and D, 68% in NC subregions B and C, 57% in the South and 55% in the West. These differences from the national average may reflect regional reporting differences or actual differences.

The one parameter which is varied to fit the AIDS incidences in heterosexual partners of

IVDUs is the average number of new heterosexual partners per month. This value is usually about 0.06, but is 0.076 in the South and 0.027 in the NE subregions A and B. These differences may be due to regional reporting differences or may reflect more heterosexual transmission by IVDUs in the South and less in the NE subregions A and B. The very low value of 0.027 new heterosexual partners per month in NE subregions A and B may be due to their reluctance to categorize men as heterosexual partners of female IVDUs. The high value of 0.076 in the South suggests that relatively more people are categorized as heterosexual partners of IVDUs in the South than in the other regions. Because the heterosexual partnership rate is multiplied by the probability of transmission per new partner in the simulation modeling and good estimates of this probability of transmission are not available, reliable estimates of turnover rates in heterosexual partners of IVDUs cannot be made.

The one parameter which is varied to fit the AIDS incidences in perinatal transmissions to children from IVDU females and female heterosexual partners of IVDUs is the fecundity, *i.e.*, the average number of children per female per month. The values of this parameter are .0059, .0067, .0058, .0054, .0045 and .0060. These values are all reasonably close together and are reasonably close to the national average of 0.0057 which corresponds to the reported value of 68.6 births per 1000 women between ages 18 and 44 per year (World Almanac, 1988). The fecundity rate of 0.0045 in the South is significantly lower than in the other regions. Thus the actual fecundity rate may be lower there or some perinatal AIDS cases may be missed by the reporting system in the South. It is noteworthy that in the South the heterosexual partnership rate is unusually high and the fecundity rate is unusually low. This suggests that some people may be misclassified as heterosexual partners.

The fits in Table 10.16 and 10.17 yield a total HIV prevalence in 1990 of 301,000 homosexual men and 163,600 IVDUs. Of course, these are only crude approximations based on fitting reported AIDS incidence data in the subregions. Since homosexual men and IVDUs constitute about 80% of the reported AIDS cases in the U.S., it is plausible that the 464,600 HIV−positive homosexual men and IVDUs constitute 80% of about 580,000 HIV−positive people in the U.S. Since all of the data used is based on reported cases and underreporting may be between 10% and 20%, the estimate above suggests that the actual number of HIV−positive people in the U.S. might have been about 700,000 in 1990. This estimate is at the low end of estimates obtained by back calculation in Table B1 in the CDC workshop report (CDC, 1990c). This estimate is somewhat less than the CDC estimate that there were approximately 800,000 to 1.2 million HIV−positive people in the U.S. in 1990. Thus our estimate is lower, but is roughly consistent with other estimates; we are not claiming that our crude estimate is more accurate than the CDC estimate of about 1 million HIV−positive people in the U.S. in 1990.

The fitting of the model to geographically aggregated data carried out in this Chapter should be regarded as a first attempt. Although the aggregations used seem reasonable, fits with more r/e subgroups in more subregions might be better. Other factors such as interactions between subregions and nonuniformity within subregions have been ignored in the modeling here, but could be important. A better geographical analysis of data should be possible after more AIDS data have accumulated.

Listing of FIT10.FOR

```
C   This program  FIT10.FOR  finds the best chi-square fit to the
C   yearly AIDS incidence estimates from 1979 to 1990.  This Fortran
C   program was coded by Herb Hethcote and Jim Van Ark.  It is used in
C   Chapter 10 of the book, "MODELING HIV TRANSMISSION AND AIDS IN THE
C   UNITED STATES", to obtain fits to AIDS data for homosexual men and
C   for IVDUs in aggregations of 15 subregions.  The AIDS incidence
C   data are given in vector form with names such as NE2TABT.M
C   corresponding to the notation in Table 10.1.  After the AIDS data
C   vector is entered, the parameter values are specified by the user
C   (see Tables 3.1 and 6.1).  For each parameter value, the user can
C   accept the default value or choose a new value.  Then the user
C   chooses two dates: the reduction starting year and month and the
C   reduction stopping year.  The nonlinear minimization program BCONF
C   from IMSL is used to obtain the values of PAS, RDN and ETA which
C   give the best chi-square fit to the AIDS incidence data.  For each
C   set of parameter values, BCONF calls the subroutine EPI, which
C   simulates the HIV epidemic and AIDS cases using the difference
C   equations corresponding to Figure 3.1.  For each set of two dates,
C   the program displays the values of the three parameter values and
C   the chi-square value corresponding to the best fit. By trying
C   different combinations of the two dates, the user can minimize the
C   chi-square value.
C
      INTEGER N
      PARAMETER (N = 3)
      DIMENSION G(20),WRH(19),IPARAM(7),RPARAM(7),P(N),PGUESS(N),
     $ PSCALE(N),PLB(N),PUB(N),DAIDS(1975:1990)
      COMMON FH,R,QV,QA,XMU,DLT,PHI,THT,M,G,QH,WRH,NYSTRT,NMSTRT,
     $ IYEAR,IMONTH,LYEAR,NYSTOP,DAIDS
      EXTERNAL EPI,U4INF,UMACH,BCONF
      CHARACTER*10 FILE0
C
C THE AIDS INCIDENCE FILE NAME IS ENTERED AND THE DATA IS STORED IN
C DAIDS
      PRINT*,'INPUT A FILENAME (IN SINGLE QUOTES) FOR AIDS INCIDENCE'
      PRINT*,'BE SURE TO INCLUDE THE .m EXTENSION'
      READ*,FILE0
      DO 2 I = 1975,1978
    2 DAIDS(I) = 0.
      OPEN(UNIT=9,FILE=FILE0,STATUS='OLD')
      READ(9,*)(DAIDS(I),I=1979,1990)
      PRINT*,'DATA IN THE AIDS VECTOR STARTING IN 1975 IS',DAIDS
C
C BASED ON DETAILED MODELING OF HOMOSEXUAL MEN IN SAN FRANCISCO, A
C CRUDE ESTIMATE OF THE EPIDEMIC STARTING DATE IS 7 YEARS BEFORE THE
C CUMULATIVE AIDS CASES REACH 40.  ALSO THE POPULATION SIZE CAN BE
C CRUDELY ESTIMATED AS 7 TIMES THE CUMULATIVE AIDS INCIDENCE THROUGH
C 1990.
      FLAG = 0
      CAIDS = 0
      DO 4 I = 1975,1990
         PRCUM = CAIDS
         CAIDS = CAIDS + DAIDS(I)
         IF (FLAG.EQ.0.AND.CAIDS.GE.40) THEN
            IYEAR = I - 7
            IMONTH = INT(12*(40-PRCUM)/(CAIDS-PRCUM)+.5)
```

```
            FLAG = 1
         ENDIF
   4     CONTINUE
         NSIZE = INT(7.0*CAIDS/10000+.5)*10000
C  IO = 6 CORRESPONDS TO MONITOR OUTPUT
         IO = 6
C  STANDARD PARAMETERS WILL BE LISTED HERE.
C  LATER THE USER WILL BE ASKED IF HE/SHE WANTS TO CHANGE THEM.
         FH = .1
         R = 10
         XMU = .000532
         DLT = .05/12.
         PHI = .05/12.
         M = 7
         G(1) = .0764
         G(2) = .0665
         G(3) = .0499
         G(4) = .0429
         G(5) = .0408
         G(6) = .0529
         G(7) = .0555
         DO 5 I = 8, 20
   5     G(I) = 0
C  THE GAMMA VALUES NEED TO BE ADJUSTED SO THAT OUR DISCRETE
C  MODEL WORKS (GAMMA IS CONTINUOUS).
         DO 10  I = 1, 7
  10     G(I) = (1 - EXP(-G(I)))
         QH = .05
         WRH(1) = 2.
         WRHA = 1
         WRHP = 1.5
         WRHM = 7.5
         LYEAR = 1990
C  SETTING PARAMETERS FOR IMSL MINIMIZATION PROGRAM BCONF
         PLB(1) = .01
         PLB(2) = .01
         PLB(3) = 0.
         PUB(1) = 10
         PUB(2) = 1.5
         PUB(3) = 1.
         PSCALE(1) = 1
         PSCALE(2) = 1
         PSCALE(3) = 1
         FSCALE = 1
         ITP = 0
         RPARAM(1) = .001
         RPARAM(2) = .001
C
         PRINT*,' '
         PRINT*,'THE DEFAULT PARAMETERS VALUES ARE LISTED BELOW;'
         PRINT*,'YOU MAY CHANGE THEM OR NOT AS YOU CHOOSE.'
         PRINT*,'ANSWER 1 FOR  change  OR 2 FOR  no change.'
         PRINT*,' '
C
C  POPULATION PARAMETER VALUES
   6     PRINT*,'THE CRUDE APPROXIMATION OF ',NSIZE,' AS THE STARTING '
         PRINT*,'POPULATION SIZE IS 7.0 TIMES THE TOTAL AIDS CASES',
        $' THROUGH 1990'
         READ*,INPUT
         IF (INPUT.NE.2) THEN
```

```
            PRINT*,'INPUT NSIZE = '
            READ*,NSIZE
      ENDIF
      PRINT*,'VERY ACTIVE FRACTION FH = ',FH
      PRINT*,'DEFAULT ACTIVITY RATIO R = ',R
      READ*,INPUT
      IF (INPUT.NE.2) THEN
            PRINT*,'INPUT FH AND R'
            READ*,FH,R
      ENDIF
      SIZE = NSIZE*1.
      QV = FH*SIZE
      QA = (1-FH)*SIZE
      PRINT*, 'XMU = ',XMU,',   DLT = ',DLT,', PHI = ',PHI
      READ*,INPUT
      IF (INPUT.NE.2) THEN
            PRINT*,'XMU , DLT, PHI = '
            READ*,XMU,DLT,PHI
      ENDIF
      THT = PHI*QV/QA
C
C READ STARTING YEAR AND MONTH, THEN ENDING YEAR
      PRINT*,'A CRUDE APPROXIMATION OF THE EPIDEMIC STARTING DATE IS '
      PRINT*,'7 YEARS BEFORE THE CUMULATIVE AIDS CASES REACH 40.'
      PRINT*,'THE STARTING YEAR IS IYEAR = ',IYEAR
      PRINT*,'THE STARTING MONTH NUMBER IS IMONTH = ',IMONTH
      READ*,INPUT
      IF (INPUT.NE.2) THEN
            PRINT*,'IYEAR, IMONTH = '
            READ*,IYEAR,IMONTH
      ENDIF
      PRINT*,'THE ENDING YEAR IS LYEAR = ',LYEAR
      READ*,INPUT
      IF (INPUT.NE.2) THEN
            PRINT*,'NEW LYEAR = '
            READ*,LYEAR
      ENDIF
C
C   M IS THE NUMBER OF INFECTIOUS STAGES IN THE MODEL,
C   WHERE STAGE 1 IS THE HIV INCUBATION PHASE, STAGES 2 to INT(M/2)
C   FORM THE ASYMPTOMATIC PHASE, STAGES INT(M/2)+1 to M-1 FORM THE
C   PRE-AIDS PHASE, STAGE M IS AIDS, AND STAGE M+1 IS DEATH.
      PRINT*,'THE NUMBER OF STAGES IS M = ',M
      READ*,INPUT
      IF (INPUT.NE.2) THEN
            PRINT*,'NEW M ='
            READ*,M
      ENDIF
C
C   G IS THE VECTOR OF EXPONENTIAL WAITING TIMES gamma FOR THE STAGES
      PRINT*,'THE VALUES FOR gamma FOR THE STAGES ARE '
      PRINT*,(G(I),I=1,M)
      READ*,INPUT
      IF (INPUT.NE.2) THEN
            PRINT*,'INPUT ',M,' NEW gamma VALUES.'
            READ*,(G(I),I=1,M)
C   THE GAMMA VALUES NEED TO BE ADJUSTED SO THAT OUR DISCRETE
C   MODEL WORKS (GAMMA IS CONTINUOUS).
            DO 15 I = 1, M
 15         G(I) = (1 - EXP(-G(I)))
```

```
C
      ENDIF
C
C  PROBABILITY OF TRANSMISSION FOR AN ASYMPTOMATIC PERSON
C  (STAGES 2 - M/2) IS QH.
      PRINT*,'THE PROBABILITY OF TRANSMISSION BY A STAGE-2',
     $' INFECTIVE IS QH = ',QH
      READ*,INPUT
      IF (INPUT.NE.2) THEN
           PRINT*,'INPUT QH = '
           READ*,QH
      ENDIF
C
C   PROBABILITY OF TRANSMISSION IN OTHER PHASES HAS W(I) FACTOR.
      PRINT*,'SINCE THE WEIGHT FACTORS W(I) AND RELATIVE ACTIVITY',
     $' FACTORS rho APPEAR ONLY AS A PRODUCT, THEY ARE INPUT THAT',
     $' WAY.  THE PRODUCTS FOR HIV INCUBATION, ',
     $'ASYMPTOMATIC PRE-AIDS, AND AIDS PHASES ARE ',
     $ WRH(1),WRHA,WRHP,WRHM
      READ*,INPUT
      IF (INPUT.NE.2) THEN
           PRINT*,'INPUT WRH(1), WRHA, WRHP, AND WRH(M) '
           READ*,WRH(1),WRHA,WRHP,WRHM
      ENDIF
C
C   OUTPUT OF PARAMETER VALUES IN THE MODEL
      WRITE(IO,*)'PROGRAM    FIT10.FOR   '
      WRITE(IO,*)'COMPUTER SIMULATION OF HIV AND AIDS IN A POPULATION'
      WRITE(IO,*)' '
      WRITE(IO,*)'THE SIZE OF THE POPULATION IS ',NSIZE
      WRITE(IO,*)'THE VERY ACTIVE FRACTION IS ',FH
      WRITE(IO,*)'THE ACTIVITY RATIO IS ',R
      WRITE(IO,*)'THE NATURAL MORTALITY RATE XMU IS',XMU
      WRITE(IO,*)'THE TURNOVER RATE DLT IS',DLT
      WRITE(IO,*)'THE CHANGE RATE PHI FROM VERY ACTIVE TO ACTIVE',
     $' IS',PHI
      WRITE(IO,*)'THE WEIGHT FACTORS FOR INFECTIVITY ARE',
     $ WRH(1),WRHA,WRHP,WRHM
      WRITE(IO,*)'THE PROBABILITY OF TRANSMISSION IS QH = ',QH
C
C   TABLE HEADING HERE
      WRITE(IO,*)' '
      WRITE(IO,*)'             ',
     $'**********************************************'
      WRITE(IO,*)' '
      WRITE(IO,900)
 900  FORMAT(8X,'M     NYSTRT   NYSTOP    PAS    RDCTN    ETA   CHISQ')
      WRITE(IO,*) ' '
C
  8   CALL U4INF(IPARAM,RPARAM)
      PRINT*,'INPUT REDUCTION STARTING DATE, NYSTRT,NMSTRT = '
      READ*,NYSTRT,NMSTRT
      PRINT*,'THE LAST YEAR OF THE REDUCTION IS NYSTOP = '
      READ*,NYSTOP
      PRINT*,'INPUT INITIAL GUESSES FOR PAS & RDCTN '
      READ*,PGUESS(1),PGUESS(2)
      PRINT*,'INPUT INITIAL GUESS FOR ETA '
      READ*,PGUESS(3)
C
C   THE HIV INCUBATION PHASE (STAGE 1) AND THE AIDS PHASE (STAGE M)
C   HAVE FIXED GIVEN TRANSITION RATES. THE STAGES IN THE ASYMPTOMATIC
```

```
C    PHASE HAVE EQUAL LENGTH, AND THE STAGES IN THE PRE-AIDS PHASE
C    HAVE EQUAL LENGTH.
     IM2 = M/2
     WRH(M) = WRHM
     DO 20 I = 2, IM2
 20  WRH(I) = WRHA
     DO 22 I = IM2+1, M-1
 22  WRH(I) = WRHP

     CALL BCONF(EPI,N,PGUESS,ITP,PLB,PUB,PSCALE,FSCALE,IPARAM,
    $ RPARAM,P,CHISQ)
     PRINT*,'NUMBER OF FUNCTION & GRADIENT EVALUATIONS = ',
    $ IPARAM(3),IPARAM(5)

950  FORMAT(1X,3I5,4F10.4)
     WRITE(IO,950)NYSTRT,NMSTRT,NYSTOP,P(1),P(2),P(3),CHISQ
     PRINT*,'DO YOU WISH TO DO IT AGAIN?  (2 = yes)'
     READ*,INPUT
     IF (INPUT.EQ.2) THEN
         PRINT*,'DO YOU WISH ONLY TO CHANGE  nystrt,nmstrt,nystop,',
    $        'pas,rdctn & eta?'
         READ*,INPUT
         IF (INPUT.EQ.2) GOTO 8
         GOTO 6
     ENDIF
     END
C
C    ********************************************************************
C
C    SUBROUTINE TO SIMULATE HIV EPIDEMIC
     SUBROUTINE EPI(N,P,CHISQ)
     DIMENSION X(20),Y(20),Z(20),DX(20),DY(20),DZ(20),G(20),
    $ WRH(19),DAIDS(1975:1990),P(N)
     COMMON FH,R,QV,QA,XMU,DLT,PHI,THT,M,G,QH,WRH,NYSTRT,NMSTRT,
    $ IYEAR,IMONTH,LYEAR,NYSTOP,DAIDS
C
     PAS = P(1)
     RDCTN = P(2)
     ETA = P(3)
     PHS = PAS/(1 + FH*(R-1))
     RDCTMO = RDCTN**(1./12.)
C
C    INITIALIZING ON IMONTH OF IYEAR
     START = 1
     DO 50 I = 1,M+1
     X(I) = 0
     Y(I) = 0
 50  Z(I) = 0
     X(1) = START
     SV = QV - X(1)
     SA = QA
C
C    STARTING THE ITERATION, WITH STEP SIZE = 1 MONTH
     NMONTH = IMONTH
     LASTK = LYEAR - IYEAR
     PRAIDS = 0
     CHISQ = 0
     DO 600 K = 0, LASTK
     NYEAR = IYEAR + K
C
```

```fortran
C    J  IS THE NUMBER OF THE MONTH
     DO  500 J = NMONTH, 12
C
C  ACTIVE HOMOSEXUALS HAVE PH PARTNERS PER MONTH
C  VERY ACTIVE HOMOSEXUALS HAVE R*PH PARTNERS PER MONTH
     IF (NYEAR.LT.NYSTRT) THEN
         PH = PHS
         ELSEIF (NYEAR.EQ.NYSTRT.AND.J.LT.NMSTRT) THEN
         PH = PHS
         ELSEIF (NYEAR.LE.NYSTOP) THEN
         PH = PHS*RDCTMO**((NYEAR-NYSTRT-1)*12+13-NMSTRT+J)
         ELSE
         PH = PHS*RDCTMO**((NYSTOP-NYSTRT)*12+13-NMSTRT)
         ENDIF
C
C  CALCULATING THE INCIDENCES
         ASUM = 0
         VSUM = 0
         DO 100 I=1,M
         ASUM = ASUM + WRH(I)*Y(I)
 100     VSUM = VSUM + WRH(I)*R*X(I)
         SUM = ASUM + VSUM
         DNM = QA - Y(M+1) + R*(QV - X(M+1))
         AINC = PH*QH*((1.- ETA)*ASUM*SA/(QA - Y(M+1)) + ETA*SUM*SA/DNM)
         VINC = PH*QH*((1.-ETA)*VSUM*SV/(QV-X(M+1)) + ETA*SUM*R*SV/DNM)
C
C  CALCULATING THE DIFFERENCES
         DSV = (DLT+XMU)*(QV-SV)-VINC-PHI*SV+THT*SA
         DSA = (DLT+XMU)*(QA-SA)-AINC+PHI*SV-THT*SA
         DX(1) = VINC-(G(1)+XMU+DLT+PHI)*X(1)+THT*Y(1)
         DY(1) = AINC - (G(1)+XMU+DLT+THT)*Y(1)+PHI*X(1)
         DZ(1) = DLT*(X(1)+Y(1))-(G(1)+XMU)*Z(1)
         DO 200 I=2,M
         DX(I) = G(I-1)*X(I-1)+THT*Y(I)-(G(I)+XMU+PHI+DLT)*X(I)
         DY(I) = G(I-1)*Y(I-1)+PHI*X(I)-(G(I)+XMU+THT+DLT)*Y(I)
 200     DZ(I) = G(I-1)*Z(I-1)+DLT*(X(I)+Y(I))-(G(I)+XMU)*Z(I)
         DZ(M) = DZ(M) - G(M-1)*Z(M-1)
         ZAIDS = ZAIDS + G(M-1)*Z(M-1)
         DX(M+1) = G(M)*X(M)+THT*Y(M+1)-(XMU+PHI+DLT)*X(M+1)
         DY(M+1) = G(M)*Y(M)+PHI*X(M+1)-(XMU+THT+DLT)*Y(M+1)
         DZ(M+1) = (DLT+XMU)*(X(M+1)+Y(M+1)) + G(M)*Z(M)
         DZ(M+1) = DZ(M+1) + XMU*(X(M) + Y(M) + Z(M))
C
C  UPDATING EACH CLASS
         SV = SV + DSV
         SA = SA + DSA
         DO 300 I=1,M+1
         X(I) = X(I) + DX(I)
         Y(I) = Y(I) + DY(I)
 300     Z(I) = Z(I) + DZ(I)
C
C  CHECKING CONSERVATION IN QV AND QA
         CKQV = SV
         CKQA = SA
         DO 400 I = 1, M+1
         CKQV = CKQV + X(I)
 400     CKQA = CKQA + Y(I)
         IF (ABS(CKQV-QV)/QV + ABS(CKQA-QA)/QA.GT.1.E-4) THEN
         PRINT*,'CONSERVATION CHECK NOT SATISFIED'
         PRINT*,QV,CKQV,QA,CKQA
```

```
      ENDIF
  500 CONTINUE
C
C YEARLY OUTPUT
      DEATHS = X(M+1) + Y(M+1) + Z(M+1)
      AIDS = DEATHS + X(M) + Y(M) + Z(M)
      AIDINC = AIDS - PRAIDS
      IF(NYEAR.GE.1978.AND.NYEAR.LE.1990)THEN
           CHISQ = CHISQ + (DAIDS(NYEAR)-AIDINC)**2 / AIDINC
      ENDIF
      PRAIDS = AIDS
  600 NMONTH = 1
      RETURN
      END



                    Listing of IVDU10.FOR

C This program  IVDU10.FOR  is used for fitting to heterosexual and
C perinatal AIDS data and also for producing tables of simulation
C values.  This program was coded by Herb Hethcote and Jim Van Ark.
C It is used in Chapter 10 of the book,  "MODELING HIV TRANSMISSION
C AND AIDS IN THE UNITED STATES",  to do fitting and to produce
C Tables 10.5, 10.6, 10.8, 10.9, 10.12 and 10.15. The program
C HOMO10.FOR for producing Tables 10.2, 10.3, 10.4, 10.7, 10.10,
C 10.11, 10.13 and 10.14 for homosexual men is similar, but simplier
C since there are no heterosexual partners. For an aggregated
C population, the AIDS incidence data from 1979 to 1990 for IVDUs,
C heterosexual cases and perinatal cases are input to the program as
C vectors such as NE2TABT.M, NE5TABT.M AND NECTABT.M.  After the
C parameter values found by FIT10.FOR for the best fit to the AIDS
C data for IVDUs are entered into this program, the user runs the
C program in terminal mode to find the value of the parameter PAP,
C the average number of new heterosexual partners per month, which
C gives the best fit.  This PAP value is found by a user-directed
C iterative search to minimize the chi-square value of the fit to the
C heterosexual AIDS data.  After the value of PAP has been found, the
C fecundity FC is found by a user-directed iterative search to
C minimize the chi-square value of the fit to the perinatal AIDS
C data.  When the best fitting values of PAP and FC have been found,
C then the printer mode is used to produce a table of parameter
C values followed by simulation values for the HIV epidemic and AIDS
C cases in IVDUs (I), their heterosexual partners (P), and perinatal
C cases in children (C).  The program also produces external files of
C the bimonthly HIV and AIDS incidence values for making MATLAB
C graphs from 1974 to 1990 using the program GRIVDU10.M.
C
      DIMENSION X(20),Y(20),Z(20),DX(20),DY(20),DZ(20),GA(20),GP(20),
     $ WRH(19),DIVDU(1975:1990),DHTRO(1975:1990),DPED(1975:1990),
     $ NAIVDU(102),NHIVDU(102),NAHTRO(102),NHHTRO(102),NAPED(102),
     $ NHPED(102),YP(20),ZP(20),DYP(20),DZP(20),YC(20),DYC(20)
C
      CHARACTER*10 FILEOI,FILE1I,FILE2I,FILEOH,FILE1H,FILE2H,
     $ FILEOC,FILE1C,FILE2C
C
C THE AIDS INCIDENCE FILE NAMES ARE ENTERED AND THE DATA ARE STORED
C IN VECTORS
      PRINT*,'INPUT A FILENAME (IN SINGLE QUOTES) FOR IVDU INCIDENCE'
      PRINT*,'BE SURE TO INCLUDE THE .m EXTENSION'
```

```
      READ*,FILE0I
C  NOTE:  INPUT FILE  ALWAYS STARTS IN 1979!
      INYEAR = 1979
      DO 5 N = 1975,INYEAR-1
      DIVDU(N) = 0.
      DHTRO(N) = 0.
    5 DPED(N) = 0.
      OPEN(UNIT=9,FILE=FILE0I,STATUS='OLD')
      READ(9,*)(DIVDU(N),N=INYEAR,1990)
      PRINT*,'DATA IN IVDU VECTOR STARTING IN 1975 IS',DIVDU
      PRINT*,'INPUT THE FRACTION OF IVDUs WHO ARE WOMEN'
      READ*,PIW
C
      PRINT*,'INPUT THE FILENAME (SINGLE QUOTES) FOR HTRO INCIDENCE'
      PRINT*,'BE SURE TO INCLUDE THE .m EXTENSION'
      READ*,FILE0H
      OPEN(UNIT=9,FILE=FILE0H,STATUS='OLD')
      READ(9,*)(DHTRO(N),N=INYEAR,1990)
         PRINT*,'DATA IN HTRO VECTOR STARTING IN 1975 IS',DHTRO
      PRINT*,'INPUT THE FRACTION OF HETEROSEXUALS WHO ARE WOMEN'
      READ*,PHW
C
      PRINT*,'INPUT THE FILENAME (IN SINGLE QUOTES) FOR PED INCIDENCE'
      PRINT*,'BE SURE TO INCLUDE THE .m EXTENSION'
      READ*,FILE0C
      OPEN(UNIT=9,FILE=FILE0C,STATUS='OLD')
      READ(9,*)(DPED(N),N=INYEAR,1990)
         PRINT*,'DATA IN PED VECTOR STARTING IN 1975 IS',DPED
C
C  THE DEFAULT NAMES FOR THE EXTERNAL DATA FILES TO BE WRITTEN TO
C  ARE GIVEN HERE; ONE CAN CHANGE THESE NAMES AT THE TIME OF WRITING.
      FILE1I = 'MTGRF1.M'
      FILE2I = 'MTGRF2.M'
      FILE1H = 'MTGRF3.M'
      FILE2H = 'MTGRF4.M'
      FILE1C = 'MTGRF5.M'
      FILE2C = 'MTGRF6.M'
      DATA NAIVDU /102*0/, NHIVDU /102*0/
      DATA NAHTRO /102*0/, NHHTRO /102*0/
      DATA NAPED  /102*0/, NHPED  /102*0/
C
C  PARAMETERS WILL BE LISTED HERE.  LATER USER WILL BE ASKED ABOUT
C  CHANGING.
      NSIZE = 150000
      NSIZEP = NSIZE/2
      FH = .1
      R = 10
      XMU = .000532
      DLT = .05/12.
      PHI = .05/12.
      ETA = .5
      M = 7
      GA(1) = .0764
      GA(2) = .0665
      GA(3) = .0499
      GA(4) = .0429
      GA(5) = .0408
      GA(6) = .0529
      GA(7) = .0555
      DO 7 I = 8, 20
```

```
7      GA(I) = 0
       G1 = .4571
       G2 = .0190
       G3 = .0159
       GM = .0555
C
C  THE GAMMA VALUES NEED TO BE ADJUSTED SO THAT OUR DISCRETE MODEL
C  WORKS (GAMMA IS CONTINUOUS)
       DO 9  I=1,M
   9   GA(I)=(1-EXP(-GA(I)))
       QH = .05
       QHP = .1
       QC = .1
       WRH(1) = 2.
       WRHA = 1.
       WRHP = 1.5
       WRHM = 7.5
       NYSTRT = 1981
       NMSTRT = 1
       NYSTOP = 1986
       PAS = .7972
       RDCTN = .6889
       PAP = .0181
       FC = .0012
       A = 1.55
       PC = .34
       B = .08
       IYEAR = 1974
       IMONTH = 1
       LYEAR = 1990
       START = 1
  11   PRINT*,'INPUT 6 FOR TERMINAL OUTPUT AND 8 FOR PRINTER OUTPUT'
       READ*,IO
       PRINT*,' '
       PRINT*,'THE DEFAULT STARTING PARAMETERS WILL BE LISTED;'
       PRINT*,'YOU MAY CHANGE THEM OR NOT AS YOU CHOOSE.'
       PRINT*,'ANSWER 1 FOR  change  OR 2 FOR  no change.'
       PRINT*,' '
C
C  POPULATION PARAMETER VALUES
       PRINT*,'THE IVDU & HTRO POPULATION SIZES ARE ',NSIZE,NSIZEP
       READ*,INPUT
       IF (INPUT.NE.2) THEN
            PRINT*,'INPUT NSIZE & NSIZEP = '
            READ*,NSIZE,NSIZEP
       ENDIF
       PRINT*,'VERY ACTIVE FRACTION FH = ',FH
       PRINT*,'DEFAULT ACTIVITY RATIO R = ',R
       READ*,INPUT
       IF (INPUT.NE.2) THEN
            PRINT*,'INPUT FH AND R'
            READ*,FH,R
       ENDIF
       SIZE = NSIZE*1.
       QV = FH*SIZE
       QA = (1-FH)*SIZE
       QAP = NSIZEP*1.
       PRINT*, 'XMU = ',XMU,',   DLT = ',DLT,', PHI = ',PHI
       READ*,INPUT
       IF (INPUT.NE.2) THEN
```

```
                  PRINT*,'XMU , DLT, PHI = '
                  READ*,XMU,DLT,PHI
            ENDIF
            THT = PHI*QV/QA
C
C     M IS THE NUMBER OF INFECTIOUS STAGES IN THE MODEL, WHERE
C     STAGE 1 IS THE HIV INCUBATION PHASE, STAGES 2 to INT(M/2) FORM THE
C     ASYMPTOMATIC PHASE, STAGES INT(M/2)+1 to M-1 FORM THE PRE-AIDS
C     PHASE, STAGE M IS AIDS, AND STAGE M+1 IS DEATH.
            PRINT*,'THE NUMBER OF INFECTIOUS STAGES IS  M = ',M
            READ*,INPUT
            IF (INPUT.NE.2) THEN
                  PRINT*,'INPUT NUMBER OF STAGES, M = '
                  READ*,M
            ENDIF
C
C     ADJUSTMENT FOR gamma's FOR PEDIATRIC CASES.
C     THE HIV INCUBATION PHASE (STAGE 1) AND THE AIDS PHASE (STAGE M)
C     HAVE FIXED GIVEN TRANSITION RATES.  THE  STAGES IN THE
C     ASYMPTOMATIC PHASE HAVE EQUAL LENGTH, AND THE STAGES IN THE PRE-
C     AIDS PHASE HAVE EQUAL LENGTH. GP IS FOR PEDIATRIC gamma's.
            GP(1) = G1
            IM2=INT(M/2)
            DO 18 I = 2, IM2
   18       GP(I) = G2*(IM2-1)
            DO 19 I=IM2+1, M-1
   19       GP(I) = G3*(M-1-IM2)
            GP(M) = GM
C
C     THE GAMMA VALUES NEED TO BE ADJUSTED SO THAT OUR DISCRETE MODEL
C     WORKS (GAMMA IS CONTINUOUS)
            DO 21  I = 1, M
   21       GP(I)=(1-EXP(-GP(I)))
C
C     NOW CHECK THE ADULT gamma's.
            PRINT*,'THE gamma''s FOR ADULTS ARE ',(GA(I), I = 1, M)
            READ*,INPUT
            IF (INPUT.NE.2) THEN
                  PRINT*,'INPUT ',M,' NEW gamma VALUES.'
                  READ*,(GA(I), I = 1, M)
                  DO 23  I = 1, M
   23             GA(I)=(1-EXP(-GA(I)))
            ENDIF
C
C     PROBABILITIES OF TRANSMISSION FOR ASYMPTOMATICS ARE QH FOR
C     NEEDLE-SHARING, QHP FOR HETEROSEXUAL PARTNERS AND QC FOR CHILDREN
            PRINT*,'THE PROBABILITIES OF TRANSMISSION BY ASYMPTOMATIC',
           $' INFECTIVES ARE QH, QHP, QC = ',QH,QHP,QC
            READ*,INPUT
            IF (INPUT.NE.2) THEN
                  PRINT*,'INPUT QH, QHP & QC = '
                  READ*,QH,QHP,QC
            ENDIF
            PRINT*,'SINCE THE WEIGHT FACTORS W(I) AND RELATIVE ACTIVITY',
           $' FACTORS rho APPEAR ONLY AS A PRODUCT, THEY ARE INPUT THAT',
           $' WAY.  THE PRODUCTS FOR HIV INCUBATION, ',
           $'ASYMPTOMATIC PRE-AIDS, AND AIDS PHASES ARE ',
           $ WRH(1),WRHA,WRHP,WRHM
            READ*,INPUT
            IF (INPUT.NE.2) THEN
```

```
                 PRINT*,'INPUT WRH(1), WRHA, WRHP, AND WRH(M) '
                 READ*,WRH(1),WRHA,WRHP,WRHM
           ENDIF
           DO 20 I = 2, IM2
   20      WRH(I) = WRHA
           DO 22 I = IM2+1,M-1
   22      WRH(I) = WRHP
           WRH(M) = WRHM
C
C    MIXING BETWEEN ACTIVITY LEVELS IN PREFERRED MIXING WITH ETA AS
C    THE EXTERNAL FRACTION, AND (1 - ETA) AS THE INTERNAL FRACTION
           PRINT*,'THE EXTERNAL MIXING FRACTION IS ETA = ',ETA
           READ*,INPUT
           IF (INPUT.NE.2) THEN
                 PRINT*,'THE EXTERNAL MIXING FRACTION ETA ='
                 READ*,ETA
           ENDIF
C
C READ STARTING YEAR AND MONTH, THEN ENDING YEAR
           PRINT*,'THE STARTING YEAR IS IYEAR = ',IYEAR
           PRINT*,'THE STARTING MONTH NUMBER IS IMONTH = ',IMONTH
           READ*,INPUT
           IF (INPUT.NE.2) THEN
                 PRINT*,'IYEAR, IMONTH = '
                 READ*,IYEAR,IMONTH
           ENDIF
           PRINT*,'THE ENDING YEAR IS LYEAR = ',LYEAR
           READ*,INPUT
           IF (INPUT.NE.2) THEN
                 PRINT*,'NEW LYEAR = '
                 READ*,LYEAR
           ENDIF
C
C    THE INITIAL NUMBER OF INFECTIVES IN THE POPULATION IS START.
C    THEY WILL ALL BE PUT IN THE VERY ACTIVE CLASS EVENTUALLY.
           PRINT*,'THE INITIAL NUMBER OF INFECTIVES,  START = ',START
           READ*,INPUT
           IF (INPUT.NE.2) THEN
                 PRINT*,'START = '
                 READ*,START
           ENDIF
C
C    NEEDLE-SHARING BEHAVIOR PARAMETERS (RDCTN = YEARLY REDUCTION
C    STARTING IN NYSTRT, NMSTRT AND ENDING IN NYSTOP.)
           PRINT*,'THE STARTING TIME FOR REDUCTION(NYSTRT,NMSTRT) = ',
         $ NYSTRT,NMSTRT
           READ*,INPUT
           IF (INPUT.NE.2) THEN
                 PRINT*,'INPUT NYSTRT,NMSTRT = '
                 READ*,NYSTRT,NMSTRT
           ENDIF
           PRINT*,'THE LAST YEAR FOR THE REDUCTION IS NYSTOP = ', NYSTOP
           READ*,INPUT
           IF (INPUT.NE.2) THEN
                 PRINT*,'INPUT NYSTOP = '
                 READ*,NYSTOP
           ENDIF
   32      PRINT*,'THE AVERAGE NUMBER OF NEEDLE-SHARING PARTNERS PER',
         $' MONTH BEFORE ',NYSTRT,NMSTRT,' IS PAS = ',PAS,' AND THE',
         $' DEFAULT YEARLY REDUCTION IS RDCTN = ',RDCTN,' UNTIL DEC, ',
```

```
      $NYSTOP
      READ*,INPUT
      IF (INPUT.NE.2) THEN
          PRINT*,'NEW PAS, RDCTN = '
          READ*,PAS,RDCTN
      ENDIF
      PHS = PAS/(1+FH*(R-1))
      RDCTMO = RDCTN**(1./12.)
      PRINT*,'THE AVERAGE NUMBER OF NEW IVDU PARTNERS PER MONTH ',
     $'IS ',PAP
      READ*,INPUT
      IF (INPUT.NE.2) THEN
          PRINT*,'NEW PAP = '
          READ*,PAP
      ENDIF
C THE PROPORTION PC OF HIV CHILDREN DEVELOP AIDS EARLY FROM YCE TO
C Y(M) WITH RATE CONSTANT B.  THE OTHERS MOVE MORE RAPIDLY THROUGH
C THE M STAGES WITH G(I) MULTIPLIED BY A.
      PRINT*,'FOR 1-PC CHILDREN, gamma''s ARE MULTIPLIED BY A = ',A
      READ*,INPUT
      IF (INPUT.NE.2) THEN
          PRINT*,'NEW A ='
          READ*,A
      ENDIF
      PRINT*,'EARLY AIDS FRACTION PC & RATE CONSTANT B = ', PC,B
      READ*,INPUT
      IF (INPUT.NE.2) THEN
          PRINT*,'NEW PC,B ='
          READ*,PC,B
      ENDIF
C THE FECUNDITY OF IVDU & HETEROSEXUAL WOMEN IS FC
      PRINT*,'THE FECUNDITY IS FC = ',FC
      READ*,INPUT
      IF (INPUT.NE.2) THEN
          PRINT*,'NEW FC ='
          READ*,FC
      ENDIF
C
      NMONTH = IMONTH
C
C INITIALIZING ON IMONTH OF IYEAR
      DO 50 I = 1,M+1
      X(I) = 0
      Y(I) = 0
      Z(I) = 0
      YP(I) = 0
      ZP(I) = 0
   50 YC(I) = 0
      YCE = 0
      X(1) = START
      SV = QV - X(1)
      SA = QA
      SAP = QAP
C
C OUTPUT OF PARAMETER VALUES IN THE MODEL
      WRITE(IO,*)'TABLE'
      WRITE(IO,*)' '
      WRITE(IO,*)FILEOI,FILEOI,FILEOI,FILEOI,FILEOI
      WRITE(IO,*)'*****************************************************'
      WRITE(IO,*)'PROGRAM OUTPUT FOR IVDU10.FOR  BY H. W. HETHCOTE'
```

```
      WRITE(IO,*)'COMPUTER SIMULATION OF HIV AND AIDS IN AN',
     $' IVDU POPULATION '
      WRITE(IO,*)' '
      WRITE(IO,*)'THE IVDU & HTRO POPULATION SIZES ARE ',NSIZE,NSIZEP
      WRITE(IO,*)'THE VERY ACTIVE FRACTION IS ',FH
      WRITE(IO,*)'THE ACTIVITY RATIO IS ',R
      WRITE(IO,*)'THE NATURAL MORTALITY RATE XMU IS',XMU
      WRITE(IO,*)'THE INTERCHANGE RATE  FROM THE VERY ACTIVE',
     $' CLASS TO THE ACTIVE CLASS IS'
      WRITE(IO,*) PHI,'  AND THE TURNOVER RATE IS DLT = ',DLT
      WRITE(IO,*)'THE NUMBER OF INFECTIOUS STAGES IS  M = ',M
      WRITE(IO,*)'THE G PARAMETERS FOR THE TRANSFER BETWEEN',
     $' ADULT STAGES ARE ',(GA(I), I = 1, M)
      WRITE(IO,*)'THE WEIGHTS OF TRANSMISSION PER INFECTIOUS ',
     $'PARTNER TIMES THE FRACTION STILL'
      WRITE(IO,*)'SEXUALLY ACTIVE FOR THE STAGES ARE WRH(I) = ',
     $ (WRH(I), I = 1, M)
      WRITE(IO,*)'THE PROBABILITIES OF TRANSMISSION ARE QH, QHP &',
     $' QC = ',QH,QHP,QC
      WRITE(IO,*)'THE EXTERNAL MIXING FRACTION IS ETA = ',ETA
      WRITE(IO,*)'THE AVERAGE NUMBER OF NEEDLE-SHARING PARTNERS PER ',
     $'MONTH IS ',PAS,'   BEFORE ',NYSTRT,NMSTRT,', THEN IT IS ',
     $'REDUCED EACH YEAR BY A FACTOR OF ',RDCTN,' UNTIL DEC, ',NYSTOP
      WRITE(IO,*)'THE FRACTION OF IVDU WHO ARE WOMEN IS ',PIW
      WRITE(IO,*)'THE FRACTION OF HETEROSEXUALS WHO ARE WOMEN IS ',PHW
      WRITE(IO,*)'THE AVERAGE NUMBER OF IVDU PARTNERS OF HETERO',
     $'SEXUALS PER MONTH IS',PAP
      WRITE(IO,*)'THE FRACTION',PC,' OF CHILDREN PROGRESS RAPIDLY TO',
     $' AIDS WITH RATE    CONSTANT',B,'. OTHERS MOVE THROUGH M STAGES',
     $' WITH SPEED FACTOR',A
      WRITE(IO,*)'THE FECUNDITY FC (CHILDREN/MONTH) IS',FC
      WRITE(IO,*)'THE STARTING YEAR AND MONTH ARE ',IYEAR,IMONTH
      WRITE(IO,*)'THE STARTING NUMBER OF VERY ACTIVE INFECTIVES IS',
     $ START
C
C  TABLE HEADING HERE
      WRITE(IO,*)'**************************************************'
      WRITE(IO,*)' '
      WRITE(IO,*)'THE SIMULATED INCIDENCES ARE GIVEN ON THE NEXT PAGE'
      WRITE(IO,850)
  850 FORMAT('1')
      WRITE(IO,*)FILEOI,FILEOI,FILEOI,FILEOI,FILEOI
      WRITE(IO,*)'**************************************************'
      WRITE(IO,900)
  900 FORMAT(1X,'YEAR        HIV      HIV   FRACTNAL_PREV ',
     $' YR AIDS INC   AIDS(SIMULATION)')
      WRITE(IO,901)
  901 FORMAT(1X,'       CLASS    INC    PREV  ALL  V_A  ACT ',
     $' DATA    SIM    PREV  DTHS OUTSF')
      WRITE(IO,*) ' '
C
C  STARTING THE ITERATION, WITH STEP SIZE = 1 MONTH
      LASTK = LYEAR - IYEAR
      PRAIDS = 0
      PRDTHS = 0
      PRZAID = 0
      ZAIDS = 0
      CHISQ = 0
      PRAIDP = 0
      PRDTHP = 0
```

```
      PRZAIP = 0
      ZAIDSP = 0
      CHISQP = 0
      PRAIDC = 0
      PRDTHC = 0
      CHISQC = 0
      DO 600 K=0,LASTK
      SUMAIN = 0
      SUMVIN = 0
      SUMAIP = 0
      SUMAIC = 0
      NYEAR = IYEAR + K
C
C  J IS THE NUMBER OF THE MONTH
      DO 500 J=NMONTH,12
C
C  ACTIVE IVDU'S HAVE PH PARTNERS PER MONTH
C  VERY ACTIVE IVDU'S HAVE R*PH PARTNERS PER MONTH
      IF (NYEAR.LT.NYSTRT) THEN
          PH = PHS
      ELSEIF (NYEAR.EQ.NYSTRT.AND.J.LT.NMSTRT) THEN
          PH = PHS
      ELSEIF (NYEAR.LE.NYSTOP) THEN
          PH = PHS*RDCTMO**((NYEAR-NYSTRT-1)*12+13-NMSTRT+J)
      ELSE
          PH = PHS*RDCTMO**((NYSTOP-NYSTRT)*12+13-NMSTRT)
      ENDIF
C
C  CALCULATING THE MONTHLY INCIDENCES
      ASUM = 0
      VSUM = 0
      SUMP = 0
      SUMC = 0
      DO 100 I=1,M
      ASUM = ASUM + WRH(I)*Y(I)
      VSUM = VSUM + WRH(I)*R*X(I)
      SUMP = SUMP + WRH(I)*(X(I)+Y(I))
  100 SUMC = SUMC + WRH(I)*YP(I)
      SUM = ASUM + VSUM
      DNM = QA - Y(M+1) + R*(QV - X(M+1))
      AINC = PH*QH*((1.-ETA)*ASUM*SA/(QA-Y(M+1))+ETA*SUM*SA/DNM)
      VINC = PH*QH*((1.-ETA)*VSUM*SV/(QV-X(M+1))+ETA*SUM*R*SV/DNM)
      AINCP = PAP*QHP*SUMP*SAP/(QAP-YP(M+1))
C  PIW OF IVDU & PHW OF HETEROSEXUALS ARE WOMEN
      AINCC = FC*QC*(PIW*SUMP+PHW*SUMC)
      SUMAIN = SUMAIN + AINC
      SUMVIN = SUMVIN + VINC
      SUMAIP = SUMAIP + AINCP
      SUMAIC = SUMAIC + AINCC
C
C  FIRST LOAD THE VECTORS FOR GRAPHING !
C  {NOTICE THAT THIS ROUTINE WILL LOAD DATA ON THE EVEN MONTHS.}
      IF (NYEAR.GE.1974.AND.NYEAR.LE.1990) THEN
         IF(INT(J/2)*2.EQ.J) THEN
         N4 = (NYEAR - 1974) * 6 + INT(J/2)
         NAIVDU(N4)=GA(M-1)*(X(M-1)+Y(M-1))
         NHIVDU(N4) = AINC + VINC
         NAHTRO(N4)=GA(M-1)*YP(M-1)
         NHHTRO(N4) = AINCP
         NAPED(N4)=A*GP(M-1)*YC(M-1)+B*YCE
```

```
              NHPED(N4) = AINCC
           ENDIF
        ENDIF
C
C   CALCULATING THE DIFFERENCES
        DSV = (DLT+XMU)*(QV-SV)-VINC-PHI*SV+THT*SA
        DSA = (DLT+XMU)*(QA-SA)-AINC+PHI*SV-THT*SA
        DSAP = (DLT+XMU)*(QAP-SAP)-AINCP
        DX(1) = VINC-(GA(1)+XMU+DLT+PHI)*X(1)+THT*Y(1)
        DY(1) = AINC - (GA(1)+XMU+DLT+THT)*Y(1)+PHI*X(1)
        DZ(1) = DLT*(X(1)+Y(1))-(GA(1)+XMU)*Z(1)
        DYP(1) = AINCP - (GA(1)+XMU+DLT)*YP(1)
        DZP(1) = DLT*YP(1)-(GA(1)+XMU)*ZP(1)
        DYC(1) = (1-PC)*AINCC - A*GP(1)*YC(1)
        DO 200 I=2,M
        DX(I) = GA(I-1)*X(I-1)+THT*Y(I)-(GA(I)+XMU+PHI+DLT)*X(I)
        DY(I) = GA(I-1)*Y(I-1)+PHI*X(I)-(GA(I)+XMU+THT+DLT)*Y(I)
        DZ(I) = GA(I-1)*Z(I-1)+DLT*(X(I)+Y(I))-(GA(I)+XMU)*Z(I)
        DYP(I) = GA(I-1)*YP(I-1)-(GA(I)+XMU+DLT)*YP(I)
        DZP(I) = GA(I-1)*ZP(I-1)+DLT*YP(I)-(GA(I)+XMU)*ZP(I)
  200   DYC(I) = A*GP(I-1)*YC(I-1) - A*GP(I)*YC(I)
        DZ(M) = DZ(M) - GA(M-1)*Z(M-1)
        ZAIDS = ZAIDS + GA(M-1)*Z(M-1)
        DZP(M) = DZP(M) -GA(M-1)*ZP(M-1)
        ZAIDSP = ZAIDSP +GA(M-1)*ZP(M-1)
        DX(M+1) = GA(M)*X(M)+THT*Y(M+1)-(XMU+PHI+DLT)*X(M+1)
        DY(M+1) = GA(M)*Y(M)+PHI*X(M+1)-(XMU+THT+DLT)*Y(M+1)
        DZ(M+1) = (DLT+XMU)*(X(M+1)+Y(M+1)) + GA(M)*Z(M)
        DZ(M+1) = DZ(M+1) + XMU*(X(M) + Y(M) + Z(M))
        DYP(M+1) = GA(M)*YP(M)-(XMU+DLT)*YP(M+1)
        DZP(M+1) = (DLT+XMU)*YP(M+1) + GA(M)*ZP(M) + XMU*(YP(M)+ZP(M))
        DYC(M) = DYC(M) + B*YCE
        DYC(M+1) = A*GP(M)*YC(M)
C
C   UPDATING EACH CLASS
        SV = SV + DSV
        SA = SA + DSA
        SAP = SAP + DSAP
        DO 300 I=1,M+1
        X(I) = X(I) + DX(I)
        Y(I) = Y(I) + DY(I)
        Z(I) = Z(I) + DZ(I)
        YP(I) = YP(I) + DYP(I)
        ZP(I) = ZP(I) + DZP(I)
  300   YC(I) = YC(I) + DYC(I)
        YCE = YCE + PC*AINCC - B*YCE
C
C   CHECKING CONSERVATION IN QV AND QA
        CKQV = SV
        CKQA = SA
        CKQAP = SAP
        DO 400 I = 1, M+1
        CKQV = CKQV + X(I)
        CKQA = CKQA + Y(I)
  400   CKQAP = CKQAP + YP(I)
        IF (ABS(CKQV-QV)/QV + ABS(CKQA-QA)/QA.GT.1.E-5) THEN
           PRINT*,'CONSERVATION CHECK NOT SATISFIED (IVDU)'
           PRINT*,QV,CKQV,QA,CKQA
        ENDIF
        IF (ABS(CKQAP-QAP)/QAP.GT.1.E-5) THEN
```

```
          PRINT*,'CONSERVATION CHECK NOT SATISFIED (HETERO)'
          PRINT*,QAP,CKQAP
        ENDIF
  500 CONTINUE
C
C  YEARLY OUTPUT
        SUMINC =  SUMAIN + SUMVIN
        SUMINP = SUMAIP
        XPREV = 0
        YPREV = 0
        ZPREV = 0
        YPREVP = 0
        ZPREVP = 0
        PREVC = YCE
        DO 550 I = 1, M
        XPREV = XPREV + X(I)
        YPREV = YPREV + Y(I)
        ZPREV = ZPREV + Z(I)
        YPREVP = YPREVP + YP(I)
        ZPREVP = ZPREVP + ZP(I)
  550 PREVC = PREVC + YC(I)
        PREV = XPREV + YPREV
        IF (QV.GT.0) FXPREV = XPREV / QV
        IF (QA.GT.0) FYPREV = YPREV / QA
        FPREV = PREV / NSIZE
        PREVP = YPREVP
        FPPREV = YPREVP / NSIZEP
        DEATHS = X(M+1) + Y(M+1) + Z(M+1)
        AIDPRV =   X(M) + Y(M) + Z(M)
        AIDS = DEATHS + AIDPRV
        YRDTHS = DEATHS - PRDTHS
        AIDINC = AIDS - PRAIDS
        OUTINC = ZAIDS - PRZAID
        DEATHP = YP(M+1) + ZP(M+1)
        AIDPRVH =   YP(M) + ZP(M)
        AIDSP = DEATHP + AIDPRVH
        YRDTHP = DEATHP - PRDTHP
        AIDINP = AIDSP - PRAIDP
        OUTINP = ZAIDSP - PRZAIP
        DEATHC = YC(M+1)
        AIDPRVC = YC(M)
        AIDSC = DEATHC + AIDPRVC
        YRDTHC = DEATHC - PRDTHC
        AIDNCC = AIDSC - PRAIDC
  910 FORMAT(1X,I4,1X,A4,2F8.0,3F5.2,F7.0,5F7.0)
  911 FORMAT(1X,I4,1X,A4,2F8.0,3F5.2,'   ****',5F7.0)
  912 FORMAT(7X,A4,2F8.0,F5.2,'  -    -  ',5F7.0)
  913 FORMAT(7X,A4,2F8.0,F5.2,'  -    -    ****',5F7.0)
  914 FORMAT(7X,A4,2F8.0,'  -    -    -  ',5F7.0)
  915 FORMAT(7X,A4,2F8.0,'  -    -    -    ****',5F7.0)
        IF (NYEAR.GE.1975.AND.NYEAR.LE.1990.AND.AIDINC.GE.1.E-5) THEN
            CHISQ = CHISQ + (DIVDU(NYEAR)-AIDINC)**2 / AIDINC
            WRITE(IO,910) NYEAR,'IVDU',SUMINC,PREV,FPREV,FXPREV,FYPREV,
     $                  DIVDU(NYEAR),AIDINC,AIDPRV,YRDTHS,OUTINC
          ELSE
            WRITE(IO,911) NYEAR,'IVDU',SUMINC,PREV,FPREV,FXPREV,FYPREV,
     $                  AIDINC,AIDPRV,YRDTHS,OUTINC
        ENDIF
        IF (NYEAR.GE.1975.AND.NYEAR.LE.1990.AND.AIDINP.GE.1.E-5) THEN
            CHISQP = CHISQP + (DHTRO(NYEAR)-AIDINP)**2 / AIDINP
```

```
            WRITE(IO,912) 'HTRO',SUMINP,PREVP,FPPREV,DHTRO(NYEAR),
      $                   AIDINP,AIDPRVH,YRDTHP,OUTINP
         ELSE
            WRITE(IO,913) 'HTRO',SUMINP,PREVP,FPPREV,AIDINP,AIDPRVH,
      $                   YRDTHP,OUTINP
         ENDIF
         IF (NYEAR.GE.1975.AND.NYEAR.LE.1990.AND.AIDNCC.GE.1.E-5) THEN
            CHISQC = CHISQC + (DPED(NYEAR)-AIDNCC)**2 / AIDNCC
            WRITE(IO,914) 'PED',SUMAIC,PREVC,DPED(NYEAR),
      $                   AIDPRVC,AIDNCC,YRDTHC
         ELSE
            WRITE(IO,915) 'PED',SUMAIC,PREVC,AIDNCC,AIDPRVC,YRDTHC
         ENDIF

         PRDTHS = DEATHS
         PRAIDS = AIDS
         PRZAID = ZAIDS
         PRDTHP = DEATHP
         PRAIDP = AIDSP
         PRZAIP = ZAIDSP
         PRDTHC = DEATHC
         PRAIDC = AIDSC
  600    NMONTH = 1
         WRITE(IO,*)' '
         WRITE(IO,*)'CHISQD = ',CHISQ
         WRITE(IO,*)'CHISQP = ',CHISQP
         WRITE(IO,*)'CHISQC = ',CHISQC
         CHISQT = CHISQ + CHISQP + CHISQC
         WRITE(IO,*)'SUM OF CHISQ-D,P,C =',CHISQT
C
C     CHECK TO SEE IF THE DATA IS TO BE USED FOR GRAPHING.
         PRINT*,'WOULD YOU LIKE TO WRITE DATA FILES TO EXTERNAL '
      $'(GRAPHING) FILES? 2 = YES.'
         READ*,INPUT
         IF (INPUT.EQ.2) THEN
            PRINT*,'THE DEFAULT NAMES FOR IVDU FILES ARE ',FILE1I,FILE2I
            READ*,INPUT
            IF (INPUT.NE.2) THEN
               PRINT*,'INPUT NEW DATA FILE NAMES (IN SINGLE QUOTES)'
               READ*,FILE1I,FILE2I
            ENDIF
            OPEN(UNIT=10,FILE=FILE1I)
            WRITE(10,*)NHIVDU
            OPEN(UNIT=10,FILE=FILE2I)
            WRITE(10,*)NAIVDU
C
            PRINT*,'THE DEFAULT NAMES FOR HTRO FILES ARE ',FILE1H,FILE2H
            READ*,INPUT
            IF (INPUT.NE.2) THEN
               PRINT*,'INPUT NEW DATA FILE NAMES (IN SINGLE QUOTES)'
               READ*,FILE1H,FILE2H
            ENDIF
            OPEN(UNIT=10,FILE=FILE1H)
            WRITE(10,*)NHHTRO
            OPEN(UNIT=10,FILE=FILE2H)
            WRITE(10,*)NAHTRO
C
            PRINT*,'THE DEFAULT NAMES FOR THE PED FILES ARE ',FILE1C,FILE2C
            READ*,INPUT
            IF (INPUT.NE.2) THEN
```

```
      PRINT*,'INPUT THE NEW DATA FILE NAMES (IN SINGLE QUOTES)'
      READ*,FILE1C,FILE2C
      ENDIF
      OPEN(UNIT=10,FILE=FILE1C)
      WRITE(10,*)NHPED
      OPEN(UNIT=10,FILE=FILE2C)
      WRITE(10,*)NAPED
      ENDIF
C
      PRINT*,'INPUT 1 TO STOP, OR 2 TO DO IT AGAIN'
      READ*,INPUT
      IF (INPUT.NE.2) GOTO 999
      DO 700 I=1,102
      NHIVDU(I)=0
      NAIVDU(I)=0
      NHHTRO(I)=0
      NAHTRO(I)=0
      NHPED(I)=0
  700 NAPED(I)=0
      GO TO 11
  999 END
```

Listing of GRIVDU10.M

```
%  The program  GRIVDU10.M  is a MATLAB graphing program using pre-
%  generated vectors for the estimated and simulated HIV and AIDS
%  incidence from 1974 to 1990.  The AIDS incidence data vector names
%  (such as NE2TABT, NE5TABT, NECTABT) are entered first.  Then the
%  simulation vectors for HIV and AIDS pre-generated by the Fortran
%  program IVDU10.FOR with default names mtgrf#.m  (# =1 to 6)  are
%  entered.  This program then produces the graphs of the AIDS
%  incidence data and the HIV and AIDS simulation incidences for the
%  IVDUs, heterosexual partners and perinatally-infected children.
%  This program was coded by Herb Hethcote and Jim Van Ark.  It is
%  used in Chapter 10 of the book, "MODELING HIV TRANSMISSION AND
%  AIDS IN THE UNITED STATES", to produce Figures 10.18, 10.19,
%  10.26, 10.27, 10.43 and 10.54.
%
   n = 3
%
%  Input the names of the vectors for inputing data and labeling the
%  graphs.
   m1 = input('Input the vector name for IVDUs (in single-quotes) ');
   l1 = [m1,' solid'];
         m2 = input('Input the vector name for HTRO ');
         l2 = [m2,' dashed'];
               m3 = input('Input the vector name for PED  ');
               l3 = [m3,' dashdot'];
%
%  Y0, Y0H, Y0C are yearly AIDS data for IVDU, HTRO & PED from  CDC
   file0 = m1;
   eval(['load ',file0,'.m'])
   eval(['Y0 = ',file0,';'])
   Y0 = Y0*(1/12);
   Y0 = Y0(:);
   file0H = m2;
   eval(['load ',file0H,'.m'])
```

```
      eval(['YOH = ',fileOH,';'])
      YOH = YOH*(1/12);
      YOH = YOH(:);
      fileOC = m3;
      eval(['load ',fileOC,'.m'])
      eval(['YOC = ',fileOC,';'])
      YOC = YOC*(1/12);
      YOC = YOC(:);
%
%   These matrices contain the x - entries for the data points
      XO = 1979+1/2:1:1990+1/2;
      X = 1974:1/6:1991 - 1/12;
%
%   Load the simulation vectors for IVDU
      disp('Use 2 to accept or 1 to change.   ');
      inp = input('the default names for IVDU are mtgrf1 & mtgrf2   ');
      if inp == 1
         file1 = input('Input file1 name (in single quotes)   ');
         file2 = input('Input file2 name   ');
      else
         file1 = 'mtgrf1';
         file2 = 'mtgrf2';
      end;
      eval(['load ',file1,'.m']);
      eval(['load ',file2,'.m']);
      eval(['Y1 = ',file2,';'])
      eval(['Z1 = ',file1,';'])
      Y1 = Y1';
      Z1 = Z1';
      Y1 = Y1(:);
      Z1 = Z1(:);
%
%   Load the simulation vectors for HTRO
         inp = input('the defaults for HTRO are mtgrf3 & mtgrf4   ');
               if inp == 1
                  file3 = input('input file3 name   ');
                  file4 = input('Input file4 name   ');
               else
                  file3 = 'mtgrf3';
                  file4 = 'mtgrf4';
               end;
               eval(['load ',file3,'.m']);
               eval(['load ',file4,'.m']);
               eval(['Y2 = ',file4,';'])
               eval(['Z2 = ',file3,';'])
               Y2 = Y2';
               Z2 = Z2';
               Y2 = Y2(:);
               Z2 = Z2(:);
%
%   Load the simulation vectors for PED
         inp = input('the defaults for PED are mtgrf5 & mtgrf6   ');
               if inp == 1
                  file5 = input('input file5 name   ');
                  file6 = input('Input file6 name   ');
               else
                  file5 = 'mtgrf5';
                  file6 = 'mtgrf6';
               end;
               eval(['load ',file5,'.m']);
```

```
        eval([′load ′,file6,′.m′]);
        eval([′Y3 = ′,file6,′;′])
        eval([′Z3 = ′,file5,′;′])
        Y3 = Y3′;
        Z3 = Z3′;
        Y3 = Y3(:);
        Z3 = Z3(:);
%
   pack
%
%   Plotting
  plot(X0,Y0,′:′,X0,Y0,′x′,X0,Y0H,′:′,X0,Y0H,′x′,X0,Y0C,′:′,X0,...
    Y0C,′x′,X,Y1,′-′,X,Y2,′--′,X,Y3,′-.′,X,Z1,′-′,X,Z2,′--′,X,Z3,′-.′)
        title(′MONTHLY INCIDENCES′)
        xlabel(′Year′)
        ylabel(′Incidence′)
        text(.2,.82,11,′sc′)
        text(.2,.76,12,′sc′)
        text(.2,.7,13,′sc′)
        text(.6,.8,′HIV′,′sc′)
        text(.7,.4,′AIDS′,′sc′)
        pause
        ni = input(′do you wish to print this?(1 = yes)   ′);
        if ni == 1
            print
        end;
    end
```

REFERENCES

Ahlgren DJ, Gorny MK and Stein AC (1990). Model–based optimization of infectivity parameters: a study of the early epidemic in San Francisco. *JAIDS* 3 #6, 631–643.

Allain J–P (1986). Prevalence of HTLV–III/LAV antibodies in patients with hemophilia and their sex partners in France. *N Eng J Med* 315, 517.

Anderson RM, Ed. (1982). *Population Dynamics of Infectious Diseases: Theory and Applications.* Chapman and Hall, New York.

Anderson RM (1988a). The epidemiology of HIV infection: variable incubation plus infectious periods and heterogeniety in sexual activity. *J R Stat Soc A* 151, 66–93.

Anderson RM (1988b). The role of mathematical models in the study of HIV transmission and the epidemiology of AIDS. *JAIDS* 1, 241–256.

Anderson RM and May RM, Eds.(1982). *Population Biology of Infectious Diseases.* Springer-Verlag, New York.

Anderson RM and May RM (1988). Epidemiological parameters of HIV transmission. *Nature* 333, 514–519.

Anderson RM and May RM (1982). Directly transmitted infectious diseases: Control by vaccination. *Science* 215, 1053–1060.

Anderson RM and May RM (1983). Vaccination against rubella and measles: Quantitative investigations of different policies. *J Hyg Camb* 90, 259–325.

Anderson RM and May RM (1985). Vaccination and herd immunity to infectious diseases. *Nature* 318, 323–329.

Anderson RM and May RM (1991). *Infectious Diseases of Humans.* Oxford Science Publications, Great Britain.

Anderson RM, May RM and McLean AR (1988). Possible demographic consequences of AIDS in developing countries. *Nature* 332, 228–234.

Anderson RM, Medley GP, May RM and Johnson AM (1986). A preliminary study of the transmission dynamics of the human immunodeficiency virus, the causative agent of AIDS. *IMA J Math Appl Med Biol* 3, 229–263.

Andrews EB, Creagh–Kirk T, Pattishall K, and Tilson HH (1990). Number of patients treated with zidovudine in the limited distribution system, March–September, 1987. *JAIDS* 3, 460.

Auger I, Thomas R, DeGruttola V et al. (1988). Incubation periods for paediatric AIDS patients. *Nature* 336, 575–577.

Bacchetti P (1990). Estimating the incubation period of AIDS comparing population infection and diagnosis pattern. *J Am Stat Assn* 85, 1002–1008.

Bacchetti P and Moss AR (1989). Incubation period of AIDS in San Francisco. *Nature* 338, 251–253.

Bailey NTJ (1975). *The Mathematical Theory of Infectious Diseases,* Second Edition. Hafner, New York.

Bailey NTJ and Duppenthaler J (1985). Sensitivity analysis in the modeling of infectious disease dynamics. *J Math Biol* 10, 113–131.

Bartlett MS (1960). *Stochastic Population Models in Ecology and Epidemiology.* Methuen, London.

Battjes RJ, Pickens RW and Amsel Z (1989). Introduction of HIV infection among intravenous drug abusers in low prevalence areas. *JAIDS* 2, 533–539.

Becker N (1989). *Analysis of Infectious Disease Data.* Chapman and Hall, New York.

Becker MH and Joseph JG (1988). AIDS and behavioral change to reduce risk: A review. *AJPH* 78 #4, 394–410.

Berkelman R, Karon J, Thomas P et al (1989). AIDS incidence and mortality. Abstract WAO 13, V International Conference on AIDS, Montreal.

Black JL, Dolan MP, DeFord HA et al. (1986). Sharing of needles among users of iv drugs. *N Eng J MED* 314, 446–447.

Bloom BR (1987). AIDS vaccine strategies. *Nature* 327, 193.

Blower SM, Hartel D, Dowlatabadi H et al. (1991). Drugs, sex and HIV: a mathematical model for New York City. *Phil Trans R Soc Lond B* 321, 171–187.

Blythe SP and Anderson RM (1988). Heterogeneous sexual activity model of HIV transmission in male homosexual populations. *IMA J Math Appl Med Biol* 5, 237–260.

Blythe SP and Castillo–Chavez C (1989). Like with like preference and sexual mixing models. *Math Biosci* 96, 221–238.

Brauer F, Blythe SP and Castillo–Chavez C (1992). Demographic recruitment in sexually transmitted disease models, preprint.

Broder S (1987). *AIDS: Modern Concepts and Therapeutic Challenges.* Marcel Dekker, New York.

Brookmeyer R and Damiano A (1989). Statistical methods for short term projections of AIDS incidence. *Stat in Med* 8, 23–34.

Brookmeyer R and Gail MH (1986). Minimum size of the acquired immunodeficiency virus syndrome epidemic in the U.S. *Lancet ii*, 1320–1322.

Brookmeyer R and Gail MH (1988). A method for obtaining short–term projections and lower bounds on the size of the AIDS epidemic. *J Am Stat Assn* 83, 301–308.

Brookmeyer R, Gail MH and Polk BF (1987). The prevalent cohort study and the acquired immunodeficiency virus syndrome. *Am J Epidem* 26 #1, 14–24.

Burke DS, Brundage JF, Herbold JR et al. (1987). Human immunodeficiency virus infections among civilian applicants for U.S. military service, Oct 1985 to March 1986. *N Eng J Med* 317 #3, 131–136.

Burke DS, Redfield RR, Fowler A, and Oster C (1989). Increased "viral burden" in late stages of HIV infection. Abstract ThAP 93, V International Conference on AIDS, Montreal, Canada.

Busenberg S and Castillo–Chavez C (1989). Interaction, pair formation and force of infection terms in sexually transmitted diseases. In Castillo–Chavez C, Ed., *Mathematical and Statistical Approaches to AIDS Epidemiology*, Lecture Notes in Biomathematics 83, 289–300.

Busenberg S and Castillo–Chavez C (1991). A general solution of the problem of mixing of subpopulations and its application to risk– and age–structured epidemic models for the spread of AIDS. *IMA J Math Appl Med and Biol* 8, 1–29.

Bye L (1987). Designing an effective AIDS prevention campaign strategy for San Francisco: Results from the fourth probability sample of an urban gay male community. Prepared by *Communication Technologies* for The San Francisco AIDS Foundation.

Byers RH Jr., Morgan WM, Darrow WW et al. (1988). Estimating AIDS infection rates in the San Francisco cohort. *AIDS* 2, 207–210.

Cardell NS and Kanouse DE (1989). Modeling heterogeneity in susceptibility and infectivity for HIV infection. In: *Mathematical and Statistical Approaches to AIDS Epidemiology*, C Castillo–Chavez, Ed., Lecture Notes in Biomathematics 83, Springer–Verlag, Germany, 138–156.

Carlson JR, Bryant ML, Hinrichs SH et al. (1985). AIDS serology testing in low– and high–risk groups. *JAMA* 253 #23, 3405–3408.

Carne CA, Weller IVD, Johnson AM et al. (1987). Prevalence of antibodies to human immunodeficiency virus, gonorrhea rates, and the changed sexual behavior in homosexual men in London. *Lancet* 8534, 656–658.

Castillo–Chavez C, Ed. (1989). *Mathematical and Statistical Approaches to AIDS Epidemiology*. Lecture Notes in Biomathematics 83, Springer–Verlag, Germany.

Castillo–Chavez C, Cooke KL, Huang W, and Levin SA (1989). On the role of long incubation periods in the dynamics of AIDS Part 2: Multiple group models. In: *Mathematical and Statistical Approaches to AIDS Epidemiology*, Lecture Note in Biomathematics 83, C Castillo–Chavez, Ed., Springer–Verlag, 200–217.

Cates W, Jr, Handsfield HH (1988). HIV counseling and testing: does it work? *AJPH* 78, 1533–1534.

Centers for Disease Control (1981a). Pneumocystis pneumonia – Los Angeles. MMWR 30, 250–252.

Centers for Disease Control (1981b). Kaposi's sarcoma and *Pneumocystis* pneumonia among homosexual men – New York City and California, MMWR 30, 305–308.

Centers for Disease Control (1981c). Follow–up on Kaposi's sarcoma and *Pneumocystis* pneumonia, MMWR 30, 409–410.

Centers for Disease Control (1982). Update on Acquired Immune Deficiency Syndrome (AIDS) – United States. MMWR 31, 507–14.

Centers for Disease Control (1984). Declining rates of rectal and pharangeal gonorrhea among males – New York City, MMWR 33, 295–297.

Centers for Disease Control (1985a). Update: Acquired immune deficiency syndrome – United States, MMWR 34, 245–248.

Centers for Disease Control (1985b). World Health Organization workshop: conclusions and recommendations on the acquired immune deficiency syndrome, MMWR 34, 275–276.

Centers for Disease Control (1985c). Revision of the case definition of the acquired immune deficiency syndrome for national reporting – United States, MMWR 34, 373–375.

Centers for Disease Control (1985d). Heterosexual transmission of HTLV–III/LAV, MMWR 34, 561–563.

Centers for Disease Control (1985e). Update: AIDS in the San Francisco cohort study, 1978–1985. MMWR 34, 573–575.

Centers for Disease Control (1985f). Self–reported behavioral change among gay and bisexual men – San Francisco. MMWR 34, 613–615.

Centers for Disease Control (1986a). Update: The acquired immune deficiency syndrome – United States, MMWR 35, 17–21.

Centers for Disease Control (1986b). Additional recommendations to reduce sexual– and drug abuse – related transmission of HTLV–III/LAV, MMWR 35, 152–155.

Centers for Disease Control (1986c). AIDS in correctional facilities: a report of the National Institute of Justice and the American Correctional Association, MMWR 35, 195–199.

Centers for Disease Control (1986d). Classification system for HTLV–III/LAV infections, MMWR 35, 334–339.

Centers for Disease Control (1986e). HTLV–III/LAV antibody prevalence in United States military recruit applicants, MMWR 35, 421–424.

Centers for Disease Control (1986f). AIDS among blacks and hispanics – United States, MMWR 35, 655–666.

Centers for Disease Control (1986g). Surveillance of hemophilia–associated AIDS MMWR 35, 669–671.

Centers for Disease Control (1986h). Update: AIDS – United States, MMWR 35, 757–766.

Centers for Disease Control (1987a). Survey of non–U.S. Hemophilia Treatment Centers for HIV seroconversions following therapy with heat – treated factor concentrates, MMWR 36, 121–124.

Centers for Disease Control (1987b). HIV infection in transfusion recipients and their family members, MMWR 36, 137–140.

Centers for Disease Control (1987c). Antibody to HIV in female prostitutes, MMWR 36, 157–161.

Centers for Disease Control (1987d). Self–reported changes in sexual behaviors among homosexual and bisexual men from the San Francisco city clinic cohort. MMWR 36, 187–189.

Centers for Disease Control (1987e). Trends in human immunodeficiency virus infection among civilian applicants for military service – United States, Oct '85 – Dec '86, MMWR 36, 273–280.

Centers for Disease Control (1987f). Update: AIDS – United States, MMWR 36, 522–526.

Centers for Disease Control (1987g). HIV infection and pregnancies in sexual partners of HIV–seropositive hemophiliac men – United States, MMWR 36, 593–595.

Centers for Disease Control (1987h). HIV infection in the United States, MMWR 36, 801–804.

Centers for Disease Control (1987i). Human Immunodeficiency Virus in the United States: A review of current knowledge, MMWR 36, #S–6.

Centers for Disease Control (1987j). Revision of the CDC surveillance case definition for AIDS. MMWR 36, 3S–15S.

Centers for Disease Control (1988). Increase in pneumonia mortality among young adults and the HIV epidemic—New York City, United States, MMWR 37, 593–596.

Centers for Disease Control (1989a). Update: Acquired immunodeficiency syndrome associated with intravenous–drug use—United States, 1988, MMWR 38, 165–170.

Centers for Disease Control (1989b). AIDS and human immunodeficiency virus infection in the United States: 1988 update. MMWR 38, #S–4.

Centers for Disease Control (1990c). Update: Acquired Immunodeficiency Syndrome – United States, 1989. MMWR 39, 81–86.

Centers for Disease Control (1990d). Estimates of HIV Prevalence and Projected AIDS Cases: Summary of a Workshop, October 31–November 1, 1989, MMWR 39, 110–112, 117–119.

Centers for Disease Control (1990e). HIV prevalence estimates and AIDS case projections for the United States: Report based on a workshop. MMWR 39, #RR–16: 1–31.

Centers for Disease Control (1991a). Update: Acquired immunodefficiency syndrome – United States, 1981 – 1991, MMWR 40, 357–363.

Centers for Disease Control (1991b). Summary of Notifiable Diseases, United States, 1990, MMWR 39.

Centers for Disease Control (1992). HIV/AIDS Surveillance Report, January, 1–22.

Chaisson RE, Bacchetti P, Osmond D et al. (1989). Cocaine use and HIV infection in intravenous drug users in San Francisco. JAMA 261, 561–565.

Chaisson RE, Moss AR, Onishi R, et al (1987). Human immunodeficiency virus in heterosexual drug users in San Francisco. AJPH 77 #2, 169–172.

Chu SY, Peterman TA, Doll LS, et al. (1992). AIDS in bisexual men in the United States: epidemiology and transmission to women. AJPH 82 #2, 220–224.

Coates TJ, Morin SF and McKusick L (1987). Behavioral consequences of AIDS antibody testing among gay men. JAMA 258 #14 1889.

Colgate SA, Stanley EA, Hyman JM et al. (1988). A behavior based model of the initial growth of AIDS in the United States. Preprint.

Collier AC, Meyers JD, Murphy VL et al.(1987). Relationship between antibodies to LAV/HTLV–III and the natural course of subclinical cellular immune dysfunction in homosexual men. STD 14 #1, 1–8.

Consensus Conference (1986). The impact of routine HTLV–III antibody testing of blood and plasma donors on public health. JAMA 256 #13, 1778–1783.

Coolfont Report (1986). Pub Health Rep 101 #4, 341–348.

Curran JW, Jaffe HW, Hardy AM et al. (1988). Epidemiology of HIV infection and AIDS in the United States. Science 239, 610–616.

Curran JW, Lawrence DN, Jaffe H et al. (1984). Acquired immunodeficiency syndrome (AIDS) associated with transfusion. N Eng J Med 310, 69–75.

Curran JW, Morgan WM, Hardy AM, et al. (1985). The epidemiology of AIDS: current status and future prospects. Science 229, 1352–1357.

Darrow WW (1989). Personal communication.

Darrow WW, Echenberg DF, Jaffe HW et al. (1987). Risk factors for human immunodeficiency virus infection in homosexual men. AJPH 77 #4, 479–483.

De Gruttola V and Lagakos SW (1987). The value of doubling time in assessing the course of the AIDS epidemic, preprint.

De Gruttola V, Mayer KH (1987). Assessing and modeling heterosexual spread of the human immunodeficiency virus in the United States. Rev Inf Dis 10 #1, 138–150.

Denning PJ (1987). Computer models of AIDS epidemiology, Am Scientist July–Aug, 347–352.

Des Jarlais DC and Friedman SR (Ed. review)(1987). HIV infection among intravenous drug users: epidemiology and risk reduction. AIDS 1 #2, 67–76.

Des Jarlais DC, Friedman SR, Marmor M et al. (1987). Development of AIDS, HIV seroconversion, and potential cofactors for T4 cell loss in a cohort of intravenous drug users. *AIDS* 1 #2, 105–111.

Des Jarlais DC, Friedman SR, and Stoneburner RL (1988). HIV infection and intravenous drug use: critical issues in transmission dynamics, infection outcomes, and prevention. *Rev Inf Dis* 10 #1, 151–158.

Diekmann O, Heesterbeek JAP and Metz JAJ (1990). On the definition and the computation of the basic reproduction ratio R_0 in models for infectious diseases in heterogeneous populations. *J Math Biol* 28, 365–382.

Dietz K. (1988). On the transmission dynamics of HIV. *Math Biosci* 90, 397–414.

Dietz K and Hadeler KP (1988). Epidemiological models for sexually transmitted diseases. *J Math Biol* 26, 1–25.

Dietz K and Schenzle D (1985a). Mathematical models for infectious disease statistics. In: *A Celebration of Statistics.* Atkinson AC and Fienberg SE, Eds., New York, Springer–Verlag, 167–204.

Dietz K and Schenzle D (1985b). Proportionate mixing models for age–dependent infection transmission. *J. Math. Biol.* 22, 117–120.

Dolan MP, Black JL, Deford HA et al. (1987). Characteristics of drug abusers that discriminate needle–sharers, *Pub Health Rep* July–August, 395–398.

Doll LS, Darrow WM, Jaffe H et al (1987). Self–reported changes in sexual behaviors in gay and bisexual men from the San Francisco City Clinic Cohort. III International Conference on AIDS, Washington D.C.

Doll LS (1988). Personal communication.

Downs AM, Ancelle RA, Jager HJC and Brunet J–B (1987). AIDS in Europe: current trends and short–term predictions estimated from surveillance data, Jan 1981–June 1986. *AIDS* 1 #1, 53–57.

Drucker E (1986). AIDS and addiction in New York City. *Am J Drug Alc Abuse* 12, 165–181.

Ebbesen P. (1986). The global epidemic of AIDS, *AIDS Res* 2 supp 1, s23–s28.

El–Sadr W, Marmor M, Zolla–Pazner S et al. (1987). Four–year prospective study of homosexual men: correlation of immunilogical abnormalities, clinical status, and serology to human immunodeficiency virus. *J Inf Dis* 155 #4, 789–793.

Eyster ME, Gail MH, Ballard JO et al. (1987). Natural history of human immunodeficiency virus infections in hamophiliacs: effects of T–cell subsets, platelet counts, and age. *Ann Int Med* 107, 1–6.

Fischl MA, Dickinson GM, Scott GB et al. (1987). Evaluation of heterosexual partners, children, and household contacts of adults with AIDS. *JAMA* 257 #5, 640–644.

Fischl MA, Richman DD, Grieco MH et al. (1987). The efficacy of A.Z.T. in the treatment of patients with AIDS and AIDS–related complex. *N Eng J Med* 317 #4, 185–191.

Fischl MA, Dickinson GM, Flanagan S, and Fletcher MA (1987). Human Immunodeficiency Virus (HIV) among female prostitutes in Southern Florida. III International Conference on AIDS, Washington D.C.

Fleming DW, Cochi SL, Steece RS, and Hull HF (1987). AIDS in low–incidence areas: how safe is safe sex? *JAMA* 258 #6, 785–787.

Fox R, Eldred LJ, Fuchs EJ et al. (1987). Clinical manifestations of acute infection with H.I.V. in a cohort of gay men. *AIDS* 1 #1, 35–38.

Francis DP and Chin J (1987). The prevention of AIDS in the U.S. *JAMA* 257 #10, 1357–1366.

Friedland GH and Klein RS (1987). Transmission of the human immunodeficiency virus. *N Eng J Med* 317, 1125–1135.

Furth PA (1987). Heterosexual transmission of AIDS by male drug users. *Nature* 327, 193.

Fusaro RE, Jewell WW, Hauch DC et al. (1989). An annotated bibliography of quantitative methodology relating to the AIDS epidemic. *Stat Sci* 4, 264–281.

Gail MH, Rosenberg PS, and Goedert JJ (1990). Therapy may explain recent deficits in AIDS incidence. *JAIDS* 3 #4, 296–306.

Gail MH and Brookmeyer R (1988). Methods for projecting course of acquired immunodeficiency syndrome epidemic. *J Nat Cancer Inst* 80 #12, 900–911.

Gallo RC (1986). The first human retrovirus. *Scientific American*, Dec '86, 88–98.

Gallo RC (1987). The AIDS virus. *Scientific American* Jan '87, 47–56.

Gallo RC and Montagnier L (1987). The chronology of AIDS research. *Nature* 326, 435–436.

General Accounting Office (1989), *AIDS Forecasting: Undercount of Cases and Lack of Key Data Weaken Existing Estimates*. GAO/PEMD–89–13, Washington D.C.

Goedert JJ, Eyster ME, Biggar RJ and Blattner WA (1987). Heterosexual transmission of human immunodeficiency virus: association with severe depletion of T–helper lymphocytes in men with hemophilia. *AIDS Res Human Retrov* 3 #4, 355–361.

Goedert JJ, Kessler CM, Aledort LM et al. (1989). A prospective study of human immunodeficiency virus type 1 infection and the development of AIDS in subjects with hemophilia. *N Eng J Med* 321 #17, 1141–1148.

Goedert JJ, Biggar RJ, Weiss SH et al.(1986). Three–year incidence of AIDS in five cohorts of HTLV–III–infected risk group members. *Science* 231, 992–995.

Goedert JJ, Biggar RJ, Melbye M et al. (1987). Effect of T4 count and cofactors on the incidence of AIDS in homosexual men infected with human immunodeficiency virus. *JAMA* 257 #3, 331–334.

Goldsmith JM, Variakojis D, Phair JP and Green D (1987). The spectrum of HIV infection in patients with factor IX deficiency (Christmas disease). *Am J Hematology* 25, 203–210.

Goldsmith JM, Kalish SB, Ostrow DG et al. (1987). Antibody to HTLV–III: Immunological status of homosexual contacts of patients with the acquired immunodeficiency syndrome and AIDS–Related Conditions. *STD* 14 #1, 44–47.

Goldsmith MF (1987). Sex in the age of AIDS calls for common sense and 'condom sense'. *JAMA* 257 #17, 2261–2266.

Grant RM, Wiley JA and Winkelstein W (1987). Infectivity of the human immunodeficiency virus: estimates from a prospective study of homosexual men. *J Inf Dis* 156 #1, 189–193.

Greenberg WM (1987)(letter). On HIV transmission in homosexual/bisexual men. *AJPH* 77 #12, 1552.

Guinan ME and Hardy A (1987). Epidemiology of AIDS in women in the U.S. *JAMA* 257 #15, 2039–2042.

Hadeler KP, Waldstätter R and Wörz–Busekros A (1988). A model for pair formation in bisexual populations. *J Math Biol* 26, 635–649.

Hahn BH, Gonda MA, Shaw GM et al. (1985). Genomic diversity of the AIDS virus HTLV–III: different viruses exhibit greatest divergence in their envelope genes. *Proc Nat Acad Sci* 82, 4813–4817.

Hahn BH, Shaw GM, Taylor ME et al. (1986). Genetic variations in HTLV–III/LAV over time in patients with AIDS or at risk for AIDS. *Science* 232, 1548–1553.

Hardy AM, Starcher ET III, Morgan WM et al.(1987). Review of death certificates to assess completeness of AIDS case reporting. *Pub Health Rep* July–August, 386–391.

Harris J.E.(1987). The AIDS epidemic: looking into the 1990's. Technology Review 90 #5, 59–64.

Healy MJR and Tillett HE (1988). Short–term extrapolation of the AIDS epidemic. *J R Stat Soc A* 151, 50–61.

Hessol NA, Lifson A, O'Malley P et al. (1990). Prevalence, incidence, and progression of human immunodeficiency virus infection in homosexual and bisexual men in hepatitis B vaccine trials, 1978 – 1988. *Am J Epidem* 130 #6, 1167–1175.

Hessol NA, O'Malley P, Lifson A et al. (1989). Incidence and prevalence of HIV infection among homosexual and bisexual men, 1978 – 1988. Abstract M.A.O. 27, V International Conference on AIDS, Montreal, Canada.

Hethcote HW (1976). Qualitative analysis for communicable disease models. *Math Biosci* 28, 335–356.

Hethcote HW (1978). An immunization model for a heterogeneous population. *Theor Pop Biol* 14, 338–349.

Hethcote HW (1983). Measles and rubella in the United States, *Am J Epidem* 117, 2–13.

Hethcote HW (1987). AIDS modeling work in the United States. In: *Future Trends in AIDS*, Her Majesty's Stationary Office, London, 35–46.

Hethcote HW (1988). Optimal ages of vaccination for measles. *Math Biosci* 89, 29–52.

Hethcote HW (1989a). Three basic epidemiological models. In: *Applied Mathematical Ecology*, L Gross, TG Hallam and SA Levin, Eds., Springer–Verlag, New York, 119–144.

Hethcote HW (1989b) Rubella. In: *Applied Mathematical Ecology*, L Gross, TG Hallam and SA Levin, Eds., Springer–Verlag, New York, 212–234.

Hethcote HW (1989c). A model for HIV transmission and AIDS. In: *Mathematical Approaches to Problems in Resource Management and Epidemiology*, C Castillo–Chavez, SA Levin and C Shoemaker, Eds., Lecture Notes in Biomathematics 81, Springer–Verlag, Germany, 164–176.

Hethcote HW and Levin SA (1989). Periodicity in Epidemiological Models. In: *Applied Mathematical Ecology*, L Gross, TG Hallam and SA Levin, Eds., Springer-Verlag, New York, 193–211.

Hethcote HW, Stech HW and van den Driessche P (1981). Periodicity and stability in epidemic models: A survey. In: *Differential Equations and Applications in Ecology, Epidemics, and Population Problems*, S Busenberg and KL Cooke, Eds. Academic Press, New York, 65–82.

Hethcote HW and Tudor DW (1980). Integral equation models for endemic infectious diseases. *J Math Biol* 9, 37–47.

Hethcote HW and Van Ark JW (1987). Epidemiological models for heterogeneous populations: proportionate mixing, parameter estimation, and immunization programs. *Math Biosci* 84, 85–118.

Hethcote HW and Van Ark JW (1992). Weak Linkage between HIV epidemics in homosexual men and intravenous drug users in New York City. In: *AIDS Epidemiology: Methodological Issues*, N Jewell, K Dietz and V Farewell, Eds., Birkhauser–Boston, Boston, to appear.

Hethcote HW, Van Ark JW and Karon JM (1991). A simulation model of AIDS in San Francisco: II. Simulations, therapy, and sensitivity analysis. *Math Biosci* 106, 223–247.

Hethcote HW, Van Ark JW and Longini IM Jr (1991). A simulation model of AIDS in San Francisco: I. Model formulation and parameter estimation. *Math Biosci* 106, 203–222.

Hethcote HW and Waltman P (1973). Optimal vaccination schedules in a deterministic epidemic model. *Math Biosci* 18, 365–381.

Hethcote HW and Yorke JA (1984). *Gonorrhea Transmission Dynamics and Control.* Lecture Notes in Biomathematics 56, Heidelberg, Springer–Verlag.

Hethcote HW, Yorke JA and Nold A (1982). Gonorrhea modeling: a comparison of control methods. *Math Biosci* 58, 93–109.

Ho DD, Pomerantz RJ and Kaplan JC (1987). Pathogenesis of infection with human immunodeficiency virus. *N Eng J Med* 317 #5, 278–286.

Horn RA and Johnson CR (1985). *Matrix Analysis.* Cambridge University Press, New York.

Huminer D, Rosenfeld JB and Pitlik SD (1987). AIDS in the pre–AIDS era. *Rev Inf Dis* 9 #6, 1102–1108.

Hyman JM and Stanley EA (1988). Using mathematical models to understand the AIDS epidemic. *Math Biosci* 90, 415–473.

Hyman JM and Stanley EA (1989). The effects of social mixing patterns on the spread of AIDS, In: *Mathematical Approaches to Problems in Resource Management and Epidemiology* C Castillo–Chavez, SA Levin and C Shoemaker, Eds.,, Lecture Notes in Biomathematics 81, Springer–Verlag, Germany.

Isham V (1987). Mathematical modeling of the transmission dynamics of HIV infection and AIDS: a review. *J R Stat Soc A* 151 #1:5–30. (Discussion pp. 44–9, response pp. 120–3).

Jacquez JA, Simon CP and Koopman J (1989). Structured Mixing. In: *Mathematical and Statistical Approaches to AIDS Epidemiology,* C Castillo–Chavez, Ed., Lecture Notes in Biomathematics 83, Springer–Verlag, Germany, 301–315.

Jacquez JA, Simon CP, Koopman J et al. (1988). Modeling and the analysis of HIV transmission: the effect of contact patterns. *Math Biosci* 92, 119–199.

Jaffe HW, Darrow WW, Echenberg DF et al. (1985). The acquired immune deficiency syndrome in a cohort of homosexual men. *Ann Int Med* 103 #2, 210–214.

Jager HJC and Ruitenberg EJ (1987). The statistical analysis and mathematical modelling of AIDS, *AIDS* 1, 129–130.

Jason J, Holman RC, Dixon G et al. (1986). Effects of exposure to factor concentrates containing donations from identified AIDS patients. *JAMA* 256 #13, 1758–1762.

Jason JM, McDougal JS, Dixon G et al. (1986). HTLV–III/LAV antibody and immune status of household contacts and sexual partners of persons with hemophilia. *JAMA* 255 #2, 212–215.

Jay K and Young A (1979). *The Gay Report,* Summit Press, New York.

Johnson AM (1988). Social and behavioral aspects of the HIV epidemic: a review. *J R Stat Soc A* 151 #1, 99–114. (Discussion pp 115–119, response p 125.)

Jones CC, Waskin H, Gerety B et al. (1987). Persistence of high–risk sexual activity among homosexual men in an area of low incidence of the acquired immunodeficiency syndrome. *STD* 14 #2, 79–82.

Judson FN (1983). Fear of AIDS and gonorrhea rates in homosexual men. *Lancet ii*, 159–160.

Kaplan EH and Lee YS (1990). How bad can it get? Bounding worst case epidemic heterogeneous mixing models of HIV/AIDS. *Math Biosci* 99, 157–180.

Kaplan EH, Crampton PC and Paltiel AD (1989). Nonrandom mixing models of HIV transmission. In: *Mathematical and Statistical Approaches to AIDS Epidemiology*, C. Castillo–Chavez, Ed., Lecture Notes in Biomathematics 83, Springer–Verlag, Berlin, 58–88.

Kaplan LD, Wofsy CB and Volberding PA (1987). Treatment of patients with acquired immunodeficiency syndrome and associated manifestations. *JAMA* 257 #10, 1367–1374.

Karon JM and Berkelman RL (1991). The geographic and ethnic diversity of AIDS incidence trends in homosexual/bisexual men in the United States. *JAIDS* 4 1179–1189.

Karon JM, Devine OJ and Morgan WM (1989). Predicting AIDS incidence by extrapolation from recent trends. In: *Mathematical and Statistical Approaches to AIDS Epidemiology*, C. Castillo–Chavez, Ed., Lecture Notes in Biomathematics 83, Springer–Verlag, Berlin, 58–88.

Karon JM, Dondero TJ, and Curran JW (1988). The projected incidence of AIDS and estimated prevalence of HIV infection in the United States. *JAIDS* 1, 542–550.

Kaslow RA and Francis DP, Eds. (1989). *The Epidemiology of AIDS*. Oxford University Press, New York.

Kaslow RA, Ostrow DS, Detels R et al. (1987). The multicenter AIDS cohort study: rationale, organization, and selected characteristics of the participants. *Am J Epidem* 36 #2, 310–318.

Kegeles SM, Catania JA, and Coates TJ (1988)(letter). Intentions to communicate HIV – antibody status to sex partners. *JAMA* 259 #2, 216–217.

Kellogg TA, Marelich WD, Wilson MJ, et al (1990). HIV prevalence among homosexual and bisexual men in the San Francisco Bay area: evidence of infection among young gay men. Abstract FC548, VI International Conference on AIDS, San Francisco.

Kessler HA, Blaauw B, Spear J et al. (1987). Diagnosis of human immunodeficiency virus infection in seronegative homosexuals presenting with an acute viral syndrome. *JAMA* 258 #9, 1196–1199.

Kingsley LA, Detels R, Kaslow R et al. (1987). Risk factors for seroconversion to H.I.V. among male homosexuals. *Lancet* 8529, 345–349.

Kinsey AC, Pomeroy WB and Martin CE (1948). *Sexual Behavior in the Human Male*. W.B. Saunders, Philadelphia.

Knox EG (1986). A transmission model for AIDS. *Eur J Epidem* 2 #3, 165–177.

Kohn R (1990). personal communication.

Kolata G.(1987). Mathematical models predict AIDS spread. *Science* 235, 1464–1465.

Koopman JS, Simon CP and Jacquez JA (1989). Selective contact within structured mixing groups; with an application to the analysis of HIV transmission risk from oral and anal sex. In: *Mathematical and Statistical Approaches to AIDS Epidemiology*, C Castillo–Chavez, Ed., Lecture Notes in Biomathematics 83, Springer–Verlag, Germany, 316–348.

Kozel NJ and Adams EH (1986). Epidemiology of drug abuse: an overview. *Science* 34, 970–974.

Lajmanovich A and Yorke JA (1976). A deterministic model for gonorrhea in a nonhomogeneous population. *Math Biosci* 28, 221–236.

Lambert, B (1988). Halving of estimate on AIDS is raising doubts in New York. *New York Times*, July 20, 1–28.

Lang W, Anderson R, Perkins H et al. (1987). Clinical, immunological, and serological findings in men at risk for acquired immunodeficiency syndrome (The San Francisco Men's Health Study). *JAMA* 257 #3, 326–330.

Lang W, Osmund D, Samuel M, et al. (1991). Population based estimates of zidovudine and aerosol pentamidine use in San Francisco, 1987–1989. *JAIDS* 4, 713–716.

Lange JMA, Paul DA, Huisman H–G et al. (1986). Persistant HIV antigenaemia and decline of HIV core antibodies associated with transition to AIDS. *Br Med J* 293, 1459–1462.

Laurence J (1986). AIDS: definition, epidemiology, and etiology. *Lab Med* 17 #11, 659–663.

Lemp GF (1990). Effect of therapy on AIDS patient survival. Abstract FB85, VI International Conference on AIDS, San Francisco.

Lemp G (1991). Personal communication.

Lemp GF, Payne SF, Rutherford GW et al. (1990). Projections of AIDS morbidity and mortality in San Francisco. *JAMA* 263 #11, 1497–1501.

Lifson AR, Hessol NA, Rutherford GW et al. (1990). The natural history of HIV infection in a cohort of homosexual and bisexual men: clinical and immunilogical outcomes, 1977 – 1990. Abstract ThC33, VI International Conference on AIDS, San Francisco.

Lin X (1991). Qualitative analysis of an HIV transmission model. *Math Biosci* 104, 111–134.

Lindan C, Rutherford GW, Payne S et al. (1989) Decline in rates of new AIDS cases among homosexual and bisexual men in San Francisco. Abstract WAP24, V International Conference on AIDS, Montreal.

Longini IM Jr, Ackerman E and Elveback LR (1978). An optimization model for influenza A epidemics. *Math Biosci* 38, 141–157.

Longini IM, Clark WS, Byers RH, et al. (1989). Statistical analysis of the stages of HIV infections using a Markov model. *Stat in Med* 8, 831–843.

Longini IM, Clark WS, Gardner LI, and Brundage JF (1991). The dynamics of CD4⁺ T–lymphocyte decline in HIV–infected individual: A Markov modeling approach. *JAIDS* 4 #11, 1141–1147.

Longini IM, Clark WS, Haber M et al. (1990) The stages of HIV infection: Waiting times and infection transmission probabilities. In: *Mathematical and Statistical Approaches to AIDS epidemiology*, C Castillo–Chavez, Ed., Lecture Notes in Biomathematics 83, Springer–Verlag, Germany, p. 111–137.

Ludwig D (1974). *Stochastic Population Theories*. Lecture Notes in Biomathematics 3, Springer–Verlag, Berlin.

Lui K–J, Darrow WW, Rutherford GW III (1988). A model–based estimate of the mean incubation period for AIDS in homosexual men. *Science* 240, 1333–1335.

Machado SG, Gail MH and Ellenberg SS (1990). On the use of laboratory markers as surrogates for clinical endpoints in the evaluation of treatment for HIV infection. *JAIDS* 3, 1065–1073.

Magura S, Grossman JI, Lipton S et al. (1989). Determinants of needle–sharing among intravenous drug users. *A J Pub Health* 79, 459–462.

Mann JM (1987). The global AIDS situation. *World Health Stat Quar* 40, 185–192.

Mann JM, Francis H, Quinn T et al. (1986). Surveillance for AIDS in a central African city. *JAMA* 255 #23, 3255–3259.

Mann JM, Francis H, Quinn TC et al. (1986). HIV seroprevalence among hospital workers in Kinshasa, Zaire. *JAMA* 256 #22, 3099–3102.

Marlink RG and Essex M (1987). Africa and the biology of HIV. *JAMA* 257 #19, 2632–2633.

Marmor M, Des Jarlais DC, Cohen H et al. (1987). Risk factors for infection with H.I.V. among intrvenous drug abusers in New York City. *AIDS* 1 #1, 39–44.

Martin JL (1987). The impact of AIDS on gay male sexual behavior patterns in New York City, *AJPH* 77 #5, 578–581.

Martin K, Katz BZ and Miller G (1987). AIDS and antibodies to human immunodeficiency virus in children and their families. *J Inf Dis* 155 #1, 54–63.

Matthews GW and Neslund VS (1987). The initial impact of AIDS on public health law in the United States – 1986. *JAMA* 257 #3, 344–352.

May RM (1981). The transmission and control of gonorrhea. *Nature* 291, 376–377.

May RM (1988). HIV infection in heterosexuals. *Nature* 331, 655–656.

May RM and Anderson RM (1987). Transmission dynamics of HIV infection. *Nature* 326, 137–142.

May RM and Anderson RM (1989). The transmission dynamics of human immunodeficiency virus (HIV). *Phil Trans R Soc London B* 321, 565–607.

McEvoy M and Tillet HE (1985). Some problems in the prediction of future numbers of cases of the acquired immunodeficiency syndrome in the United Kingdom. *Lancet* 7 Sept, 541–542.

McGrady GA, Jason JM and Evatt BL (1987). The course of the epidemic of AIDS in the United States hemophilia population. *Am J Epidem* 26 #1, 25–30.

McKusick L, Horstman W, and Coates TJ (1985). AIDS and sexual behavior reported by gay men in San Francisco. *Am J Pub Health* 75 #5, 493–496.

Medley GF, Anderson RM, Cox DR, Billard L (1987). Incubation period of AIDS in patients infected via blood transfusion. *Nature* 328, 719–721.

Meyer KB and Pauker SG (1987). Screening for HIV: can we afford the false positive rate? *N Eng J Med* 317 #4, 238–241.

Miller RK and Michel AN (1982). *Ordinary Differential Equations.* Academic Press, New York.

Mitsuya H. and Broder S.(1987). Strategies for antiviral therapy in AIDS. *Nature* 325, 773–778.

Mode CJ, Gollwitzer HE and Herrman W (1989). A methodological study of a stochastic model of an AIDS epidemic. *Math Biosci* 92, 201–229.

Morgan WM and Curran JW (1986). AIDS: current and future trends. *Pub Health Rep* 101 #5, 459–465.

Moss AR, Bacchetti P, Osmund D, et al. (1988). Seropositivity for HIV and the development of AIDS or AIDS related condition: three year follow up of the San Francisco General Hospital Cohort. *Br Med J* 296, 745–750.

Moss AR, Osmond D, Bacchetti P et al. (1987). Risk factors for AIDS and HIV seropositivity in homosexual men. *Am J Epidem* 125 #6, 1035–1047.

Mulleady G and Green J (1985). Syringe sharing among London drug abusers. *Lancet* 8469, 1425.

Nasell I (1985). *Hybrid Models of Tropical Infections*, Springer–Verlag, Berlin.

National Heart, Lung, and Blood Institute Division of Blood Diseases and Resources (1977). *Study to Evaluate the Supply–Demand Relationships for AHF and PTC Through 1980.* US Dept. HEW, PHS, NIH, 86 pages. (pub # NIH 77–1274, contract # 1–HB–6–2965.)

National Heart, Lung and Blood Institute (1985). *The Nation's Blood Resource: A Summary Report.* U.S. Dept. HHS, PHS, NIH (call #HE20.3002:B62/20).

Nelkin D (1987). AIDS and the social sciences: review of useful knowledge and research needs. *Rev Inf Dis* 9 #5, 980–986.

New York City Dept Health AIDS Surveillance (1986). The AIDS epidemic in New York City, 1981–1984, *Am J Epidem* 123, 1013–1025.

Nold A (1980). Heterogeneity in disease transmission modeling. *Math Biosci* 52, 227–240.

Osmund D, Bacchetti P, Chaisson RE et al. (1988). Time of exposure and risk of HIV infection in homosexual partners of men with AIDS. *AJPH* 78 #8, 944–948.

OSTP (1988). *A National Effort to Model AIDS Epidemiology*, Report of a workshop held at Leesburg, Virginia, July 25–29, 1988, Office of Science and Technology Policy, Executive Office of the President, Washington D.C., 20506.

Padian NS (1987). Heterosexual transmission of AIDS: International perspectives and national projections. *Rev Inf Dis* 9 #5, 947–960.

Padian N, Marquis L, Francis DP et al. (1987). Male–to–female transmission of human immunodeficiency virus. *JAMA* 258 #6, 788–790.

Padian NS, Shiboski SC and Jewell NP (1991). Female–to male transmission of human immunodeficiency virus. *JAMA* 266 #12, 1664–1667.

Pagano M, De Gruttola V, MaWhinney S and Tu XM (1991). The HIV epidemic in New York City: Statistical Methods for projecting AIDS incidence and prevalence. In: *AIDS Epidemiology: Methodological Issues.* N Jewell, K Dietz, and V Farewell, Eds., Birkhauser, Boston, to appear.

Payne SF, Lemp GF, Rutherford GW et al. (1989). Effect of multiple disease manifestations on length of survival for AIDS patients in San Francisco. Abstract WAP80, V International Conference on AIDS, Montreal.

Payne SF, Rutherford GW, Lemp GF, and Clevenger AC (1990). Effect of the revised case definition on AIDS reporting in San Francisco: evidence of increased reporting in intravenous drug users. *AIDS* 4 #4, 335–339.

Peterman TA and Curran JW (1986). Sexual transmission of HIV. *JAMA* 256 #16, 2222–2226.

Peterman TA, Drotman DP and Curran JW (1985). Epidemiology of the acquired immune deficiency syndrome. *Epidem Rev* 7, 1–21.

Peterman TA, Jaffe HW, Feorino PM et al. (1985). Transfusion–associated AIDS in the United States. *JAMA* 254 #20, 2913–2917.

Peterman TA, Lang GR, Mikos NJ et al. (1986). HTLV–III/LAV infection in hemodialysis patients. *JAMA* 255 #17, 2324–2326.

Peterman TA, Stoneburner RL, Allen JR et al. (1988). Risk of HIV transmission from heterosexual adults with transfusion–associated infection. *JAMA* 259 #1, 55–58.

Pickering J, Wiley JA, Padian NS et al. (1986). Modeling the incidence of A.I.D.S. in San Francisco, Los Angeles, and New York. *Math Modeling* 7, 661–688.

Piot P, Kreiss JK, Ndinya–Achola JO et al. (1987). Heterosexual transmission of HIV. *AIDS* 1 #4, 199–206.

Potterat JJ, Muth JB, and Markewich GS (1986). Serological markers as indicators of sexual orientation in AIDS virus–infected men. *JAMA* 256 #6, 712.

Potterat JJ, Dukes RL, and Rothenberg RB (1987). Disease transmission by heterosexual men with gonorrhea: an empirical estimate. *STD* 14 #2, 107–110.

PHS (1987). *AIDS: information/education plan to prevent and control AIDS in the United States.* the U.S. Department of Health and Human Services.

Quinn TC, Piot P, McCormick JB et al. (1987). Serological and immunological studies in patients with AIDS in North America and Africa. *JAMA* 257 #19, 2617–2621.

Quinn TC, Glasser D, Cannon RO et al. (1987). Human immunodeficiency virus infection among patients attending clinics for sexually transmitted diseases. *N Eng J Med* 318 #4, 197–203.

Rabkin CS, Thomas PA, Jaffe HW and Schultz S (1987). Prevalence of antibody to HTLV–III/LAV in a population attending a sexually transmitted disease clinic. *STD* 14 #1, 48–51.

Rauch KJ, Rutherford GW, Echenberg DF, et al. (1989). Surveillance of acquired immunodeficiency syndrome in San Francisco: evaluation of the completeness of reporting. 114th *Annual Meeting of the American Public Health Association*, Abstract WAP24, Washington.

Redfield R. and Burke D.(1987). Shadow on the land: the epidemiology of HIV infection. *Viral Immun* 1, 69–81.

Redfield RR, Wright DC and Tramont EC (1986). The Walter Reed staging classification for HTLV–III/LAV infection. *N Eng J Med* 314, 131–132.

Rees M (1987). The sombre view of AIDS. *Nature* 326, 343–345.

Rezza G and Greco D (1987). AIDS: Drug addicts, homosexual males and international travel. *AIDS* 1 #3, 191.

Robert–Guroff M, Weiss SH, Giron JA, et al. (1986). Prevalence of antibodies to HTLV–I, –II, and –III in intravenous drug abusers from an AIDS endemic region. *JAMA* 255 #22, 3133–3137.

Sattenspiel L and Simon CP (1988). The spread and persistence of infectious diseases in structured populations. *Math Biosci* 90, 341–366.

Schechter MT, Boyko WJ, Craib KJP et al. (1987). Effects of long–term seropositivity to H.I.V. in a cohort of homosexual men. *AIDS* 1 #2, 77–82.

Schuster CR (1988). Intravenous drug use and AIDS prevention. *Pub Health Rep* 103, 1125–1135.

Schwager SJ, Castillo–Chavez C and Hethcote HW (1989). Statistical and Mathematical Approaches in HIV/AIDS Modeling. In: *Mathematical and Statistical Approaches to AIDS Epidemiology*, C Castillo–Chavez, Ed., Lecture Notes in Biomathematics 83, Springer–Verlag, Germany, 2–35.

Scitovsky AA, Cline M and Lee PR (1986). Medical care costs of patients with AIDS in San Francisco. *JAMA* 256 #22, 3103–3106.

Seligmann M, Pinching AJ, Rosen FS et al. (1987). Immunology of human immunodeficiency virus and the acquired immune deficiency syndrome. *Ann Int Med* 107 #2, 234–242.

Selik RM, Castro KG and Pappaioanou M (1988). Racial/ethnic differences in the risk of AIDS in the United States. *AJPH* 78 #12, 1539–1545.

Selwyn PA, Feiner C, Cox CP et al. (1987). Knowledge about AIDS and high–risk behavior among intravenous drug users in New York City. *AIDS* 1 #4, 247–254.

Shilts R (1987). *And the Band Played On.* St. Martin's Press, New York.

Simon CP and Jacquez JA (1992). Reproduction numbers and the stability of equilibria of SI models for heterogeneous populations, *SIAM J Appl Math* 52 #2, 541–576.

Sivak SL and Wormser GP (1985). How common is HTLV–III infection in the United States? *N Eng J Med* 313, 1352.

Stehr–Green JK, Holman RC, Jason JM and Evatt BL (1988). Hemophilia–associated AIDS in the United States: 1981 to September 1987. *AJPH* 78 439–442.

Stevens CE, Taylor PE, Zang EA, et al. (1986). HTLV type III infection in a cohort of homosexual men in New York City. JAMA 255 #16, 2167–2172.

Stoneburner RL, Des Jarlais DC, Benezra D et al. (1988). A larger spectrum of severe HIV–1–related disease in intravenous drug users in New York City. *Science* 242, 916–919.

Tan WY (1991). Some general stochastic models for the spread of AIDS and some simulation results. *Math and Computer Modelling* 15, 19–39.

Tan WY (1992). *Mathematical Models of AIDS Epidemiology.* Marcel Dekker, New York, to appear.

Turner CF, Miller HG and Moses LE, Eds. (1989). *AIDS: Sexual Behavior and Intravenous Drug Abuse.* National Academy Press, Washington D.C.

U.S. Bureau of the Census (1987). Statistical Abstract of the United States: 1980 (108th edition). Washington D.C.

U.S. Bureau of the Census (1989). Current Population Reports, Series P–25, No. 1040–RD–1, Population Estimates by Race and Hispanic Origin for States, Metropolitan Areas and Selected Countries, 1980 to 1985. U.S. Government Printing Office, Washington, D.C.

van Griensven GJP, Tielman RAP, Goudsmit J et al. (1987). Risk factors and prevalence of HIV antibodies in homosexual men in the Netherlands. *Am J Epidem* 125 #6, 1048–1057.

von Reyn CF, Clements CJ, and Mann JM (1987). HIV infection and routine childhood immunisation. *Lancet* 8560, 669–672.

Walker BD, Chakrabarti S, Moss B et al. (1987). HIV–specific cytotoxic T–lymphocytes in seropositive individuals. *Nature* 328, 345–348.

Ward JW, Deppe DA, Samson S et al. (1987). Risk of HIV infection from blood donors who later developed AIDS. *Ann Int Med* 106 #1, 61–62.

Weber JN, Clapham PR, Weiss R et al. (1987). HIV infection in two cohorts of homosexual men: neutralizing sera and association of anti–GAG antibody with prognosis. *Lancet* 8525, 119–122.

Wendt D, Sadowski L, Markowitz N, and Saravolatz L (1987). Prevalence of serum antibody to human immunodeficiency virus among hospitalized intravenous drug abusers in a low—risk geographical area. *J Inf Dis* 155 #1, 151—152.

Wickwire KH (1977). Mathematical models for the control of pests and infectious diseases: a survey. *Theor Pop Biol* 8, 182—238.

Windom RE (1987). The third international AIDS conference — reflections, *Pub Health Rep* 102 #5, 461—462.

Winkelstein W and Levy J (1986). Potential for transmission of AIDS — associated retroviruses from bisexual men in San Francisco to their female sexual contacts. *JAMA* 225 #7, 901.

Winkelstein W, Lyman DM, Padian N et al.(1987) Sexual practices and risk of infection by the human immunodeficiency virus. *JAMA* 257 #3, 321—325.

Winkelstein W, Samuel M, Padian NS et al. (1987). The San Francisco Men's Health Study: III. Reduction in human immunodeficiency virus transmission among homosexual/bisexual men 1982—1986. *AJPH* 76 #9, 685—689.

Winklestein W, Wiley JA, Padian N and Levy J (1986). Potential for transmission of AIDS—associated retrovirus from bisexual men in San Francisco to their female sexual contacts. *JAMA* 255 #7, 901.

Winkelstein W, Wiley JA, Padian N et al. (1988). The San Francisco Men's Health Study: Continued decline in HIV seroconversion rates among homosexual/bisexual men. *AJPH* 78 #11, 1472—1474.

World Almanac (1988). Newspaper Enterprise Assn, Inc, New York.

World Health Organization (1991). *World AIDS Day Newsletter #2*, WHO Global Programme on AIDS, October/November.

Yorke JA, Hethcote HW and Nold A (1978). Dynamics and control of the transmission of gonorrhea. *STD* 5, 51—56.

Zagury D, Leonard R, Fouchard M et al. (1987). Immunization against AIDS in humans, *Nature* 326, 249—250.